Children and
Young People's Nursing

Children and Young People's Nursing

PRINCIPLES FOR PRACTICE

Editors

Ruth Davies RGN, RSCN, RHV, MA PhD PG CertEd.
Senior Lecturer in Children and Young People's Nursing,
Swansea University, Swansea, UK

Alyson Davies RGN, RSCN, BSc, MN PG Cert Ed.
Lecturer in Children and Young People's Nursing, Swansea
University, Swansea, UK

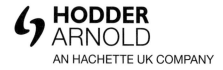

HODDER
ARNOLD

AN HACHETTE UK COMPANY

First published in Great Britain in 2011 by
Hodder Arnold, an imprint of Hodder Education, an Hachette UK company
338 Euston Road, London NW1 3BH

http://www.hodderarnold.com

© 2011 Hodder & Stoughton Ltd

Hachette UK's policy is to use papers that are natural, renewable and recyclable products and made from wood grown in sustainable forests. The logging and manufacturing processes are expected to conform to the environmental regulations of the country of origin.

Whilst the advice and information in this book are believed to be true and accurate at the date of going to press, neither the author[s] nor the publisher can accept any legal responsibility or liability for any errors or omissions that may be made. In particular, (but without limiting the generality of the preceding disclaimer) every effort has been made to check drug dosages; however it is still possible that errors have been missed. Furthermore, dosage schedules are constantly being revised and new side-effects recognized. For these reasons the reader is strongly urged to consult the drug companies' printed instructions before administering any of the drugs recommended in this book.

British Library Cataloguing in Publication Data
A catalogue record for this book is available from the British Library

Library of Congress Cataloging-in-Publication Data
A catalog record for this book is available from the Library of Congress

ISBN-13   978-1-444-107845

1 2 3 4 5 6 7 8 9 10

Commissioning Editor:	Naomi Wilkinson
Project Editor:	Joanna Silman
Production Controller:	Jonathan Williams
Cover Design:	Lynda King
Index:	Lisa Footitt

Cover image © Alamy images

Typeset in 11 on 14pt Minion Pro by Phoenix Photosetting, Chatham, Kent
Printed and bound in the UK by MPG Books, Bodmin

What do you think about this book? Or any other Hodder Arnold title?
Please visit our website: www.hodderarnold.com

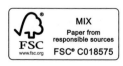

To Tom (17th April 1987 – 3rd August 2006)
and
To Gwilym and Megan who make each day wonderful

Instructions for companion website

This book has a companion website available at:
http://www.hodderplus.co.uk/childrensnursing

To access the PowerPoint presentations and MCQs included on the website, please register using the following access details:

Serial number: tzw731yh56km

Once you have registered, you will not need the serial number but can log in using the username and password you will create during registration.

Contents

Contributors

Dave Barton PhD, MPhil, BEd, DipN, RGN, RNT
Academic Lead for Nursing, College of Human and Health Sciences, Swansea University, Swansea, UK

Pat Colliety PhD, MA, BSc(Hons), PGCEA, RN(Adult), RN(Child), RHV
Senior Tutor, Faculty of Health and Medical Sciences, University of Surrey, UK

Alyson Davies RGN, RSCN, BSc, MN, PG CertEd.
Lecturer in Children and Young People's Nursing, College of Human and Health Sciences, Swansea University, Swansea, UK

Ruth Davies RGN, RSCN, RHV, MA PhD PG Cert Ed.
Senior Lecturer in Children and Young People's Nursing, College of Human and Health Sciences, Swansea University, Swansea, UK

Carwen Earles MSc(Econ.), BSc, RGN, HV, RSCN, PG Cert.(FE)
Academic Lead, Department of Public Health and Policy Studies, College of Human and Health Sciences, Swansea University, Swansea, UK

Richard Griffith LLM, BN, DipN, PgDLaw, RMN, RNT, CertEd.
Lecturer in Health Law, College of Human and Health Sciences, Swansea University, Swansea, UK

Sue Higham RSCN, RGN, DPSN, BSc, PGCEA, MA
Lecturer in Children's Nursing, The Open University, Milton Keynes, UK

Jill E John BSc, MA, RGN, RSCN, Specialist Community Nurse, tHE(PGCE)
Tutor in Children and Young People's Nursing, College of Human and Health Sciences, Swansea University, Swansea, UK

Susan Jones BSc(Hons), SCPHN(SN), RN
Lead Nurse School Health Nursing, Abertawe Bro Morgannwg University Health Board, Port Talbot, UK

Jeremy Jolley BN, MA, PhD, PGCEA, PGCTheol, RGN, RSCN
Senior Lecturer, Paediatric Nursing, Faculty of Health and Social Care, The University of Hull, Hull, UK

Katrina McNamara-Goodger RN(General), RN(Child), RHV
Head of Policy and Practice, ACT The Association for Children's Palliative Care, UK

Catherine Powell RGN, RSCN, RHV, BNSc(Hons) PhD
Consultant Nurse, Safeguarding Children, NHS Portsmouth and Visiting Senior Lecturer, School of Health Sciences, University of Southampton, UK

Gary Rolfe PhD, MA, BSc, RMN, PGCEA
Professor of Nursing, College of Human and Health Sciences, Swansea University, Swansea, UK

Julia Terry MSc, BSc(Hons), DipHE, PGCE, RMN
Mental Health Nurse Tutor, College of Human and Health Sciences, Swansea University, Swansea, UK

Alison Twycross MSc, DMS, CertEd(HE), RGN, RMN, RSCN
Reader in Children's Nursing, Kingston University–St George's University of London, UK

Sally Williams BN, MSc Nursing, RN(Child), Post Grad Cert tHE
Tutor, Children and Young People's Nursing, College of Human and Health Sciences, Swansea University, Swansea, UK

Vasso Vydelingum PhD, PGDip, Ed, BSc(Hons), RN, DN, RHV
Senior Lecturer, Faculty of Health and Medical Sciences, University of Surrey, UK

Foreword

Challenging boundaries of practice is not something you usually expect from a standard textbook. Chapter upon chapter of 'how to' is something practitioners have come to expect. But this is no ordinary textbook. It is a book which challenges current practice in children and young people's nursing and encourages the new generation of children's nurses to become critical thinkers.

Edited by two highly experienced children's nurses who have worked in higher education for a number of years, this book includes chapters from nurse practitioners, researchers and academics, covering issues most pertinent to children's lives today. Chapters on safeguarding, child and adolescent mental health, participation and school nursing among others are interspersed with case studies from visionary practitioners. It also reflects upon the long and colourful history of the profession – from the establishment of the first children's hospital in 1852 to the introduction of Project 2000 which saw student nurses given a full student status – and acknowledges that children and young people are a group of patients with particular needs, entitled to expertly crafted care.

More than anything else, this book details how children and young people are at the heart of healthcare planning and delivery and how the rights-based approach to children and young people's nursing should help ensure all developments and decisions are centred on the child. Members of this distinct group of patients are no longer seen as 'future adults' but instead 'current present persons'. As Wales's 'children's champion' I can but warmly welcome this approach.

Whilst this book has intentionally engaged with controversial issues, the real measure of its success is whether children and young people are being given a voice, a choice and that a rights-based approach to nursing is being implemented fully and consistently across the country.
This book is timely. It is the twenty-first anniversary of the United Nations Convention on the Rights of the Child this year and although there seems to be a real commitment to this international standard in certain areas of the UK, much more needs to be done to ensure children's rights are effectively championed and safeguarded.

Children and young people's nurses have challenging, stimulating and rewarding careers. They play a vital role not only in providing direct care but also in promoting physical health and well-being. I think that this should be on the must-read list not just of undergraduate and postgraduate nursing students but of all existing practitioners working with children and young people.

Keith Towler, Children's Commissioner for Wales

Preface

Children and Young People's (CYP) nursing has made great strides over the last twenty years in consolidating its own body of knowledge and developing its own evidence base. Whilst it continues to be an evolving discipline it remains committed to the ideal that children and young people are a distinct group of patients and clients with their own particular needs who are entitled to expertly crafted care. This is a point worth making as the discipline remains threatened by the generalist agenda from a number of angles including the constant drive to change the education and training of nurses, policy drivers, and a changing political landscape. For all these reasons, it is imperative to identify our principles of practice, showcase initiatives within CYP nursing and explore how we are changing the boundaries of practice to meet the ever changing and complex needs of patients and clients whether in hospital or community settings through the promotion of good physical and mental health as well as 'hands on nursing'. We hope this book will promote CYP nursing as a dynamic area of practice which benefits children and young people, their families and the communities in which they live and in so doing so offers a rewarding career to the individual CYP nurse in whatever setting they may practice.

Both editors of this book are CYP nurses who have worked in Higher Education for a number of years and have witnessed direct entry at pre-registration level for CYP nurses in the 1990s as well as the move towards all graduate entry which has been achieved in our own country, Wales, and which will be finally rolled out across the United Kingdom over the next few years. This will not only give nursing educational parity with other health professions but bring it in line with the rest of the developed world. We believe that children and young people as well as their families will ultimately benefit from graduate nurses who are educated to be critical thinkers and therefore question and develop practice as well as research it. As our existing knowledge is refined and new knowledge emerges which is added to our theoretical and clinical evidence base so we need to discuss and analyse the implications of using such evidence. There is a need to be critical in the most positive sense and to constantly question and analyse the discipline of CYP nursing. This should be viewed not as a threat to people's integrity or to their knowledge and activity but as an opportunity to 'push the boundaries' and to create and stimulate debate and new ways of working that benefit children and young people.

This book sets out to accomplish this task, to stimulate the reader to not only consider the information presented to them but to critically analyse and engage with some of the key principles and debates within CYP nursing. The approach taken within the writing is often deliberately controversial in order to develop new and innovative ways of thinking and of viewing practice, education and research. As a profession and discipline we need to debate our core principles and values in a challenging yet informed discourse. This book contains chapters designed to do this and contributors discuss their own field of expertise by providing reflection points and case studies designed to provoke debate and discussion of the sometimes controversial and awkward issues in CYP nursing. For the sake of brevity and consistency we have used the nomenclature Children and Young People's (CYP) nursing to reflect the age group (0–19 plus) that we care for.

The aim of Part 1 of this book is to put children and young people's (CYP) nursing in context and so begins with Jeremy Jolley's chapter which sets out some pertinent historical facts about our development as a distinct area of practice. Appropriately, this emphasises a fundamental principle of practice, that is, the continuing need for us to retain our 'genuine care' for children and young people and ends on a contentious note by questioning whether it is sensible for CYP nurses to specialise first without obtaining a general qualification. Although, as editors, we do not agree with this position, we do of course respect his right to express it. This is a timely question, given the recent consultation by the (NMC) Nursing and Midwifery Council into pre registration nursing education, and the debate surrounding this is something we return to in the final chapter of this book. In Chapter 2, Sue Higham discusses the concept of Family-Centred Care (FCC) and the importance of fathers when children and young people are sick. She questions the reality of whether fathers are truly regarded as partners in care and suggests that more can be done to address real shortcomings in how they are treated in the care process. She highlights the fact that the term FCC is often equated with the role of the mother acting as the main carer and that this has been perpetuated by research which has focused heavily on the maternal role. Sue Higham argues that the role of the father should assume equal importance within research and clinical practice as children need and value their father's perspectives and care. She calls for a careful consideration of how practice might develop to understand not only the father's experiences and needs whilst caring for a sick child but those of the wider family too – siblings and grandparents.

Such consideration of the wider family is discussed in Chapter 3 by Vasso Vydelingum and Pat Colliety who consider the issues facing children and young people from ethnic minorities when engaging with the health care system. It is shown that they still face discriminatory practice despite the UK being a multi-cultural society and Vasso Vydelingum and Pat Colliety argue persuasively that care must always be culturally sensitive. This chapter highlights that CYP nurses cannot make assumptions about the needs of children and young people from ethnic minorities, assumptions which may limit the range and scope of care and services provided. Rather, a careful assessment through listening and discussion is vital if inclusion and participation is to be a reality and they are to be given the care and services as well as the respect and dignity they are entitled to.

The aim of Part 2 is to identify, using a rights-based approach, why and how the interests of children and young people must be respected and safeguarded. This begins with Chapter 4, by Jill John and Richard Griffiths, which examines the evidence surrounding whether children and young people's right to participate in their own healthcare is actually upheld. Their overview of present practice, and the legal position with regard to this, raises important issues for, as they argue, whilst there is now a benchmark in place for children's rights, there has been a failure by many countries, including the United Kingdom (UK), to incorporate these into domestic law. Whilst the appointment of Children's Commissioners in the UK, as well as other parts of Europe, has done much to raise the profile of children and young people and to monitor, promote and safeguard their rights there is still much that remains to be done if their autonomy is to be truly respected and upheld in actual practice. In this connection, children and young people have the right to be safe and protected from harm and in Chapter 5, Catherine Powell has, based on her work as a Consultant Nurse, Safeguarding Children, clearly set out professional roles and responsibilities in relation to this. Her use of key messages from serious case reviews serves to remind us all too well of the need to learn from these and be forever vigilant. Chapter 6 explores a hitherto under researched issue, namely the use of restraint on children and young people. Sally William's chapter poses some disturbing questions about how we treat some of the most vulnerable children and young people in society and will no doubt be the subject of much heart-searching debate as well as research in the future. The final chapter in this section, by Alison Twycross, highlights the issues involved in managing children and young people's pain. She discusses the challenges in ensuring that their right to have their pain managed effectively in upheld in actual practice. Alison Twycross argues that poor pain management affects all areas of their development and recovery and may have profound and lasting effects which can persist into adulthood. She clearly demonstrates that barriers to effective pain management focus on socialisation, beliefs about children's pain, knowledge deficits and role modelling. She posits that best practice guidelines and current research provide a solid foundation base upon which effective, efficient pain management can be delivered.

Children and Young People's (CYP) nurses are just as involved in the promotion of physical health and well being as they are in the giving direct 'hands of care' across a range of settings as highlighted throughout this section. Chapter 8, by Carwen Earles and Susan Jones, identifies how the role of the school nurse has evolved over the last 140 years and the vital role they currently play in public health and health promotion. In doing so they draw attention to the fact that despite a number of government recommendations to increase school nursing provision it continues to be under resourced. A regrettable fact given, as they note, that so many children and young people in the UK continue to live in poverty and school nurses can do so much to help them attain good health which not only has a positive effect on their life chances but educational attainment as well. In the following chapter, Ruth Davies, in a similar vein, also draws attention to the fact that Children's Community Nursing (CCN) services across the United Kingdom is also under resourced despite a plethora of government reports over the last fifty years which have recommended that children and young people with acute and complex care needs should be cared for at home rather than in hospital. Her historical overview of the care of sick children makes the point that care outside of the home and the institutionalisation of sick children is a relatively new development and that most children and young people would prefer to be cared for and indeed even die in the family home. Both chapters call upon CYP nurses, practising as school nurses and CCNs, to work at a political level to increase provision by identifying how further expansion of their services will benefit children and young people as well as their families and communities.

CYP nursing practice is developing rapidly with care being delivered in diverse settings. Thus children and young people's nurses are faced by a number of challenges on an individual level. Rather than being consumed by the pressures of a rapidly changing health service and meeting targets it is often the immediate practice of delivering individual, personalised care in those diverse settings which focuses the attention and mind of the CYP nurse. Therefore, this section of the book focuses on such challenges – the need to consider the whole family as well as the physical, psychological and cultural needs of the children and young people we care for and also on how to engage in best practice in order to deliver the highest quality care.

This issue of accessing knowledgeable and appropriate care is reiterated by Julia Terry and Alyson Davies in Chapter 10 in which they highlight the increase in the incidence of mental health issues in children and young people. The rising incidence is multi-factorial and is due in part to enhanced awareness of the mental health issues which affect the younger population. Increased academic and societal pressures, chronic illness, a shifting society and home life also lead to increasing levels of stress and affect the ability to cope. As a result more children, young people and families are being seen within the health care system and they are entitled to be seen and cared for by knowledgeable practitioners. The authors argue that mental health care is no longer the domain of the specialist nurse but is now part of the role of every CYP nurse who provides holistic care.

Building on their previous chapter, Alyson Davies and Julia Terry in Chapter 11 draw attention to the increasing incidence of complex mental health problems in children and young people with a particular focus on suicide, self harm, anorexia nervosa, ASD (Autistic Spectrum Disorder) and Attention Deficit Hyperactivity Disorder (ADHD). As they rightly point out, all CYP nurses come into contact with or care for these children and young people so it is essential that they have insight and knowledge about these so that they may provide appropriate, sensitive and holistic care. As this chapter highlights CYP nurses also need to work collaboratively with Children and Adolescent Mental Health Services (CAMHS), the multi-disciplinary team as well as voluntary agencies so that the child or young person who is in mental distress is able to receive the high quality care and support they so desperately need.

Katrina McNamara-Goodger, in her poignant chapter on the transitional care pathway for children and young people with life-limiting and life-threatening conditions also stresses the need for knowledgeable and appropriate care. She stresses that young people have needs which are very different to those of younger children and adults which must be valued. Care must be holistic and delivered sensitively at a time when the transition from child oriented services to adult based care can be bewildering and complex. She also highlights that all too often transitional care is poorly managed with noticeable gaps in the care packages provided. She reiterates that involvement and participation in the process by the young person and their family leads to their need being understood and met. Care should be co-ordinated, based upon openness with clear communication and continuity of care being hallmarks of the experience of transition. It is a crucial period where nurses must face the challenges involved in providing care which engenders the confidence of the young person and family in the experience of transitional care.

It would appear that if children and young people's nursing is to continue developing, those who deliver the care must continue to be innovative, creative and flexible in shaping the delivery of that care. This will mean rigorously exploring our current practice and critically analysing how those boundaries can be challenged to ensure that children and young people remain at the heart of health care planning and the delivery of services which must always meet their needs and be centred on the individual child, young person and their family. This theme will be expanded upon in section four of this book.

Throughout this book it has been our intention to promote CYP nursing as a stimulating and rewarding career for high achievers by identifying the many roles performed by them in different spheres including school nursing, hospital nursing, community children's nursing and, as will be shown in our penultimate chapter, advanced nursing practice. In doing so, we have shown how the Skills for Health Framework (Chapter 9) is linked to educational attainment so the novice CYP nurse may plan his/her career and continue to progress. In this connection, whatever their level of practice the CYP nurse is well advised to develop a professional portfolio for, as Chapter 13 by Alyson Davies and Gary Rolfe shows, these are increasingly being used by practitioners for professional and personal development. This chapter shows how a portfolio may give the CYP nurse the freedom to explore his or her own knowledge base and knowledge acquisition as well as the application of these to practice. Portfolios may also be used by the individual CYP nurse in career progression planning and to identify the specific knowledge, competencies and skills required to deliver high quality care to children and young people and their families. Indeed, as the authors claim, this may be used effectively to help them articulate their own particular contribution to care as a CYP nurse. This particular observation would seem appropriate in the context of this book for, if CYP nursing is to survive and indeed flourish as a distinct branch of the family of nursing we must make plain and manifest the high quality and expertly crafted care we can and do provide for children and young people in whatever setting they may be cared for.

The final chapter by Dave Barton, Alyson Davies and Ruth Davies is perhaps the most contentious one within this book debating as it does Advanced Nursing Practice (ANP). After tracing the history of ANP and putting their present scope of practice and educational attainment into context they pose the question 'Who are the ANPs and who are treating children and young people?' and ask whether these should be generalist or CYP nurses. Both sides of the debate are presented and the reader is invited to engage in this through a series of reflection points. We leave the reader to decide!

We hope that a new generation of student CYPs, whether undertaking study at pre- or post-registration level or studying at diploma or graduate level, will find this a stimulating and thought provoking book. In putting our final touches to this in November 2010 we are mindful of the significance of this year in relation to our most famous nurse Florence Nightingale (1820–1910), and so we end with her words spoken to her nurses all those years ago but which are still applicable to us in a new century and a very different world as we continue to care for children and young people:

'Little children, love one another. Remember we are not so many selves, but members of a community'.

Florence Nightingale

March 2011
Ruth Davies and Alyson Davies,
Department of Nursing, Swansea University

Acknowledgements

Ruth and Alyson would like to gratefully thank:

All the contributors to this book who have given of their time and have written in order to share their knowledge and expertise.

Keith Towler, The Children's Commissioner for Wales, for his kindness in taking the time to write an excellent foreword for the book.

The All Wales Community Children's Nurse Forum for their help, kindness and expertise in providing practice exemplars.

Christopher Griffiths, Consultant Nurse Learning Disabilities/Lecturer, Abertawe Bro Morgannwg University Health Board for his kindness, expertise and help in providing practice exemplars.

Paula Phillips, Community Nurse, Learning Disabilities Abertawe Bro Morgannwg University Health Board for her kindness, expertise and help in providing practice exemplars.

Jacquie Taylor, APNP, Kirkcaldy, Scotland for her kindness, help and expertise in providing practice exemplars.

Mervyn Townley, Consultant Nurse Specialist CAMHS, Aneurin Bevan Health Board Gwent, for his kindness, expertise and help in providing practice exemplars.

Our families who have shared in and supported us in the process of writing and compiling the book.

Our academic colleagues at the College of Human and Health Sciences, Swansea University for their support during the writing of this book.

Our colleagues at Hodder Education who have provided invaluable support and guidance throughout this process.

PART I
Children and young people's nursing in context

Chapter 1

The development of children's nursing

Jeremy Jolley

Overview

This chapter will provide an overview of the historical development of child nursing. The chapter will focus on the key elements of child nursing and the characteristics that make it distinct from adult nursing and from medicine. It will be seen that child nursing is both ancient and new. Its ancient history is intermingled with that of medicine and adult nursing. Its modern history is unique, and it is distinguished both by its focus on the care of children and by its unique mix of science and romanticism. Child nurses care for children not just because they can, not just because the work is fascinating but because they 'care', i.e. they 'feel' for the child and are willing to develop an emotional bond with the child and his or her family. This is not a new characteristic; it can be traced back to Victorian nursing and back even further into history. However, other healthcare disciplines have come to embrace science and objectivity to the point where 'care' has become synonymous with 'management'. In contrast, child nursing has both retained and developed what can be regarded as 'genuine care' with important elements of romanticism and affection for the child and for childhood. It will be argued that such a notion of care has nothing whatsoever to do with 'management' but is concerned with a relationship with the child that is based on affection, perhaps even love.

Why history?

One of the reasons that professions have prestige is that they have been around for a long time. Professions are rather like a good cheese, they need time to mature. Perhaps you are keen on a decent piece of cheese with a glass or two of nice wine. If so, you may well want to know where your choice of delicacy came from; you will want to know something about its history. So it is with the professions – they have history. What they are today is composed to some extent of what they have been. In fact, it is sometimes difficult for the professions to shake off their history. As a result, barristers still wear wigs and academics dress in ancient garb for degree ceremonies. The understanding we have of nursing is formed only partly from current experiences of nursing. An important part of people's perception of what nursing is derives from our knowledge of the past, of Florence Nightingale, of war films showing brave, caring nurses and of more light-hearted films, such as *Carry on Nurse*, which gave us the image of the bossy, authoritative ward sister (Thomas 1959). These 'images' from the past provide us with a colourful mix of somewhat disparate characteristics; because of this, the nurse today may be seen as dedicated, courageous *and* bossy.

History both gives child nursing its pedigree and colours our understanding of it. If we ignore history, we will also fail to understand what nursing really 'is' and what that history can teach us. The result could be that child nursing would 'go round in circles', failing to learn from its mistakes and failing to build on its progress. It is necessary that nursing should be able to recall its past, learn from that past and build on its past.

So history is important, but it is also interesting and fun. History is full of such amazing things as 'human ventilators' (the first ventilators were medical students who would manually inflate patients' lungs) and 'mechanical students' (the machines which replaced the medical students); we still use the term 'mechanical ventilation' (Jolley 2008a). The red and white striped pole sometimes seen outside a barber's shop comes from the day when surgeons (barber surgeons) were tradespeople (Ellis 2001). The barber–surgeons would perform surgery and use rags to mop up the blood. These rags would then be hung on a plain, white pole. The wind wound the bloody rags around the pole – and so we have our red and white pole. And now you know why surgeons are called 'Mr', the one-time title for a qualified tradesperson or businessman. It is to honour the surgeons' history and respect the time when surgery was a rather messy high street trade. Our history is full of amazing facts. Nursing and medicine have a rich and colourful history, reflecting, no doubt, the rich and colourful nature of our practice.

So:

- History demonstrates that child nursing is an important and enduring activity and that it is a professional orientation to the care of sick children that itself demands our care.
- We have a duty to look after our profession and to make it fit for the next generation. Lastly, history is not just something that happened in the past. You will be making history – in your practice, now and in the years to come. Indeed, this is your responsibility, the responsibility that a professional has to their profession.
- In time, history will come to judge you for what you manage to do with the discipline of child nursing, for your contribution to the ever-developing history of child nursing.

The beginning: the nurse–doctor

The care of the young is something which characterizes most animal species, and it characterizes us. In a sense then, people have always nursed sick children. However, when we talk of 'child nursing' we are referring to a professional activity, the employment of a range of skills which were acquired through learning and through experience. In this way, child nursing is a focused activity, a service provided by a group of people defined by their training. To find the beginning of child nursing, we need to look at when this first existed as a discipline. Perhaps we can define this beginning as the moment when individuals first saw themselves as child nurses and were able to recognize others who undertook similar roles. Child nursing, then, is not something that one person does in isolation; rather, it is an organization, a discipline.

It might be thought that the discipline of nursing is derived from the older discipline of medicine; however, this view deserves to be challenged. The history of medicine, as it is traditionally understood, can be found in the ancient civilizations. We know that there were large and enduring civilizations in ancient Greece, Arabia, Rome (Naraghi 1996) and elsewhere (David 2008). We know that these civilizations produced medical knowledge which remained current at least into the nineteenth century (Still 1931). Most of this material has been seen as part of the history of medicine but much of it is both holistic and orientated to care in a way that makes it sit very awkwardly with modern medicine. The Greek philosopher Hippocrates (460–370 BC) is marked out by medical historians (Still 1931) as the 'father' of medicine, a kind of early pioneer of medicine, someone chiefly responsible for taking medicine out of 'philosophy' and making it a subject of study in its own right.

Hippocrates did write about health and healing and also about midwifery, nutrition and ethics (Bruhn 2005). So what has this got to do with nursing? Two things, really. First, medicine's hold on science was, at least in the beginning, a very tenuous thing indeed. Hippocrates was not averse to relying on 'wisdom', as interpreted through his maxims or aphorisms (Hippocrates 2004). Second, what Hippocrates was concerned with was not so much medicine as a separate discipline from nursing but a single caring and therapeutic discipline, ethically modelled on the interests of the patient (Jolley 2008b). This history, rich and diverse, is as much nursing's as it is medicine's. Through the ages, our shared history has had little to do with science; rather, practitioners of nursing–medicine have employed wisdom, traditional 'knowledge', experience and faith (Porter 1997a).

Today, nursing and medicine claim to be separate disciplines. They have a separate training and separate professional bodies. However, we see nurses and doctors working together. In university bookshops, nurses purchase books written for doctors and medical students. Doctors write books for nurses (Young and Martin 1979), perhaps because they want nurses to understand the doctor's perspective on things so that nurses can be more helpful to them. Lastly, courses exist for child nurses to undertake the work of doctors (Ashington Audit Group 2004; Jolley 2007a). Today, the two disciplines can argue that they are separate, but history suggests otherwise. The public probably views nursing and medicine as being pretty much the same occupational discipline, and the public is pretty much right.

The public's perception of nursing and medicine as a more or less single occupational discipline may serve both disciplines well. In the past, some of the respect in which nursing has been held has probably derived from its close association with medicine. After all, not everyone could work so closely with surgeons and physicians; such nurses would have been seen to have been skilled and to have been accepted by doctors. However, the association probably did medicine much good too. Nursing was the caring face of medicine. Without nursing, medicine might well have appeared hard, remote and even brutish. This was, indeed, an association that was mutually beneficial, and the blurring of the occupational boundaries between the two disciplines was both real and really useful. Much of this is true even now. Today, the high level of respect with which nurses are viewed has made it remarkably easy for them to take on roles such as 'nurse consultant' and 'advanced nurse practitioner'. Nursing has been able to adapt to the increasing complexity of modern healthcare. Nursing has also been able to develop roles that employ the highest level of independent and critical thinking. Patients have been happy to accept nurses' intervention for practices that in the past would have been squarely within the doctors' domain. This has been even more remarkable in child nursing, in which parents have allowed nurses to practise advanced skills on their most precious possession, on the person they love more than themselves – their child. This is an astonishing degree of trust which has, in part at least, come about because of the way in which nursing–medicine has been seen as a single occupational group.

Reflection point

★ Historically, the development of nursing and medicine as separate disciplines is a very recent one. Arguably, there is still an 'interface' between the two disciplines, the nature of which is quite extraordinary. Try to think of any other two disciplines which work as closely together as do nursing and medicine today.

We have seen that the history of medicine is also the history of nursing. This means that for most of history we cannot discern or 'tease out' something that is nursing. Nursing–medicine, like most great human achievements, tended to develop during periods that were relatively ordered – during the times of the great civilizations such as those in ancient Greece, the Roman empire and in ancient Egypt (Ellis 2001). For this reason, we should not expect to see a great deal happening in Britain for much of the last two millennia. Indeed, we see medicine developing from the eighteenth century, but not a great deal happening before that. It is not for nothing that much of British history from the fall of Rome (*c*.476 AD) to the enlightenment (seventeenth–eighteenth centuries) has been known as 'the Dark Ages'. It is perhaps only the monastic movement which provided some degree of nursing–medical practice and learning. However, there is little evidence that nursing–medicine developed much in this period. The monastic movement was very good at producing beautiful copies of books but seems to have done little in respect of developing new knowledge. Even in the eighteenth century, most of the medical texts (Cadogan 1748; Nelson 1753) were little more than 'reprints' of much earlier Greek and Arabic books.

However, even if nursing–medicine as a discipline did not develop much until perhaps the reformation (sixteenth century), there are several examples of individual practitioners working as nurse–doctors. We should bear in mind that, throughout history, there would have been people who took an interest in healthcare or who earned their living by practising one or more aspects of healthcare. The reason we know so little about such people is either that they did not document what they did or such written evidence has been lost. We do know about the work of a few individuals because records about them have survived.

Individuals working as nurse–doctors may have used magic, faith, herbal remedies and a range of skills and traditional knowledge. These 'healers' may not have had a degree in medicine or nursing but they were recognized by others as being healers. Some of these people will have earned their living as a healer; others would have practised largely out of interest and fulfilment. It is perhaps too easy to see these people developing into what we would now regard as a physician or a surgeon. However, the notion of 'care' was very much part of what these healers practised. Their work was more holistically driven than is that of the typical doctor today. In addition, much of the work of these healers was rooted in the spiritual; this might have been magic or faith but it was spiritual rather than scientific. Perhaps we can argue that these healers fashioned part of the foundations of nursing.

Mary Webb: surgeoness

Wyman (1984) provides an account of Mary Webb, who, in 1729, became apprenticed to Mrs Anne Saint of Shoreditch. This 7 year apprenticeship was to teach Mary Webb the craft of 'surgeoness'. Today, the word 'surgeon' conjures up an image of well-educated doctors in an operating theatre. However, the fact that your GP works from a 'surgery' indicates to us that the word might have a wider meaning. In fact, a surgeon was probably someone who treated a wide range of ailments. In any case, the lack of anaesthesia and antibiotics limited any 'surgical intervention' to setting fractures and healing external wounds (Ellis 2001).

We do not know exactly what Mary Webb practised. We know that she was a woman whose education would have given her a very practical slant on the practice of healthcare. Nurses today value the practical nature of their work. Nurses help to treat wounds and do many other things with which Mary Webb would have been familiar.

For the most part, the history of nursing is inextricably mixed up with the history of healthcare in general and of the other professions, such as surgery, pharmacy and medicine which were to come out of this cauldron of work. However, we know very little indeed about what work was done with children. It does seem likely that there were few, if any, people who confined their practice to child health. Indeed, children may have seemed particularly difficult to treat and the course of their disease inevitable given the high infant and child mortality rate.

Key points

- The history of nursing is inextricably mixed with other strands of medicine, surgery and healthcare.
- While we know of some individuals who focused their work on children, there was no occupation group which did so, at least prior to the inception of the children's occupational dispensaries in the eighteenth century.
- There was no child nursing occupational group prior to the founding of the children's hospitals from the mid-nineteenth century.

Thomas Phaer's text (Bowers 1999) on the treatment of children, written in 1544, offers unusual insight into the work of a practitioner with a specific focus on the treatment of children. In this extract from his book, Phaer discusses the treatment of childhood smallpox and measles (these 'evell affections' (Bowers 1999, p. 68)). The account is more about nursing than it is of medicine (Bowers 1999, pp. 68–9):

The best and most sure helpe in this case is not to meddle with any kynde of medicine, but to let nature woorke her operation. Notwythstandynge, yf they be too slowe in commynge oute it shall be good for you to gyve the chylde to drynke sodden mylke and saffron, and so to kepe hym close and warme whereby they maye the soner issue forth [the impurities in the child's body were thought to 'come out' as a rash] … Yf the wheles be outragyous and great, with moche corrosion and venim, some make a decoction of roses and plantayne in the water of oke, and dissolve it in a lytle Englysh honye and camphor … Moreover, it is good to droppe in the pacientes eyes, .v or .vi tymes a daye, a little rose or fenel water to comforte the sight, lest it be hurte by contynuall renning of matter … The same rose water is also good to gargle in hys mouthe, if the chylde be then payned in the throte.

It can be seen that there is 'care' here; Phaer is interested in the child's suffering, even when there is no clear treatment for the condition. In common with his contemporaries, Phaer is using herbs and other materials which would be at hand in any country household. However, Phaer would have understood little of 'science'. His evidence came from experience and from ancient texts which had been updated little over hundreds of years. It is also the case that Phaer was happy to use charms, for, to the sixteenth century practitioner, God had provided objects with curative powers in exactly the same way as He had done with plants and herbs:

I fynde that manye thynges have a naturall vertue agaynste the fallyng evell, not of any quality elemental but by a simgular propertie, or rather an influence of heaven, whyche almyghtye God hath gyven into thynges here in earth … [he goes on to recommend such things as red coral, sapphires and the stone found in the belly of swallows and that they should be hung around the neck of the ill child as an amulet] These, or one of them, hanged about the necke o the childe saveth and preserveth it from the sayde syckenes.

(Bowers 1999, p. 41)

So, just like Hippocrates centuries before him, Phaer was no scientist. Phaer used the understanding of his day, just as we do in our day. Phaer looked for evidence to support his practice, but he was faced with a mountain of ignorance, just as we are today. Nevertheless, Phaer considered himself to be a learned man:

… my purpose is here to do them good that have moost nede, that is to say chyldren, and to shewe the remedyes that God hath created for the use of man to distrybute in Englysshe to them that are unlerned part of the treasure that is in other languages, to provoke them that are of better lernying to utter theyr knowledge in suche lyke attemptes, finallye to declare that to the use of many which ought not to be secrete for lucre of a fewe, and to communicat the frute of my labours to them that wyl gently and thankefully receyve them.

(Bowers 1999, p. 27)

Reflection point

Do you think Phaer's care did any good? How might it have helped people?

My guess is that Phaer's care did do good. It gave families hope; it assured them that all that could be done was being done. Sometimes that is all we have to offer today; indeed, perhaps such things are some of the most important things we do today. We call such things 'care' and we call such things 'nursing'. We do these things because the child and the family matter, and their comfort in times of distress matters. Perhaps this is what nursing is and perhaps Thomas Phaer was the UK's first nurse (Jolley 2006a).

So far, we have discerned that:

- Nursing, up the Tudor period, was really just part of a more-or-less single healthcare discipline.
- Those disciplines that might have considered themselves nurses, including some monastic orders such as the Order of St John (now St John Ambulance), did also practise medical and surgical intervention (Evans 2004).
- Other people's practice might have been more orientated to medical treatment. From this, both apothecaries (pharmacists) and physicians would eventually emerge.
- However, most or all of these people also practised 'care', i.e. they sought to 'comfort' the patient and not just treat disease or injury.
- We can be clear that nursing was not a predominantly female activity, for there were female surgeons (Wyman 1984) and male nurses (Brooke 1997; Brown 2000; Evans 2004; Cook 2005). It would take Florence Nightingale, in the mid-nineteenth century, to fashion nursing as a female-only discipline (Mackintosh 1997).

We have discerned something else about our history. Although it is possible to map the history of nursing through time, child nursing hardly seems to have existed at all. It is probably the case that child nursing, as a discipline, was not much in existence before the children's hospitals were built in the second half of the nineteenth century. We have noted the work of Thomas Phaer but he seems to have been unusual in focusing his work on child illness. It is possible that so many children died that their conditions were largely seen as untreatable. Certainly Armstrong (1777)[1] complains bitterly that children's diseases had been largely ignored because they were not thought worth treating. In his book of 1777, he complains about:

> The absurd notion, which has too long, and too universally prevailed, that there is little or nothing to be done in the complaints of children has prevented many parents from applying to physicians for advise.

(Armstrong 1777, p. vii)

The children's hospital and the advent of child nursing

Let us look at the time when the treatment of children first began to be seen as a legitimate activity. There were no children's hospitals in Britain until 1852, when the Hospital for Sick Children in Great Ormond Street, London, UK, opened. There were general hospitals before this time, though there is little evidence that they cared for many children (Lomax 1996). It is important to understand that the nineteenth century 'hospital' tended to be a place for the deserving poor, and not for everyone. The deserving poor were those working people who could not afford medical treatment. Both the well-off and the destitute could, on the whole, not access the nineteenth century hospitals (including the children's hospitals).

In wider Europe, there were children's hospitals, including some that were state funded. Perhaps the most well known of these was l'Hôpital des Enfants Malades in Paris, France, which formally became a hospital in 1802. In the UK, the first real evidence we have of a provision of healthcare to children were the children's dispensaries; the first one was opened in 1769 by George Armstrong in Red Lion

---

[1] George Armstrong founded the first children's dispensary in the UK.

Square, London. The dispensaries were rather like hospital outpatient departments. The poor could take a sick child to see a physician or an apothecary. A diagnosis would be made and medicine dispensed. The dispensaries were active until perhaps the end of the nineteenth century when more and more hospitals were being built and (arguably) the dispensaries were no longer needed. When children's hospitals became available, they were better able to attract charitable funding and the dispensaries found that they had become unsustainable. This is perhaps the first sign of the success of the hospital movement. Hospitals were successful because they provided an image of 'care'; for example, Florence Nightingale cooling the patient's fevered brow. Such an image requires a bed and it requires a nurse. The wealthy would give money to the hospitals because hospitals became associated with the romantic image of the nurse caring for the patient.

The development of medicine as a discipline meant that it needed continuous access to the patient; the hospital was the doctor's perfect model. Remember that the advance of the hospital movement in the nineteenth century would have been nothing without nursing. Of course, doctors needed nurses to care for the patient throughout the day and to deliver the treatment ordered by the doctor. The hospital was 'the' way in which medicine was able to develop beyond independent practice, offered from the doctor's family home. In this way, the hospital was at least as good for medicine as it was for the sick person (Porter 1997b) and, in every way, the development of the hospital and therefore of medicine required nurses.

Key points

- Hospitals enabled doctors to develop their practice in ways which had never been possible before, simply because doctors could see the patient's response to treatment over time.
- Hospitals needed nurses who were skilled, educated and disciplined. As such, the rise of the hospital movement in the nineteenth century was chiefly responsible for modern nursing.

We have already touched on another contribution made by nurses. The hospitals were charitable affairs; they depended on public subscription and on wealthy benefactors. The nineteenth century was a period of intense religious fervour. There were wide differences between the rich and the poor, social unrest was feared and most feared of all was an English copy of the French Revolution. Fear of social unrest and a keen notion that Hell awaited the ungodly caused society to invest heavily in the poor. The writing of Charles Dickens (1984) brought the lot of the Victorian poor into the heart of the reading rooms of the middle and upper classes. Factory Acts (Hendrick 1994; Cunningham 1995) dealt with some of the more inhumane aspects of industrial life. The Education Act of 1870 brought initial education to the masses, and also ensured that the streets were clear of unemployed children with too much time on their hands. All this meant that people with money wanted to give some of their wealth to the less well-off. What better – indeed, what more romantic – image of dutiful benefaction surpassed that of the hospital. Here was duty, discipline and care. The hospital carried middle-class values to the deserving poor. There was

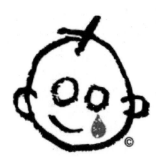

Figure 1.1
Logo of the Great Ormond
Street Hospital Charity's
Wishing Well Appeal.
Image copyright of Great
Ormond Street Hospital
for Children.

cleanliness, new knowledge which epitomized the success of Victorian society and there was romantic 'care'. It is likely that hospitals were successful chiefly because of the caring image provided by nurses. Without nurses and the romantic image of care with which they had become so closely associated, the hospital movement might have failed and medicine would still be operating out of the doctor's family home.

Today, some hospitals are funded charitably (the children's hospices). Some NHS hospitals have associated charities to enable them to improve and advance the level of care they can offer. Figure 1.1 shows the logo used in the Wishing Well Appeal by the Great Ormond Street Hospital Charity, which was launched by the Prince and Princess of Wales in 1984 and has funded a new building and new units over the years.

The image shown in Fig. 1.1 is 'romantic' in that it seeks to cause us to 'feel' for the child and for the hospital. It creates a strong sense of a child needing care. Perhaps the image makes you want to look after the crying child; you cannot but you could donate to the hospital to enable it to care for sick children. An image of a doctor operating on a child would probably not have the same emotional impact. Most of us do not have an urge to use a scalpel; images of 'caring', on the other hand, or the need for care do have an effect on us.

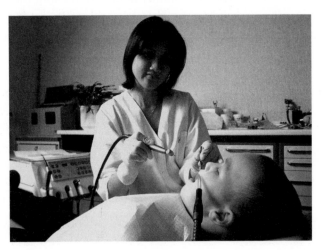

Figure 1.2 Operating on a child. ©Imagestate Media

> **Reflection point**
>
> Would the picture shown in Fig. 1.2 cause you to donate money to the hospital?

The hospital movement in the nineteenth century and indeed the development of medicine itself were dependent on the image of nursing, i.e. the image of 'care'. Even today, if we were to ask nurses what it is that differentiates their discipline from medicine, their answer would include the word 'care'. To the charity-donating public of the nineteenth and twentieth centuries, 'care' was all important. The hospital movement owes much of its success to this 'care', provided by the image of the nurse ministering to the patient.

Nurses as servants

It is clear that hospital nurses were a new occupational group. Most 'nurses' were recruited from the servant classes. Many domestic servants would have had a role in caring for children in the family. Usefully, servants were also skilled at cleaning clothes, bed linen, brasses and just about everything else within the domestic household. Domestic servants were also familiar with preparing at least the more simple meals and of cooking for the sick. Perhaps most useful of all, the domestic servant knew how to do what she was told; in other words, she was a disciplined creature. Discipline was important in any well-ordered household. Discipline preserved the important social distinction between the family and the servants. Discipline also maintained standards, especially those related to hygiene and cleanliness, upon which the health of the family depended.

> *Household servants would wear a cap to keep their hair out of the way. A white pinafore would be worn to protect the uniform from getting soiled and to enable the employer to see that the servant washed it frequently enough. These were the clothes of the nurse, at least until fairly recently.*

> (Pearson et al. *2001*)

Reflection point

★ Think of images you have seen of nurses' uniform from the nineteenth century to the present day. How do you think that the changing style of uniform reflects changes in society and in child nursing itself?

It was not just the uniform which kept alive the association with servanthood; nurses were treated as servants too. Nurses were expected to do practical and often menial work and to put the needs of their workplace above their own needs. Because of this, people sometimes still see nurses as being 'dedicated' and hard-working people.

Case study

A letter from a nurse working at Yorkhill, Glasgow, UK, between 1924 and 1928 indicates the conditions under which paediatric nurses had to work at that time (Edwards 1980).

It was a gruelling business, rules and regulations were very strict. Lights out at 10pm sharp no matter what you were doing … Personal belongings were checked … Sisters were strict and generally unfriendly. To be ill was a crime … The food was poor and the off duty never made up until the day you had it, so it was impossible to keep in touch with your friends. Phone calls in or out were not allowed … In spite of this we did get some fun, I suppose we ganged together against the monstrous establishment … many a tear was shed and a resolve to leave but everyone suffered and so carried on.

This new occupational group (nurses) emerged from the needs of the new nineteenth century hospitals. Perhaps the role of household servant and nurse has always been a little confused. Today, who tidies up the ward at the end of the shift? Do the doctors do that, the physiotherapists, the hospital cleaners? Perhaps it is still the case that nurses are expected to tidy up, to prepare at least the lighter meals and to take orders from doctors concerning the patients' treatment. These might not be aspects of the nurses' work that we consider central to the role, but they are there all the same.

A new history of nursing commenced with the establishment of the nineteenth century hospitals. Medicine would make most use of the hospitals, and medical practice developed both in complexity and in authority. The hospital provided doctors with a new throne, and from it they would take command of almost every aspect of healthcare. Gone would be the healers of past centuries – the bone setters (Adams 1997), the surgeoness, the barber–surgeons and the independent birth attendants (midwives). Already gone were the nurses, male and female, who spent their lives in monasteries and religious orders. Hospitals brought a new and quite distinct profession of medicine, characterized by a university education and membership of either the Royal College of Medicine or the Royal College of Surgery. Medicine had achieved what Hardyment (1995) called 'occupational closure' – it had ensured that only doctors could practise medicine and that they had control over the whole arena of healthcare.

The new hospitals needed a new kind of disciplined and dedicated nurse. The creation of this new model of nursing is widely seen to be the work of Florence Nightingale (Mackintosh 1997; Evans 2004). It was also Nightingale who ensured that nursing would be a female-only discipline. Men would be allowed to work in mental health, but general nursing (and child nursing) would be the exclusive domain of the female. There can be little doubt that this helped to reinforce the hierarchical position of doctor and nurse. For, at this time, men were considered superior in the workplace and a woman's role was to support her male superior. As late as 1927, Ashdown (1927, p. 1) commented that:

> *A nurse must be punctual, good tempered, obedient and loyal to all rules as the foundation of her work. She must also be active, yet quiet and deft; methodical, reliable, careful, clean and neat; observant, intelligent and economical; possessed of self control, persevering gentleness, tact, sympathy, and common sense; careful to respect professional etiquette, remembering what is due to those in authority; courteous in manner and in attention to visitors and patients' friends (a duty that nurses in the pressure of their work are apt to overlook); careful to wear her uniform with spotless cleanliness, neatness and simplicity, with hair tidy, no jewellery, her general bearing that of military smartness; careful to be guarded in her behaviour towards doctors and students.*

By the beginning of the twentieth century, nursing and medicine were quite separate disciplines, but they were disciplines which worked intimately together. Doctors were ready to build on their success, for they had hospitals to work in and a ready source of female, well-disciplined labour to support them. Now every large town had a hospital and the advance of medicine must have seemed inevitable.

The first children's hospital

The first children's hospital was opened in 1852 by Charles West in Great Ormond Street, London. There was a considerable amount of snobbery among the more successful physicians who consulted for the general hospitals. Medical education was expensive and, to obtain a sufficiently sound reputation in medicine, one had to come from the 'right part' of society. For this reason, it was difficult for some people to become doctors. For women, this was almost impossible; however, it was difficult for some men as well. Charles West came from a non-Anglican background. This meant that he had to conduct much of his clinical education abroad. On his return to England, West found that a career in the general hospitals was not available to him.

Britain was a deeply religious country at this time and the dominant religion was Anglicanism. Other religions were tolerated but still distrusted. Nurses themselves would have had to be Anglican and be able to recite the Lord's Prayer; they would certainly be expected to lead the prayers in the ward.

Robinson (1972) provides evidence of evening prayers and grace being said by the ward sister at Yorkhill in the nineteenth century. In 1892 (Yorkhill Hospitals Archive 1883–91) nurses are reported to have provided simple religious instruction. This appears to have been common practice at the time and indicates that nurses did not confine their focus to the child's physical needs.

West found himself frustrated by an inability to secure a suitable position. What West did in response was to found a new hospital. Indeed, this was a time when specialist hospitals were springing up in other disciplines, such as in ophthalmology, orthopaedics and hospitals for women. These hospitals, too, often arose because of an individual's disenfranchisement with the medical establishment.

West's hospital in Great Ormond Street experienced opposition from the local general hospitals (Lomax 1996) and from Florence Nightingale herself (Nightingale 1860). A children's hospital was a new idea and there were fears that it would cause the spread of infectious diseases. Florence Nightingale felt that sick children were better cared for in adult wards where the patients could look after them (Atkinson 1981). Nightingale was also concerned that it would simply not be possible to recruit enough nurses able to care for sick children. However, West ensured that he had a group of powerful supporters, including Charles Dickens and Queen Victoria. In addition, West ensured that his hospital would be seen as a caring place. West made certain that the nurses were always kind to the children (West 1854). West's new hospital was to be a place that could always receive wealthy visitors who might provide the finance needed for the hospital to survive in the long term.

Charles West provided the template for children's hospitals across the UK (West 1854; Lomax 1996). It is known, for example, that his list of 'rules' for The Hospital for Sick Children, Great Ormond Street, were widely copied by the children's hospitals that opened after 1852. West identified the proper role and philosophical underpinning of the new child nurse. West determined that child nurses had to be able to keep children happy, they had never to be cruel or harsh, and they had to be caring people (West 1854). Arguably, this is a model that exists to the present day.

It was easy to see what child nursing was – it was the nursing of sick children in hospital. Child nurses may not have had the training and education available to doctors but they were still fairly well educated. Even in the 1860s and 1870s, most child nurses would have had an initial education and would have been able to read and write. Hospitals would admit nurses as 'probationers' (students) and would offer a training programme which was usually 3 years long. So, child nurses were 'trained' people who looked after sick children, almost exclusively in hospital.

The problem was, however, that child nurses were not the only people nursing children. The general hospitals competed with the children's hospitals and admitted at least small numbers of children. By the end of the nineteenth century, most general hospitals had opened children's wards and, here, most of the staff were general nurses. Other specialist hospitals also trained their own staff so that orthopaedic hospitals, which traditionally had catered largely for children, were staffed by orthopaedic and not child nurses. Infectious disease hospitals also catered for a large proportion of children in hospital but they too tended not to employ child nurses. In practice, each hospital trained and employed its own nurses. When nurses did wish to move to another hospital, they would tend to find it easier to get employment in the same 'type' of hospital as the one in which they had trained. This meant that child nursing did not have occupational closure. It must have seemed as if anyone could nurse children. This lack of occupational closure would continue to trouble child nursing and arguably troubles it still.

Twentieth century troubles

The nineteenth century had been a romantic time for nursing. Child nurses were seen as brave, dedicated souls who were offering themselves up to the service of God and his children. Child nurses worked hard, long hours and were paid very little. Perhaps it was the way in which nurses lived in the hospital and in which they were largely divorced from normal life outside the hospital which endeared them to the public and which made them appear 'dedicated'. Children's hospitals were places of 'care', largely open to the scrutiny of those who were considering the provision of funds. Nurses had high standards and these were oriented to the needs of the child patient. It is clear that, at least in the years before *c*.1920, children's need for emotional or psychological care was understood (Lindsay 2001a). Yapp (1915) in her 'lectures to probationers' wrote at length of the provision of play, the need to develop an empathic understanding of child life and the provision of 'love and understanding':

> The successful children's nurse must have a real love for children, little children cannot be loved too much but they must be loved wisely. The nurse must possess sufficient imagination to enable her to put herself in her little charge's place. She must have a sympathetic understanding of child life, an abundant patience in dealing with children, and keen observation.

> (Yapp 1915, p. 107)

Yapp (1915, p. 8) was also clear about children's need for their own family:

> Probably most of you think that these children must be happier with us than they are in their own homes. Now, they are certainly in a healthier environment, but I am not at all sure that they are happier. However poor the house they have come from, it is their home, and that is what the ward can rarely be … [At home] mother is there to caress and soothe when pains gnaw at

one, and things are becoming more than one small person can bear alone. …
There is a quality of happiness in these very homes which we cannot in the
nature of things realise. The family of the working man are so closely drawn
together that they instinctively cling to one another, and whenever there is self
sacrifice, which is inevitable in their condition, there is the essence of love. It is
in the power of every nurse to make these children feel that they are not
'unwanted' and to see that at any rate they will never feel 'un-mothered' in the
wards of a poor law infirmary. No one with motherly instincts will ever allow a
child to go to sleep unhappy.

Reflection points

★ How does Yapp's statement (above) compare with the modern child nurses' orientation to his or her work?

★ How does Yapp's statement relate to the modern, finance and business-orientated National Health Service? Try to relate Yapp's statement to the increase in patient throughput and the continuing development of hospital day-case admissions. Indeed, try to relate Yapp's statement to the notion of a patient as a 'case'.

The twentieth century was to see a sea change in the way in which child nursing was orientated. Gone would be the romanticism expressed by Yapp (above) and by others of influence in the Victorian era (Wood 1888) and in its place would come 'science' and 'professionalism'.

The romanticism was all but gone by 1920. In its place was a much harder stance in which the child was seen from a medical- and disease-related perspective. Here was a more 'objective' approach to care. It was an approach to care which emphasized the superiority of the nurse over the family. The nurse knew better than did the family; she was an expert in caring, the family was not. The nurse worked closely with doctors, and this closeness to medicine gave nurses a new prestige.

Today, there is a well-understood 'balance' between the rights and responsibilities of the family and the duties of the health services. The family and the health services try to work together so that both their needs can be met while the child receives the most appropriate care and treatment. What was different about the years from *c.*1920 is that the 'power' in this relationship was held chiefly by the health professions (Hardyment 1995). This imbalance of power and the new emphasis on objectivity and professionalism caused the family to be excluded from the care of hospitalized children. Parents were often forbidden from visiting their child or were limited to visiting for perhaps half an hour a week. When parents did visit, they were sometimes limited to observing their child through a one-way glass. Often, parents had to stay outside in the cold and try to communicate through a closed window. Even when parents could meet with their child, they were discouraged from holding and cuddling the child (Jolley 2007b). Good nursing and medical care were being provided but there was a price to pay; the balance of power was now in the hands of nurses and doctors and families had to do what was thought best for them. The case studies below illustrate this.

Case study

The following is a transcript from an elderly gentleman recalling his stay in hospital in the 1930s (Jolley 2007b, p. 22):

When the matron did her rounds, you know she would come down the centre of the ward … with her entourage and cape flowing and everybody was in fear and I really mean fear [emphasis] the nurses as well. I can see the old battle-axe now, coming down and criticising this, that and another. I can remember being in fear of the matron, I was in fear of everything really. You were nearly in fear of [pause] moving off your bed or moving in bed really because everything had to be kept … like that board [pointing], so straight. You know, I can't remember much laughing. I don't know why I'm like this [cries].

- Consider what this account tells us about the nursing care this gentleman received and the impact that care had on him.

Parents were simply 'not needed' and were expected to cope with the separation because this was considered to be in the interest of the child; after all, the child was being looked after by skilled and professional people.

Case study

Here, an elderly lady recalls the admission of her child to hospital in the 1950s (Jolley 2007b, p. 22):

Anyway, they X-rayed her and they told her what had happened. And they said [to the parent], 'now you go home now and ring up about midnight' (because we had to sign that she could have an anaesthetic). And [child's name] was crying for me [painfully], but they wouldn't let us … The last thing I remember was that they were cutting her Wellingtons off. I left her and … I often wake up in the night and I can hear her.

- Consider what this account tells us about the mother's separation from her child and how it affected her.

Notice that the elderly lady still claimed to wake up in the night, hearing her child calling for her. The transcript was taken 45 years after the child's admission to hospital. This is evidence of psychological trauma and is typical of the accounts from this period (Jolley 2004). The 'trauma' of separation did not just affect hospitalized children, it affected the parents and siblings and grandparents too. It is the same with love, which is something that unites two or more people and in a sense makes them into a single emotional entity. It is appropriate, then, that the modern notion of 'family-centred care' accepts that parents and grandparents and siblings and school friends are all a legitimate focus of the nurse's attention.

Case study

An experienced nurse looks back at her time in the 1960s as a student on a children's ward (Jolley 2004, participant B). This student had admitted a toddler whose mother, of course, had been sent home.

And so this Toddler that by now was distraught, sobbing, I went to pick him up, because he was just, he was just left on the cot to break his heart and sob, so I went to pick him up and just as I did, he was like a little monkey, his arms around me, and [laugh] I can still see him today, his little fingers … I'm going to get upset again [crying] hanging up to me. [crying] [pause] [pause] It was awful [crying] [pause]. And so [crying] the good children's nurse came and put a harness on him and fastened him down [emphasis] [pause] and sob, sob, sob [meaning the child] it was awful. I think, one of the worst things and he was just left to get on with it [pause]. And I don't know why, I don't know why, I don't know why, I don't know why [emphasis].

- Consider what this account tells us about the nursing practice on a children's ward in the 1960s and how this would have affected the student nurse.

It was not just the child and family who were traumatized, nurses were traumatized too. Nurses were caught up in a 'culture' which emphasized a behaviouristic approach to the understanding of childhood and which argued that emotion was unscientific (Watson 1928). At the same time, nurses were controlled by a culturally derived system of discipline and hierarchy which prevented them from openly questioning established practice. Consider this quote from a nursing textbook:

… it is an accepted fact that the former [doctor] takes precedence over the latter [nurse] … no doctor can be expected to recognise socially the nurse who is working for him, and she must wait for acknowledgement from him first.

(Vivian 1919, pp. 56–7)

It was a cultural 'norm' that nurses were subordinate to doctors. Here is a doctor's view on the matter (Lindsay 2001b, p. 7):

A good modern nurse is wholly feminine, full of vitality, ordered in service, faithful and un-weary in well doing, a fine responsive devoted instrument, willingly placed in the hands of medicine for the service of the sick. This is common knowledge.

It was the 'common knowledge' in all of this – that children would be damaged by too much love, that they were better off in hospital without their parents and that there should be discipline in nursing – it was the common knowledge of these aspects of culture that made them so difficult to change.

Nurses knew that if children were separated from their parents they would in time (usually about 24 hours) become placid and malleable; importantly, they would stop crying. It was 'behaviour' that mattered, not the child's feelings (Watson 1928). Nurses, too, were not expected to have 'feelings'; after all, nursing was an objective science, close to medicine, and nurses were 'professional', and that meant not having feelings or concerning oneself with the feelings of others (Jolley 2004).

An explanation of impassionate nursing

These events can be explained in the way that a number of seemingly disparate events took place in society. These events were:

- the First World War (1914–1918)
- the developing acceptance of behaviourism as a key approach to the understanding of childhood
- the Nurses Act 1919
- the dominance of child nursing by adult (general) nursing.

The First World War (1914–1918)

The First World War had taken a huge toll on society. One of the many problems had been the difficulty in recruiting men who were sufficiently healthy to serve in the army (Arton 1992). This had the effect of causing the government to focus on child health and to introduce a wide range of special and residential schools, hospitals and nurseries for children funded by the state. There were residential and hospital schools for children with ringworm (Ayers 1971), tuberculosis (Anonymous 1919a) and for delicate children, etc. Here, there would be a focus on providing the children with exercise, fresh air and a nutritious diet (Anonymous 1919b). Typically, children would stay in these institutions for weeks or months. There was no thought that the child might have emotional needs and that the child's love for his or her family might cause sadness and despair when separation took place. The irony of this situation is that the people who purported to know what was best for the child had ignored one central need that all children have – to be loved by someone; for most children, the people they loved most were their parents and their brothers and sisters.

Perhaps it was the model provided by these residential hospitals for children that caused the rest of society to take the view that to separate children from their families was not only acceptable but was the best thing to do. After all, those children were ill because of a lack of good nutrition, good exercise and fresh air – all things that a good family should have provided. The professional knew best and much of childhood illness was now seen to be the fault of the family. Even the infectious diseases caused more havoc among those already weakened by poor nutrition and overcrowding at home. The modern medicine of the mid-twentieth century was as much a battle against the ignorance of the family as it was against the diseases that that ignorance had caused.

Nursing adopted an objective approach to its work. This happened easily because of nursing's now very close association with medicine. Even psychology wanted to be seen as a science. Behaviourism, with its emphasis on objectivity and research, became the key way in which children were understood. Freudian psychology had been about 'understanding' the patient (Freud and Freud 1991), but behaviourism was to put the emphasis on changing behaviour (Watson 1928). There could now be no legitimate interest in children's emotions and feelings. Cuddling children was discouraged and parents, especially mothers, were considered to be at best unnecessary and at worst harmful because they were 'emotional'. Getting the child to behave 'properly' and learn what he or she needed to learn was an objective matter – a matter for science (Cunningham 1995).

Behaviourism

Behaviourism taught that love and emotions should be no part of childhood. State intervention in the healthcare of children provided a parent-free model of child care (Maxwell 1997). Very quickly, child nursing lost its romanticism. From 1920 there was a new emphasis on professionalism and the importance of nursing knowledge and of nurses' need for a sense of discipline.

Nursing had lost its 'love'. The nurses' uniform began to take on a military appearance. Nursing confused what was written in books with 'science'. This was science that was 'learned', but which could not be critiqued (Jolley 2004). It became almost impossible for nurses to think for themselves because the established knowledge could not be questioned. This emphasis on professionalism, on the fiction that science could be read in books and on a behaviouristic image of childhood would be an enduring one. It would take another world war to force real change in nursing.

Key point

- By the 1920s the romanticism of nursing had been replaced by an objective and scientific approach to care. Unfortunately, this meant that parents and the 'love' they felt for the child was now considered superfluous to requirement and even injurious to the welfare of the sick child and his or her treatment. As such, this period in our history is characterized by sick children being separated from the people they would have felt the most need for at this time – their parents and their family.

The Nurses Act 1919

The late Victorian years had seen bitter arguments about what form nursing should take. Florence Nightingale had been against the idea of nursing being a 'profession' and had wanted nursing to be a servant-class organization characterized by discipline and effective management. Ethel Bedford Fenwick and the College of Nursing (Royal College of Nursing (RCN)) had argued that nursing should be allowed to develop into a fully fledged profession (Hector 1976). In 1919, the friction between Ethel Bedford Fenwick, the College of Nursing and Florence Nightingale was eventually settled by parliament. The 1919 Nurses Act provided for a new register of nurses to be maintained by the new General Nursing Council (GNC)[2] – nursing was to be a profession.

The setting up of the professional register in 1919 has been seen as a positive milestone in nursing's history. The 1919 Nurses Act gave nursing its professional status and enabled it to establish standards of education and practice in nursing. However, it also sent out a clear message that nursing was now a profession. It is possible that this contributed to the growing notion that nurses were experts and that they therefore knew better how to care for children than did parents. It is not surprising that nursing was enthusiastic about its new status. Romantic nursing, based on 'care' being an emotionally driven activity, could hardly be compatible with the new 'profession' of nursing.

Compounding this effect was the fact that child nursing was poorly represented on the GNC. The GNC was dominated by general (adult) nursing. Indeed, it was to be the case that child nursing came ever more closely to be seen as aligned to general nursing.

The dominance of child nursing by adult (general) nursing

Arguments had raged about which nurses should be admitted to the register (Anonymous 1919c) and, specifically, whether child nurses should be admitted to the register at all. In parliament, Sir Watson Cheyne argued that the register should contain only the names of fully trained nurses and not wet nurses and child nurses 'whose only duty it is to push perambulators' (Burdett 1919, p. 174). Dr Addison disagreed because he felt that those whose training was imperfect or incomplete should be admitted in recognition of their good work. Therefore, a supplementary register for the 'imperfect' and 'incomplete' child nurses was opened in 1919. Part of the problem was that child nurses had undergone their training in the children's hospitals and had, therefore, only got experience with babies and children. General nurses had trained in general hospitals, which were bigger and carried more political influence. General nurses had experience in many different kinds of nursing, often including children. In this way, the training received by general nurses was often considered to be superior to that obtained by child nurses (Arton 1992). It was probably also the case that, because the children's hospitals were run quite separately from the general hospitals, they were less well understood. It would have been easy to think that child nursing was a relatively simple activity which was hardly more skilled than the care carried out by domestic servants, nannies and even parents themselves. Bradley (2003, p. 362) puts it thus:

> *The history of the education of nurses to care for sick children ... is a history fraught with prejudice, threats and misapprehensions. Certain key issues recur throughout the 130 years that education of child nurses has existed: most are as familiar to professionals in this arena today as they were at the turn of the 19th century. Central to these issues is the status of child nurses within the profession. Often deemed second rate citizens in nursing spheres, relegated to a supplementary register in 1919, their skills and knowledge under-valued, the specialist needs of child nurses have often gone unrecognised. Efforts to convince general adult nurses of the equity of their value and, in the light of the differences between children and adults, the importance of specialist pre-registration education, has at times been difficult to achieve.*

[2]The equivalent organization today is the Nursing and Midwifery Council.

The RCN tried to amalgamate the child and general training with a new 'comprehensive' training scheme in which students could acquire both registrations in one course of study (Great Ormond Street Hospital Archive 1942a). However, the lobby from the children's hospitals was still a powerful one (Great Ormond Street Hospital Archive 1942b) and the decision was made to leave the Registered Sick Children's Nurse qualification alone. This infuriated the RCN, which wrote to the children's hospitals saying that it noted with 'keen disappointment' the children's hospitals' submission to the Nursing Reconstruction Committee (Horder). The RCN suggested that the children's hospitals had failed to consider the need to improve *all* nurse training (Great Ormond Street Hospital Archive 1943). In 1945, the general nurse dominated GNC[3] made it possible for general nurses working in children's hospitals for 2 years to register as child nurses by doing little more than taking the final examination for the child nursing programme (News 1945). The RCN was also dominated by general nurses, and it tried on several occasions to remove the separate part of the register for child nurses or to merge it with the general register. In 1964, the RCN (Royal College of Nursing 1964) was to state that:

> Since the principles of paediatric nursing are those of adult nursing applied to a special age group, it should be possible … to organise a course … which would prepare in three years for registration on both the General and Paediatric parts of the register.

Key point

- Historically, the training, education and practice of child nursing was problematic owing to the dominance of general nurses within the practice, management and governance of nursing. The influences served to make child nursing more and more like general nursing and sought (so far unsuccessfully) to close the part of the register for child nurses.

Over time, the general hospitals began to open wards for children and many of the smaller children's hospitals began to close. This meant that more and more general nurses were working with children. The discrimination against child nurses (Jolley 2007c) can be seen in the way in which nursing posts on children's wards were often made available only to general nurses (Birkenhead and Wirral Children's Hospital 1941); even the children's hospitals would require ward sisters to be both general and child nurses (Booth Hall Hospital for Sick Children 1940, 1956). By the 1970s and 1980s most courses in child nursing were either a combined State Registered Nurse/Registered Sick Children's Nurse programme or were designed for nurses already on the general part of the register.[4]

In many ways, the history of child nursing in the twentieth century cannot be understood outside the ways in which adult or general nursing developed. Perhaps it was that general nursing managed to influence and then control child nursing. Perhaps, too, child nursing tried too hard to match its dominant partner (general nursing) by becoming similar to it in terms of professionalism and discipline. In any case, and whatever the true cause, romanticism was lost. People no longer claimed

---

[3]The equivalent then of the NMC.

[4]The stand-alone Registered Sick Children's Nurse training was still available in Scotland.

that they were child nurses because they had a genuine love for children; indeed, the word 'love' seems to have vanished from the nurses' repertoire of words altogether. In contrast, more than a century ago, Catherine Wood (1888, p. 509) was to write of child nursing:

> *Over and above the actual skilled Nursing, it is necessary to develop in the Nurse the mother's instinct, the grand self-sacrifice and self-forgetfulness that are the outcome of the mother's love; we want each Nurse to gather her little ones into her arms with the resolve that she will spend and be spent for them. They are hers, and for a time they will look to her for a mother's love and a mother's care. They must be more than cases to her, or they will not thrive as they might in her care.*

To Catherine Wood, 'care' meant 'love'. How sad it now seems that that word, so carefully chosen by Catherine Wood, so closely linked with the notion of a mother's love, should come to mean 'organization', 'management' and perhaps everything that a nurse does. Even today, we can talk about the care of a child with intussusception and know that we mean the organization of care and the management of that child. Nursing had become brutal (Jolley 2006b) because it lacked love. Love was emotional; it signified 'involvement' in the lives of the child and parents, which was so much discouraged by general nursing. To the nineteenth century nurse, care was impossible without feeling what the child and parents were feeling, without understanding their thoughts and sharing their suffering. Only by knowing their suffering was one able to deal with it and to use nursing knowledge and skills to ameliorate that suffering. In fact, nursing was all about suffering and the desire to reduce it. It was love for the patient which caused the nurse to involve herself in the patient's suffering and to seek to make it better. The child's parents would look at the sick child in the hospital bed and want desperately to change places with the child, to take the child's suffering and even the child's death onto themselves. This was love, and it was what the nurses, unashamedly, felt for themselves.

The move to family-centred care: love returns to child nursing

> *… but a people's history of health … will show that sufferers are fertile in their resources … as patients borrow the doctors' lines … a peoples' history of suffering might restore to the history of Medicine its human face.*
>
> *(Porter 1985, p. 195)*

The First World War heralded in the years of professionalism, discipline and the separation of children from their loved ones. The Second World War would undo these changes (Jolley 2007b). The mass evacuation of children in the Second World War affected almost everyone in Britain; it was a social experiment in separating children from their families which took place on a massive scale. Almost everyone was able to see the grief and psychological trauma caused to both parents and children by the separation of children from their loved ones.

At the same time, the war was changing society; women were given the freedom and respect that came with working in factories, in the forces and elsewhere. The

British were told that they were not the jack-booted automatons of Nazi Germany but were free-thinking people. This was also the time when Britain adopted socialized medicine – the National Health Service (NHS) was born. Now the hospitals belonged to the people and people had rights to healthcare and to decide what sort of healthcare they wanted. The 1950s would see young, more affluent people; balking the traditions of dress, non-conformity was now the norm and social hierarchy was breaking down. The 1960s saw a social revolution in which the social divisions in society were finally buried. Behaviourism was replaced by the much softer Freudian psychology which emphasized the need to understand how and why people 'thought' and the importance of childhood experience (Editorial 1957).

In 1959, the Ministry of Health published what would be known as the Platt Report (Ministry of Health 1959). This signalled both the importance of paediatric nursing as a separate discipline to general nursing and the importance of the child's social and psychological needs. At last, behaviourism was dead; specifically, it suggested that:

- the emotional care of children is important
- separation could be damaging
- children should be admitted to hospital only when home care is not possible
- paediatric outpatient departments should be set up
- day care and day surgery should be encouraged
- children should not be admitted to adult wards
- physical environment should be cheerful
- children should be nursed with other children of the same age
- the sister in charge should be a child nurse
- patient allocation is used
- a paediatrician should have overall concern for all (surgical) children admitted
- nursery nurses could help with children under 5 years
- children should be prepared for admission
- there should be facilities for play
- there should be facilities for education of children
- parents should be encouraged to visit freely
- parents should stay with children under 5 years
- parents should be part of the child's care
- financial help should be available for parents to visit
- nurses, doctors and ancillary staff should be trained in the emotional needs of children.

In 1958 Robertson published a film showing a young child being admitted to hospital and experiencing separation. The film graphically portrayed the reaction of the child (Robertson 1958a,b). At around the same time, a colleague of Robertson's, John Bowlby, published his work on grief and separation in childhood (Robertson and Bowlby 1952; Bowlby 1953, 1956, 1958, 1973). Robertson also wrote an article in *The Observer* (Bradley 2001) encouraging parents to write to him about their hospital experiences, and these were published (Robertson 1962). In the same year as Robertson's article in *The Observer*, a group of mothers wrote to *The Guardian* and elicited a large number of responses from like-minded people who would come together to form the National Association for the Welfare of Children in Hospital (NAWCH), which grew very quickly in both size and political influence. Bradley

(2001) reported that by 1963 the organization had 2200 members in 40 groups and that by 1968 it had 4000 members in 58 groups. The success of NAWCH lies both in the perceived legitimacy of the debate which Robertson had initiated and in the fact that it lobbied high-ranking government ministers. Importantly, the organization provided ordinary parents with a means to speak out against the forced separation from their own sick children.

NAWCH produced a 'charter' for the care of children in hospital. Like the Platt Report, the NAWCH charter seems perfectly relevant today:

- Children shall be admitted to hospital only if the care they require cannot be equally well provided at home or on a day basis.
- Children in hospital shall have the right to have their parents with them at all times provided this is in the best interest of the child. Accommodation shall therefore be offered to all parents, and they should be helped and encouraged to stay. In order to share in the care of their child, parents should be fully informed about ward routine and their active participation encouraged.
- Children and/or their parents shall have the right to information appropriate to age and understanding.
- Children and/or their parents shall have the right to informed participation in all decisions involving their healthcare. Every child shall be protected from unnecessary medical treatment and steps taken to mitigate physical and emotional distress.
- Children shall be treated with tact and understanding and at all times their privacy shall be respected.
- Children shall enjoy the care of appropriately trained staff, fully aware of the physical and emotional needs of each age group.
- Children shall be able to wear their own clothes and have their own personal possessions.
- Children shall be cared for with other children of the same age group.
- Children shall be in an environment furnished and equipped to meet their requirements, and which conforms to recognized standards of safety and supervision.
- Children shall have full opportunity for play, recreation and education suited to their age and condition.

Reflection points

★ How relevant do you think the recommendations of the Platt Report and the NAWCH charter are today?

★ Can you improve these two sets of recommendations? Consider you were writing a 'philosophy of care' for your ward or area, what would you omit and what would you add?

It would take some years before the recommendations of the Platt Report and the NAWCH charter were fully implemented (Davies 2010). Nevertheless, behaviourism had been banished, as had the system of discipline and hierarchy that had so characterized nursing for much of the twentieth century. Nurses began to question accepted practice (Walsh and Ford 1989a–c). The development of degree courses in nursing in the 1970s and 1980s probably did much to legitimize the challenging of traditional knowledge.

The Platt Report had defended the notion that specialization in child nursing was a good thing and that the care children needed was markedly different from that required by adults. Certainly, the 1970s and 1980s were a time when child nursing as a discipline was relatively strong and also well tolerated by general nursing. This was largely because training in child nursing was undertaken either alongside training in general nursing over 4 years or as a post-registration programme over 13 months. During these years, almost all child nurses were also qualified in general nursing. This meant that there was no competition between general and child nursing. Rather, child nursing could be seen as a logical means of specializing. We were, in these two short decades of relative tranquillity, all nurses together.

Reflection point

★ Whether child nursing should be at pre-registration or post-registration level is still the subject of much debate. What are the pros and cons associated with either position and should direct entry, that is, the child branch, continue?

History now

Project 2000 (implemented 1989–1991) was designed to be a more academically orientated system of nurse education (Price 1992). For the first time, the new diploma programmes in nursing would be validated by a university. Students of nursing were at last to have full student status. At the same time, schools of nursing which had been run by NHS hospitals would now amalgamate into bigger, new 'colleges'. In time, these colleges would merge with existing universities; a situation which just about brings us up to date.

It was at this point that general nursing became known as the 'adult branch'. However, it would take more than Project 2000 to change general nursing's perspective on things, and the adult branch remained generalist in its orientation and perspective.

History teaches us that child nurses must be seen to be fully qualified as well as specialist in their area of practice. Nursing is a particularly broad discipline, and those who can practise in only one area will always be seen as less than fully qualified. Child nurses work closely with general nurses, with whom they share the same arena of work and practice. Perhaps it was never sensible for child nurses to specialize without first obtaining a general qualification. In practice, Project 2000 was a mistake which caused general nursing to look again at how it could fashion the closure of the child branch. Today, questions are being asked (Royal College of Nursing 2004) about whether there should be just one general part of the professional register (Royal College of Nursing 2007; Ellis *et al.* 2008). Project 2000 made child nurses special and different when they really needed to be extraordinary.

Child nursing's history is rich and deep. The discussion here leads us to question the nature of child nursing today and how it can continue to regard itself as unique within the wider profession of nursing. This seems a particularly important issue at the present time when child nursing may well be challenged to say why it is not in everyone's interest for there to be one kind of generalist nurse. Perhaps this would not matter much if we wished to return to the child nursing of the mid-twentieth century with its lack of romanticism and its focus on hard professionalism and objectivity. I believe that people still enter child nursing because they have a 'love' for children. Child nursing remains different from adult nursing because we seek to understand children and to share their fears, their pain and their grief. In doing this we become involved, and we suffer some of what the child and family is suffering. Perhaps this *is* the way that child nurses work and what defines them. Talk to adult nurses about 'professional love' and they will not understand us. It is this division of understanding which so clearly demonstrates the professional chasm which should and does divide us from general nursing.

Children are at once both valuable and vulnerable. Children cannot be understood on the basis of any amount of knowledge of adult nursing. Children need love; that is, they need nurses and family who would do anything to help them and would do that without condition. Love exists when one looks at a sick or dying child and recognizes the desire to change places with them. Love exists when what the child feels and experiences matters to us more than our own feelings. Love exists when we feel the child and family's pain, and when we infect ourselves with their grief, their anxiety and their joy. Love exists when the desire to help is compelling and even irrational; love is not confined to the rational and science is its servant, not its master.

Perhaps child nursing would benefit from being a post-registration entity, a true specialization. Perhaps it does not really matter. What does matter is that child nursing survives to do the work it has carried out through its long and colourful history. What does matter is that child nursing stays different from general nursing, with which its sojourn in the mid-twentieth century wreaked so much harm on sick and vulnerable children. What does matter is that the uniqueness of child nursing – its unashamed 'love' for its patients – should survive to do its work for children now and in the future.

Conclusion

In this chapter we have seen child nursing develop from centuries past when it was part of a single discipline of nursing–medicine. At this time, few people confined their practice to child nursing, but child nursing is very much discernable in what went on. Certainly, our history is ancient and fascinating.

Child nursing as we know it today began with the introduction of the children's hospitals in the mid-nineteenth century. Nurses were needed for the hospitals to work. From the beginning, nurses had 'care' as their underpinning precept. However, the twentieth century saw the notion of care become corrupted as child nursing became influenced by general nursing. The 'care' of the patient became synonymous with the 'management' of the patient. Nurses exercised emotional neutrality and emphasized their professionalism and orientation to science. To its credit, child nursing eventually broke away from the precepts of general nursing and adopted family-centred care. In doing this, child nursing rediscovered its romantic beginnings in the nineteenth century and has dared to be emotive; it has dared to 'care'. It is an historical and enduring truth that, when ill, hurting and sad, children need their family and they need to be cared for by nurses who do really care.

Today, questions are again being asked about the degree to which child nursing should be separate from general (adult) nursing and specifically whether we should keep the direct entry model brought in with Project 2000. Whatever is decided, we need to make sure that sick children receive the care that they need as children. We should also be sure that, in dealing with this and the many other issues which face child nursing today, we are indeed creating history.

Summary of principles for practice

- We must continue to retain our genuine care for children and young people.
- Understanding our history should prevent us from recreating the errors of the past; for example, our history informs us of the importance of family-centred care.
- We have good reason to be proud of our rich and fascinating history, and this should be reflected in the pride we feel for our current work.
- History is not only something that took place in the past; it is being created now, and we will be judged by others on the contribution we make today.

References

Adams J (1997) From crippledom to orthopaedic nursing: Pyrford, Surrey 1908–1945. *International History of Nursing Journal* **2**(4): 23–37.

Anonymous (1919a) A seaside hospital for tuberculous children. *Nursing Mirror and Midwives Journal* **30**(760): 37.

Anonymous (1919b) The Children's Rest, Roehampton. *Nursing Mirror and Midwives Journal* **30**(768): 195–6.

Anonymous (1919c) Nurses' Registration (no. 2) Bill: views of members of parliament and opinion of our readers. *Nursing Mirror and Midwives Journal* **30**(766): 157.

Armstrong G (1777) *An account of the diseases most incident to children, from their birth till the age of puberty; with a successful method of treating them. To which is added, An essay on nursing, also a general account of the Dispensary for the Infant Poor, from its first institution in 1769 to the present time.* London: T. Cadell.

Arton ME (1992) The development of sick children's nursing, 1919–1939. MPhil thesis, Bath University, Bath.

Ashdown AM (1927) *A complete system of nursing.* London: Waverley Book Company.

Ashington Audit Group (2004) Evaluating a nurse-led model for providing neonatal care. *Journal of Advanced Nursing* **47**: 39–48.

Atkinson BA (1981) Paediatrics past. *Nursing Times* **77**(50): ABPN 1–2.

Ayers G (1971) *England's first state hospitals and the Metropolitan Asylums Board 1867–1930.* London: Wellcome Institute for the History of Medicine.

Birkenhead and Wirral Children's Hospital (1941) Appointments. *Nursing Times* **12/04/1941**: v.

Booth Hall Hospital for Sick Children (1940) Vacancies. *Nursing Times* **27/01/1940**: v.

Booth Hall Hospital for Sick Children (1956) Appointments. *Nursing Times* **24/08/1956**: xxv.

Bowers R (1999) *Thomas Phaer and The Boke of Chyldren*. Tempe, AZ: Arizona State University.

Bowlby J (1953) *Child care and the growth of love*. Harmondsworth: Penguin.

Bowlby J (1956) The effect of mother child separation: a follow up study. *British Journal of Medical Psychology* **29**: 111.

Bowlby J (1958) The nature of the child's tie with his mother. *International Journal of Psychoanalysis* **39**: 350–73.

Bowlby J (1973) *Attachment and loss*. Vol. II. *Separation anxiety and anger*. New York: Basic books.

Bradley S (2001) Suffer the little children: the influence of nurses and parents in the evolution of open visiting in children's wards 1940–1970. *International History of Nursing Journal* **6**(2): 44–51.

Bradley SF (2003) Pride or prejudice: issues in the history of children's nurse education. *Nurse Education Today* **23**(5): 362–7.

Brooke H (1997) *Medicine women*. London: Harper Collins.

Brown B (2000) Men in nursing: ambivalence in care, gender and masculinity. *International History of Nursing Journal* **5**(5): 4–13.

Bruhn JG (2005) The lost art of the covenant: trust as a commodity in health care. *Health Care Manager* **24**(4): 311–19.

Burdett H (1919) The Nurses' Registration (No. 2) Bill. *Nursing and Midwives Journal* **30**(767): 174.

Cadogan W (1748) *Essay on the nursing and management of children*. London: John Knapton.

Cook R (2005) Male nursing reveals its peculiar history… NT centenary issue, 10 May. *Nursing Times* **101**(21): 17.

Cunningham H (1995) *Children and childhood in western society since 1500*. London: Longman.

David R (2008) The art of healing in ancient Egypt: a scientific reappraisal. *Lancet* **372**(9652): 1802–3.

Davies R (2010) Marking the 50th anniversary of the Platt Report: from exclusion, to toleration and parental participation in the care of the hospitalized child. *Journal of Child Health Care* **14**(1): 6–23.

Dickens C (1984) *A Christmas carol*. Harmondsworth: Penguin.

Editorial (1957) The mind of the young child. *Nursing Times* **15/11/1957**.

Edwards G (1980) Letter to Mrs Sacharine, 04/11/1980. Yorkhill Hospitals Archive, Glasgow.

Ellis H (2001) *A history of surgery*. London: Greenwich Medical Media.

Ellis J, Glasper EA, Horsley A, McEwing G, Richardson J (2008) NMC review of pre-registration nursing education: views of the children's and young people's nursing academic community. *Journal of Children's & Young People's Nursing* **2**(2): 56–60.

Evans J (2004) Men nurses: a historical and feminist perspective. *Journal of Advanced Nursing* **47**(3): 321–8.

Freud S, Freud A (1991) *Essentials of psychoanalysis*. Harmondsworth: Penguin.

Great Ormond Street Hospital Archive (1942a) Entries dated 09/06/1942. *Nursing Committee Record Book, Number Four: 1942*. London: Great Ormond Street Hospital Archive.

Great Ormond Street Hospital Archive (1942b) Entries dated 20/10/1942. *Nursing Committee Record Book, Number Four: 1942*. London: Great Ormond Street Hospital Archive.

Great Ormond Street Hospital Archive (1943) Entry dated 03/05/1943. *Nursing Committee Record Book, Number Four: 1942*. London: Great Ormond Street Hospital Archive.

Hardyment C (1995) *Perfect parents: baby care advice, past and present*. Oxford: Oxford University Press.

Hector W (1976) *The work of Mrs Bedford Fenwick and the rise of professional nursing*. London: Royal College of Nursing.

Hendrick H (1994) *Child welfare: England 1872–1989*. London: Routledge.

Hippocrates (2004) *Aphorisms*. Whitefish, MT: Kessinger Publishing.

Jolley MJ (2004) A social history of paediatric nursing: 1920–1970. PhD thesis, University of Hull, Hull.

Jolley MJ (2006a) The first paediatrician. *Paediatric Nursing* **18**(7): 12.

Jolley MJ (2006b) A mother's love. *Paediatric Nursing* **18**(5): 13.

Jolley MJ (2007a) Lost causes and new hope. *Paediatric Nursing* **19**(2): 12.

Jolley MJ (2007b) Separation and psychological trauma: a paradox examined. *Paediatric Nursing* **19**(3): 22–5.

Jolley MJ (2007c) Nursing's unwanted child. *Paediatric Nursing* **19**(4): 12.

Jolley MJ (2008a) Human ventilators, mechanical students and the birth of paediatric intensive care. *Paediatric Nursing* **20**(1): 12.

Jolley MJ (2008b) The NMC versus Hippocrates. *Paediatric Nursing* **20**(7): 12.

Lindsay B (2001a) Visitors and children's hospitals, 1852–1948: a re-appraisal. *Paediatric Nursing* **13**(4): 20–4.

Lindsay B (2001b) An atmosphere of recognition and respect? Sick children's nurses and medical men 1880–1930. *International History of Nursing Journal* **6**(1): 4–9.

Lomax EMR (1996) *Small and special: the development of hospitals for children in Victorian Britain.* London: Wellcome Institute for the History of Medicine.

Mackintosh C (1997) A historical study of men in nursing. *Journal of Advanced Nursing* **26**(2): 232.

Maxwell J (1997) Children and state intervention: developing a coherent historical perspective. In: Rafferty A-M, Robinson J, Elkan R (eds) *Nursing history and the politics of welfare*, pp. 225–40. London: Routledge.

Ministry of Health (1959) *The report of the committee on the welfare of children in hospital (the Platt Report).* London: HMSO.

Naraghi E (1996) The Islamic antecedents of the western Renaissance. *Diogenes* **44**(1): 73.

Nelson J (1753) *An essay on the government of children under three general heads, viz. health, manners, and education by James Nelson, apothecary, just as the twig is bent the tree's inclined.* London: Pope.

News (1945) News. *Nursing Times* **03/11/1945**: 726.

Nightingale F (1860) *Notes on nursing: what it is and what it is not.* New York: D. Appleton and Co.

Pearson A, Baker H, Walsh K, Fitzgerald M (2001) Contemporary nurses' uniforms: history and traditions. *Journal of Nursing Management* **9**(2): 147.

Porter R (1985) The patient's view: doing medical history from below. *Theory and Society* **14**: 167–74.

Porter R (1997a) *Medicine: a history of healing, ancient traditions and modern practices.* New York: Marlowe and Company.

Porter R (1997b) *The greatest benefit to mankind: a medical history of humanity from antiquity to the present.* London: Harper Collins.

Price S (1992) The child branch. *Paediatric Nursing* **4**(2): 6–8.

Robertson J (1958a) *Going to hospital with mother.* London: Tavistock Institute of Human Relations.

Robertson J (1958b) *A two year old goes to hospital.* London: Tavistock Clinic.

Robertson J (1962) *Hospitals and children: a parents' eye view.* London: Victor Gollancz.

Robertson J, Bowlby J (1952) Responses of young children to separation from their mothers. *Courrier Centre International de l'Enfance* **2**: 131–42.

Robinson E (1972) *The Yorkhill story: the history of the Royal Hospital for Sick Children, Glasgow.* Glasgow: The Board of Management for Yorkhill and Associated Hospitals.

Royal College of Nursing (1964) *First report on a special committee on nurse education; a reform of nursing education.* London: RCN.

Royal College of Nursing (2004) *The future nurse: the future of nurse education.* London: RCN.

Royal College of Nursing (2007) *Pre-registration nurse education, the NMC review and the issues.* London: RCN.

Still GF (1931) *The history of paediatrics: the progress of the study of disease of children up to the end of the XVIIIth century.* London: Royal College of Paediatrics and Child Health.

Thomas G (1959) *Carry on Nurse.* London: Carlton: 86 minutes.

Vivian MM (1919) Hospital etiquette. *Nursing Mirror and Midwives Journal* **30**(761): 56–7.

Walsh M, Ford P (1989a) *Nursing rituals, research and rational actions.* London: Heinemann.

Walsh M, Ford P (1989b) Rituals in nursing: we always do it this way … part 1. *Nursing Times* **85**(41): 26.

Walsh M, Ford P (1989c) We always do it this way: rituals in nursing in the surgical area examined in the light of research based evidence. *Nursing Times and Nursing Mirror* **85**: 26–35.

Watson JB (1928) *Psychological care of the infant and child.* London: Allen and Unwin.

West C (1854) *How to nurse sick children.* London: Longman.

Wood C (1888) The training of nurses for sick children. *Nursing Record* **1**: 507–10.

Wyman AL (1984) The surgeoness: the female practitioner of surgery 1400–1800. *Medical History* **28**: 22–41.

Yapp CS (1915) *Children's nursing: lectures to probationers*. London: Poor Law Publications.

Yorkhill Hospitals Archive (1883–1891) Reports 1883–1891. *B2/3/1*. Glasgow: Yorkhills Hospitals Archive.

Young DG, Martin EJ (1979) *Young and Weller's baby surgery*. Aylesbury: HM and M Publishers.

Chapter 2

Family-centred care and the evolving role of fathers

Sue Higham

Overview

Family-centred care is central to children and young people's nursing. As a concept, family-centred care has its origins in the development of understanding of relationships between mothers and children in the early decades of the twentieth century, yet recent years have seen increasing interest in and development of greater understanding of the importance of fathers to children's well-being. At the same time, family form and structure is becoming more diverse, as are the roles that family members play. In the UK an emphasis on father-inclusive practice has emerged in several policy strands. In this chapter, insights from these fields are drawn together and related to a critical appraisal of the evidence of current practice of child- and family-centred care, with a particular focus on acute care in hospital. Subsequently, consideration is given as to how children and young people's nursing practice might develop in future to reflect increased understanding of both fathers' and mothers' experiences and needs and encompass other family members in order to become truly child and family centred.

The meaning and origins of family-centred care

Family-centred care is widely held as the cornerstone of children's nursing practice, within the UK and across the world, yet it is argued that it is a consistently ill-defined concept (Darbyshire 1994; Hutchfield 1999; Franck and Callery 2004).

A key conceptual advance was the development of the partnership model by Casey during the late 1980s. The partnership model is based on the belief that 'the care of children, well or sick, is best carried out by their families, with varying degrees of assistance from members of a suitably qualified healthcare team whenever necessary' (Casey 1988, p. 9).

The concept of family-centred care has further developed since Casey's work, with Smith *et al.* (2002, p. 22) offering the definition of family-centred care as: 'the professional support of the child and family through a process of involvement, participation and partnership underpinned by empowerment and negotiation'.

Recently, a new terminology – 'child- and family-centred care' – has begun to emerge in policy (e.g. in the National Service Framework for Children and Young People (Department of Health 2004)) and literature in the UK (Smith and Coleman, 2010), reflecting the influence of both the children's rights agenda and consumerism on healthcare policy. Child- and family-centred care therefore incorporates the notion that children are active participants with their parents and nurses in negotiation and decision-making in healthcare (Coleman 2010).

Despite the centrality of the concepts of parents and family to children and young people's nursing practice, historically there has been limited exploration of the concepts of family or parents in children and young people's nursing literature.

Changing families

What is a family?

Family is a central concept for nurses working with babies, children and young people. Whether they practise child- and family-centred care, family-centred care or family systems nursing, family is central. Family is also a term used every day in personal life, and therefore it is easy to assume that the meaning of 'family' is obvious. However, given its centrality to children and young people's nursing practice, there is a need for children's nurses to problematize the concept.

The philosopher Archard (2003, p. 69) defines family as: 'essentially a stable multigenerational association of adults and children serving the principal function of rearing its youthful members'.

Arguably, this is the meaning with which 'family' is most usually used. Yet, thinking about this further, a group of adult siblings and their partners may regard themselves as a 'family', as might a couple without children.

Nonetheless, the social unit of adults and children has persisted across history and throughout vastly different societies and cultures (Archard 2003). Within that continuity, however, there is also considerable variation and change in family form across time and cultures.

Traditional family forms

The term 'nuclear family' has traditionally been used to refer to a heterosexual married couple and their dependent biological children (Muncie and Sapsford 1997), in which the adults adopt breadwinner/homemaker roles along traditional gender lines (Cheal 2002). This type of family has often been portrayed as an ideal and is a powerful social norm. Yet Hobson and Morgan (2002) claim that, in fact, this was the majority family type in Western Europe and the USA for only a short time during the 1950s and 1960s. This is the time at which the British welfare state was being founded. Consequently, Hearn (1998) argues, the assumption within the British welfare state has been that the nuclear family with a working father and mother at home was the norm. In reality, wars, male death rates and migration have meant that there have always been families with lone mothers, second marriages and female breadwinners (Williams 1998).

Progress in the care of children in hospital also dates from the 1950s, stemming from a growing understanding of the psychological trauma caused in part by mother–child separation in hospital (Jolley 2007), and heavily influenced by the social norm of the traditional nuclear family.

However, recent decades have seen many societal changes influencing families which have an impact on family-centred care. The key changes to family life affecting children in Britain include the following:

- the 2001 Census revealed 65% of children live with both their natural parents, 11% in a stepfamily and 23% in a lone-parent family (Office for National Statistics 2004)
- marriage rates have declined and 42% of live births are outside marriage (Office for National Statistics 2006)
- one-quarter of children are born to cohabiting couples (Cabinet Office and Department for Children, Schools and Families 2008)
- there has been an increase in the number of stepfamilies (Ferri and Smith 1998), from both marriage and cohabitation breakdown, so that one child in eight will experience living in a stepfamily by the age of 16 (Ferri and Smith 1998)
- 10% of families with dependent children are stepfamilies (Cabinet Office and Department for Children, Schools and Families 2008)
- there has been increased participation in paid work by mothers and a rapid increase in the number of families in which both parents work full time (Cheal 2002).

Social change, therefore, means that there is now considerable variation in relationships within the structure of an outwardly traditional nuclear family. The parents may be cohabiting, one or more of the children may be adopted, one adult may be a step-parent and some children may be the couple's biological children while others are stepchildren. Thus, some young people may experience multiple changes in family structure as they grow up. After divorce, many children manage life in two families, maintaining good relationships with both parents and both wider family networks (Morton *et al.* 2006). Family structure is further complicated by reproductive technologies such as egg, sperm and embryo donation, which may create outwardly traditional nuclear families in which there may be a range of genetic relationships between parents and birth children.

The most common pattern of family life in modern Britain is of families who are technically nuclear but also have extensive contact with a kin group (i.e. people to whom they are directly or indirectly related by descent) who live nearby (Muncie and Sapsford 1997). For example, one-third of working mothers cite grandparents as the most common source of informal childcare (Office for National Statistics 2009). A nationally representative survey revealed a high level of involvement with grandparents for most grandchildren in England and Wales, with a positive association between grandparental involvement and child well-being (Griggs *et al.* 2009). The authors suggest that there is a trend towards greater grandparental involvement than in the past (Griggs *et al.* 2009).

Such kinship groups have the potential to provide practical and emotional support during stressful times, such as a child's admission to hospital.

The term 'extended family' is normally used to refer to biologically related family members of three generations living together, usually grandparents, parents and children, but sometimes including others such as uncles and aunts (Dallos and Sapsford 1997). While this type of family may be traditionally associated with some minority ethnic groups, it occurs across society. Within the extended family, the child has recourse to close relationships with adults beyond his parents, and the closest child–adult relationship may not be child–parent. Responsibilities for childcare and decision-making may be shared between parents and grandparents, or parents may defer to grandparents in relation to child-rearing practices and decisions. With increasing longevity, an increasing number of four-generation families is being seen (Cheal 2002), which may mean that parents have responsibility for caring for their own grandparents as well as their children. Extended families may therefore be either a source of support for the parents of a sick child or an additional responsibility.

Non-traditional families

Lone-parent families, i.e. one parent living in a household with his or her dependent children, have always been a feature of British society, currently numbering 1.9 million parents and 3.1 million children (One Parent Families/Gingerbread 2007). Lone-parent families are more likely to experience poverty (Department for Education and Skills 2007), and poverty has negative impacts on children's health. Over half of lone parents were previously married; the median parental age is 36 years; 13% are from black or minority ethnic communities (One Parent Families/ Gingerbread 2007); 10% of lone-parent families are headed by fathers. In order to practise truly family-centred care, nurses would need to know the nature of the child's usual relationship with the non-resident parent and encompass consideration of that parent's needs into the plan of care.

A small but increasing number of families comprise same-sex couples and their dependent children, and may be biological, step, adoptive or *in vitro* in origin. There is some evidence that same-sex parents tend to balance work/home responsibilities more equally than heterosexual couples and involve more extended family networks of kin and friends in their parenting (The Scottish Government 2009). Fairtlough (2008) concluded from a literature review concerning children and young people's experiences that, although they experienced homophobia, they were predominantly positive about their parenting experiences. Yet in a Swedish study, lesbian parents were embarrassed by the assumptions of heterosexuality made by maternity healthcare professionals, who the parents also thought were embarrassed by their clients' sexuality (Röndahl *et al.* 2009).

The term 'looked after children' is used to refer to children and young people who are in the care of a local authority, which may include unaccompanied sanctuary-seeking children. In England there are approximately 60 000 looked after children at any one time, of whom approximately 70% live with foster carers and 11% in children's homes (Department for Children, Schools and Families and Department of Health 2009). The local authority acts as a corporate parent for such children, and each child or young person has a personal health plan (Department for Children, Schools and Families and Department of Health 2009). Some children and young people have continued contact with family members and others do not. Nurses need to understand an individual child or young person's circumstances and identify who has parental responsibility, and consider what information should be shared, how and with whom. As parents routinely take such active roles in the care of their children in hospital, children's nurses need to pay heed to the risk that some of the needs of unaccompanied looked after children may go unmet, and how they might compensate for the absence of parental care for some looked after children.

There are 51 000 young carers in the UK, with an average age of 12 years. While being a young carer does not necessarily have a negative impact on a young person, there is evidence that excessive care demands may have a negative impact on a young person's physical, emotional, social and educational well-being (The Children's Society and Princess Royal's Trust for Carers undated). Stigma and fear of the consequences of disclosure may make the young carer reluctant to reveal their circumstances. When young carers are themselves in need of healthcare, nurses need to be aware that there may not be someone able to fulfil the normal parental role for that young person and also that alternative caring arrangements may need to be made for the person for whom the child normally provides care.

Some parents may face particular challenges in participating in care in the way that nurses may expect and may need additional support in order to participate in care. These may include, for example, those with learning difficulties, parents with enduring mental health problems, parents with impaired mobility, parents who misuse substances, recent migrants and families who do not speak English.

Reflection points

★ To what extent do the forms and paperwork where you work demonstrate assumptions about family structure and relationships?

★ Do the questions you ask when admitting a child or meeting a family for the first time convey an assumption that every child has one mother and one father?

★ How do you adapt your negotiation of care to accommodate some parents' needs for extra support?

Mac an Ghaill and Haywood (2007) argue that 'family' is now understood as a negotiated relationship rather than an institution defined by blood and marriage ties, although its function is unchanged. Changes in family form over the last 50 years mean that membership of a 'family' today can be much more fluid and diverse, with groups of individuals defining themselves as 'a family' according to their own criteria. One size of family-centred care clearly does not fit all families; children's nurses need to treat each family as an individual unit and make no assumptions about roles and responsibilities.

Principle for practice

• If care is truly child and family centred, children and young people's nursing practice and documentation will be individualized to accommodate each family's particular circumstances, including family membership, structure, roles and responsibilities, needs and wishes.

Mothers, fathers and children

Mothers and fathers or (co)parents?

Children's nurses frequently use the term 'parents' rather than specifically talking of mothers and fathers. Again, parenting is an everyday concept, but it is worth taking time to explore what the concept really means; for example, is parenting the same as mothering or fathering?

Parenting

Parents exert a profound influence on their children's development and health (Ramchandani and McConaghie 2005). In addition to genetic health, dietary habits, lifestyle and attitudes are acquired within the family; aspects of behaviour and emotional health are dependent on relationships with parents. Hence, 'good parenting' is seen as vital for children's well-being and achievement, as defined in *Every Child Matters* (Department for Education and Skills 2003). In the Common Assessment Framework, dimensions of parenting are identified as the capacity to provide: basic care safety and protection; emotional warmth and stability; and guidance, boundaries and stimulation (Department for Children, Schools and Families 2009). Investment in support for parents, including the establishment of National Occupational Standards for people working with parents (Parenting UK 2009) and the universal availability of parenting training programmes, has become a government priority.

Much of the research on parenting has been derived from attributes of the maternal role, i.e. it has been conducted through a matrifocal lens, meaning that aspects of mothering have been regarded as the norms against which fathers' parenting is measured, resulting in what Golden (2007) has termed a 'deficit model' for fathering. Golden (2007) therefore argues that a masculine concept of care-giving needs to be developed.

Mothers

Children's nurses will be aware that the Platt Report (which began the changes that led to the development of family-centred care) on the care of children in hospital (Central Health Services Council 1959) was heavily influenced by the work of child psychiatrist John Bowlby. In 1950, Bowlby was commissioned by the World Health Organization to write a report on the effects of maternal deprivation on infant and child mental health. He says of mothers: 'What is believed essential for mental health is that an infant and young child should experience a warm, intimate and continuous relationship with his mother' (Bowlby 1965, p. 13); and of fathers: 'in the young child's eyes father plays second fiddle' and 'his value as the economic and emotional support of the mother will be assumed' (Bowlby 1965, p. 15).

Although Bowlby modified his ideas in later years, and his attachment theory has been refined to encompass a primary attachment to the father and include multiple attachments (Featherstone 2009), his understanding of the mother–child relationship was highly influential at the time.

A focus on the child's relationship with his or her mother continued in psychological and social science research for many years and is reflected in the early literature on parents in hospital. Here, the interest in parental presence has been firmly on mothers being the resident parent and performing what were described as mothering tasks, such as providing comfort, entertainment and meeting hygiene and nutritional needs (Craig and McKay 1958; Brain and Maclay 1968). However, these brief descriptive papers do show an awareness of the impact of a child's hospitalization on other family members (Moncrieff and Walton, 1952; Craig and McKay, 1958). Meadow (1964) reported an investigation into whether *mothers* wanted to stay with their child, reporting that only 44% did, with many citing their husband's needs as a reason why they could not. Brain and Maclay (1968) found only 20% of *mothers* agreed to take part in their clinical trial in which mothers accompanied children admitted for tonsillectomy.

By the 1980s researchers were using the term parent, rather than mother, although in reality their participants were almost entirely mothers (e.g. Webb *et al.* 1985; Sainsbury *et al.* 1986). This usage has continued in much of the later research until very recently. So questions arise as to whether children's nurses have taken 'parents' to mean mothers and whether, given the changing roles of fathers in family life, there is a place for fathers in family-centred care.

Fathers

Fatherhood, like motherhood, is both a biological and socially defined phenomenon. Across cultures, societies and times, the father role is seen as encompassing procreation, provision and protection (McNeill 2007). This would suggest that models of parenting derived from mothering are not appropriate for fathering. In his overview of fatherhood research, Lamb (2000) has argued that the defining aspect of fathering has shifted over decades from the provision of moral guidance through breadwinning, sex-role modelling and marital support to nurturance and the emergence of 'new fatherhood' in the 1970s. There has been growing academic interest in fatherhood and in relationships between fathers and children since that time. Early fatherhood research focused on father absence (Krampe 2009), whereas, more recently, researchers have explored the effects of fathers' personal characteristics, employment and behaviour on child development (Equal Opportunities Commission 2007). Earlier father research focused on early childhood, although more recently evidence suggests that father input during adolescence is associated with positive outcomes for young people (Videon 2005; Utting 2007).

Reflection point

★ Think about the portrayal of fathers in the media, including newspapers, magazines, television and films. What do you think the messages are from these portrayals? How have they changed since the films and television of your childhood?

In popular culture and the media, recent representations of fathers frequently fall into two categories: superdads and deadbeat dads (Utting 2007).

In constructing father roles, individuals are influenced, consciously and unconsciously, by the prevailing norms, values and expectations of what it is to be a good father in addition to their own experiences of being fathered. Attitudes and expectations among and of men are changing; for example, although Hatter *et al.* (2002) found that 25% of fathers thought mothers were the 'natural' carers of young children, 50% felt that fathers and mothers were equally capable.

Involved fatherhood

The notion of 'involved fathering' clearly underpins recent policy development and is the dominant discourse within health, social care and education. The government claims that most fathers want to be more involved in childcare (Cabinet Office and Department for Children, Schools and Families 2008). Flouri (2005) has identified involved fathering to entail: being there for children; providing for physical needs; and providing psychological support and moral guidance. Father involvement is claimed to be good for children and to lead to higher self-esteem, better friendships, more empathy, better life satisfaction, higher educational achievement, decreased risk of criminality and decreased risk of substance abuse (Layard and Dunn 2008). Videon (2005) also found involved fatherhood to have a positive influence on young people's well-being.

While involved fatherhood as a term derives from the academic/policy sphere, there is evidence that it is reflected in the values and aspirations of wider society. For example, new fathers viewed a good father as: present in the home; involved with their children; and sensitive to their needs (Henwood and Proctor 2003). A clear expectation that fathers should be 'involved' in the family was evident in research carried out by Warin *et al.* (1999), although the reality of involvement was tempered by a reluctance of both sexes to surrender traditional roles.

Social structures have an influence on individual decisions: better paid fathers have more freedom in balancing the provider role with other aspects of fathering than those who have to work long hours to provide sufficient income for their family (Marsiglio and Cohan 2000). These factors will also influence an individual father's ability to be present and involved in the care of his sick child.

Fathers' own beliefs and commitment are also important factors determining the level of involvement with children (Gaunt 2008) and these are influenced by age, race, views of gender, socioeconomic circumstances and relationships (Marsiglio and Cohan 2000). Williams (2009) also argues that white working class men and African–Caribbean fathers, who may have different understandings of masculinity and fathering, have been overlooked in fatherhood research. Within a child–adult relationship, fathering practices change as the child and father age, develop and experience different circumstances (Palkovitz and Palm 2009). Children's own perspectives on their experiences of being fathered are also under-researched.

A further factor influencing the extent of fathers' involvement is maternal gatekeeping. This is the concept that mothers regulate fathers' involvement through their own supportive or resistant behaviour (Allen and Hawkins 1999). Such gatekeeping may not be conscious or intentional (Gaunt 2008), and is in turn influenced by the mother's own beliefs and attitudes particularly in relation to gender role and beliefs about fathers (Cannon *et al.* 2008). Although the concept of maternal gatekeeping is controversial, the finding by Ellison *et al.* (2009) that more mothers than fathers held the view that childcare is primarily the mother's responsibility suggests that it may be a factor in some families. Further evidence of maternal gatekeeping was evident in Henwood and Proctor's (2003) study of new fathers, in which some men felt they were less involved in decision-making than they wanted to be or felt they had to ask mothers' permission to be involved in baby care. This highlights the point that involved fathering requires mothers to 'move over' to make space for them.

Family change means more men live apart from their children and more men are living with children to whom they are not biological fathers. An individual child may have a biological father, separated from his mother but involved in the child's life, and an unrelated male who assumes the father's role in his life. Burgess (2008) asserts that child and family services commonly fail to identify important males in children's lives and their relationships with the child, particularly when the father is living in another household. Nurses may feel awkward asking such intrusive questions, yet failing to do so can leave a child at risk or exclude a father who has a right to information about his child.

Ferri and Smith (1998) found that stepfathers were more involved in childcare than biological fathers, and Pickford (1999) found no difference between married and cohabiting fathers in their involvement or commitment to their children. Burghes et al. (1997) use the term 'social fathers' to encompass all the variations of the non-biological father–child relationship. Using such a term reminds nurses not to make assumptions about relationships based on biology alone and conveys acknowledgement that a male adult may have a significant relationship and play an important role in a child's life while having no biological or legal status.

In reality, therefore, family status and structure may make little difference in the stability, commitment to each other and relationships within the family. Ahmann (2006, p. 88) urges healthcare professionals to be open-minded and inclusive in their approach in relation to the father role in families, arguing that: 'The person or persons who see themselves in the paternal role, whether or not they are biologically related to the child, are the persons most likely to be involved participants in the child's care'.

The reality of contemporary fathers' roles in families

Strongly gendered attitudes towards family roles were revealed by Ferri and Smith (1996) in their analysis of data from the National Child Development Study; however, a study by MORI for the Equal Opportunities Commission on fathers' needs and expectations at home and work found widespread acceptance of traditional roles alongside a wide diversity of fathers' roles within families, with couples claiming to make pragmatic decisions relating to childcare and work based on earning capacity (Hatter et al. 2002).

This study and research by Warin et al. (1999) found that the majority of parents and children, but particularly fathers, saw providing an income for the family as the central aspect of fathering. Attitudes are beginning to change, however.

A large-scale national study for the Equality and Human Rights Commission revealed (Ellison et al. 2009):

- 47% of fathers thought the father's role is to provide for the family
- 23% of fathers thought that childcare is the primary responsibility of mothers
- 62% of fathers thought that fathers in general should spend more time caring for their children
- 58% believed it possible for partners to share responsibilities around work and care equally
- fathers of children with disabilities were less likely to work full time and twice as likely to say they had primary responsibility for caring for their child.

This research therefore demonstrates that attitudes are changing towards a co-parenting model; however, couples' actual decisions reflect a more traditional division of responsibilities. Although there have been changes in male and female work patterns, Dex (2003) argues that the 1.5 earner household (i.e. a father who works full time and a mother who works part time) has become the norm, with the greatest change being the increase in the number of mothers of children under 5 in paid work: 40% of mothers with young children work part time and 17% work full time (Cabinet Office and Department for Children, Schools and Families 2008). In one study, fathers in dual full-time earner households were found to be more likely to share childcare and domestic work and, in some families, shift parenting occurred where fathers were responsible for childcare while mothers worked and vice versa (Ferri and Smith 1996). However, many fathers in the Equal Opportunities Commission study described work as a welcome escape from family life (Hatter *et al.* 2002), and, in the most recent study, 75% of mothers stated that they had primary responsibility for childcare in day-to-day life (Ellison *et al.* 2009). While on specific aspects of work/parenting evidence is contradictory, trends towards more shared responsibility for earning and childcare are evident. For many parents, the day-to-day reality of bringing up children involves complex decision-making. Ellison *et al.*

Case study

Jay, aged 5, is on a children's ward with appendicitis. His mother and father both work: Sahira is a headteacher of a primary school and his father, Ramesh, is a website designer. They have no other family members in the country. They agree that Jay should have someone with him at all times, but both are also continuing to work during Jay's stay in hospital. They manage this by doing shifts. Ramesh stays with Jay during the day, arriving at 07.30, leaving at 18.00 and working at home late into the night. Ramesh also tries to work when he can on the ward during the day. Sahira comes to the ward after work at 17.30, receiving a brief 'handover' from Ramesh. Sahira, in turn, goes straight to work from the hospital at 08.00, after handing over to Ramesh.

Jay develops postoperative complications and has a prolonged stay in hospital. After 5 days, nurses have found the parents to be increasingly critical of care and irritable with each other and the staff. Sahira tells a staff nurse that she feels left out and is dependent on second-hand information because she cannot be on the ward for the surgeon's ward round. Jay seems settled and happy, although some nurses think he is 'clingy' for his age.

(2009) concluded that parenting was widely seen as a team effort and that practicalities, rather than beliefs and values, drove decision-making regarding roles and responsibilities – the person who is available at the time does what needs to be done. Therefore, parents of both sexes may experience tension between paid work, family responsibilities and the care of the child in hospital.

Reflection points

★ How would you practise family-centred care with a dual-earner two-parent family?

★ What would your personal reaction be to two working parents who both wanted to continue working while their child is ill?

★ In your workplace, how easy would it be for a parent who works 9 a.m. to 5 p.m. to speak to a senior practitioner or make a clinic appointment outside of the parent's own working hours?

★ How do your answers relate to partnership and collaboration with parents or carers?

Principles for practice

• Fathers' involvement in the care of their children in hospital will be influenced by the broader context of their normal family lives, including working patterns, their usual levels of involvement with their children and other commitments.
• Nurses need to be aware of how their own values and beliefs in relation to fathers influence their own practice.
• Maternal gatekeeping behaviour may occur in everyday life and in relation to the child's hospitalization.
• Families make decisions on a pragmatic basis rather than from their beliefs and values.

Father-inclusive policy and practice

Policy initiatives

The British government has acknowledged that increased diversity in the structure, roles and relationships within families has consequences for children and young people and therefore for policy intended to support families, however they are formed (Cabinet Office and Department for Children, Schools and Families 2008). The government has adopted a clear and consistent emphasis on the importance of families and parenting, and, more latterly, fathers' importance to their children's welfare and the need to support parents. Government activity has included setting up organizations to act as centres of expertise on parenting and policy initiatives to support families and legislation.

Key initiatives include:

- establishing the Family and Parenting Institute
- financial support for the Fatherhood Institute
- establishing the National Academy for Parenting Practitioners
- *Every Child Matters* (Department for Education and Skills 2003)
- *Every Parent Matters* (Department for Education and Skills 2007)
- the *National Service Framework for Children, Young People and Maternity Services* (Department of Health 2004)
- the introduction of 13 weeks' parental leave
- paid paternity leave
- *Healthy Lives, Brighter Futures: The Strategy for Children and Young People's Health* (Department of Health and Department for Children, Schools and Families 2009).

Some recent policy has been targeted specifically at fathers; for example, the Department for Education and Skills emphasized that fathers matter to children and public services should recognize this and seek to engage them (Department for Education and Skills 2004). *The Strategy for Children and Young People's Health* (Department of Health and Department for Children, Schools and Families 2009), developed with input from the Fatherhood Institute, asserted the significant benefits to children of paternal involvement in their lives and the Department for Children, Schools and Families ran a 'Think Fathers' campaign to encourage public services to be more inclusive of fathers (Think Fathers 2008).

Thus, there is clear support from central government in both policy and legislation for fathers to be more involved in all aspects of their children's lives, and this has an impact on health and social care practice.

Health and social care practice

There is some evidence that fathers are marginalized by health services for children, albeit unintentionally. Kerr and McKee (1981) argued that health staff assumed that, because they were rarely seen in clinics, they had little involvement at home, whereas in reality fathers were active carers for their children. The relative absence of fathers from child health-related settings such as child health clinics was noted by Lewis and O'Brien (1987). Practitioners may continue to make these assumptions. Edwards (1998) has argued that health and social care workers experience ambivalence in working with fathers. She found that workers identified lack of male partner support as a major problem for their female clients, while being unable themselves to include men in their activities unless they were the sole carers of their children. Workers would make very positive comments about men who showed an interest in their children and joke with women that their partners were 'well trained' (Edwards 1998). Marsiglio and Cohan (2000) argue that men who co-parent their children are often treated as heroic by friends and family, whereas what they do would not be considered noteworthy if done by a mother. Thus, it appears that nurses are influenced by the cultural stereotypes identified by Utting (2007), discussed earlier. Experience during a recent research project supports this. Nurses working on children's wards expressed similar views, portraying fathers who stayed overnight in hospital to care for their child with a chronic illness and went to work during the day as heroes, yet a mother who behaved in this way would be criticized for leaving her child (Higham 2009).

Research commissioned by the Department for Children, Families and Schools into how fathers can be better supported through policy identified that recognition of fathers across policy was patchy and that father-inclusive practice was not seen as mainstream in family services (Page *et al.* 2008). Lack of training among practitioners and managers in family services was a barrier to effective engagement with fathers, and health services did not engage fathers sufficiently in the early stages of fatherhood around pregnancy and birth (Page *et al.* 2008).

Practice guidance on engaging fathers has been developed for schools (Department for Education and Skills 2004), midwives (Fathers Direct 2007) and early years workers (Children in Wales 2008), but as yet there is nothing specific for children's nurses even though children's nurses are as involved in working directly with fathers as other children's professionals, if not more so.

What does this mean for children's nurses?

The demands of work and the need to provide a family income can have an impact on both fathers' and mothers' capacities to care for their ill child, either in hospital or at home. In relation to caring for sick children, evidence for father involvement is contradictory. Burghes *et al.* (1997) claim it remains largely the mother's responsibility while Burgess and Ruxton (1996) found that half of fathers in dual-earner households shared the care of sick children equally. However, working mothers saw caring for sick children at home as a key maternal role with great symbolic significance for their adequacy as mothers (Cunningham-Burley *et al.* 2006), so mothers may be reluctant to surrender this to men, adopting gatekeeping behaviour to preserve it as their own. Nurses, whether male or female, as members of society, will have their own views and expectations of what fathers do, and may subconsciously act on these to perform gatekeeping of their own.

Daniel *et al.* (2005) argued that use of the gender-neutral term 'parent' is problematic because it ignores the gendered societal context in which fathering and mothering takes place. It has been suggested that, although healthcare professionals use the term 'parent', hospitals as organizations have in the past constructed parent to mean mother (Callery 1995). A statement by the Minister for Children, Young People and Families that 'too often when we talk about engaging parents we actually only engage mothers' (Hughes 2006) implies that this is reflected in children's services more broadly. The government itself has recognized that use of 'parent' can have the effect of excluding fathers because fathers perceive the word to mean mothers, reinforced by the ingrained approaches and practices of workers (HM Treasury and Department for Education and Skills 2007).

This highlights a weakness in the nursing research on families in hospital – by and large the terms parent and family have been uncontested and undefined, with the exception of Darbyshire (1994) and Callery (1995).

The 'family' in family-centred care is taken to mean 'parents' and 'parents' equals mothers, underpinned by the assumption of a nuclear family structure. The appropriateness of family-centred care for minority ethnic families, among whom there may be more varied patterns of responsibility for childcare, has been questioned

(Ochieng 2003). If parent equals mother reflects children's nursing thinking, it could lead to the exclusion from care of individuals who are significant for the child, for example a social father, a grandparent or an older sibling.

Case study

A toddler is brought to the Accident and Emergency Department with significant scalds. He is accompanied by eight adults of different ages, none of whom appear to speak English. The adults are all distressed, shouting at each other. It is not possible to establish who, if anyone, is the child's parent. Staff assess and treat the child amid considerable noise and confusion; it is apparent that the child will need to go to the paediatric intensive care unit (PICU).

When the interpreter arrives, the relationship to the child of each adult is established. Both parents are present and insist that the child's 19 year old aunt accompanies the child to PICU as she normally cares for the child along with others in the family while the parents work. Staff try to persuade the family that it should be a parent who stays.

Reflection points

★ What is the purpose of having a resident adult with a child?

★ Who do you think should stay with the child in the case study above?

★ What are the implications for nurses if the person staying with the child is not the parent?

Childhood illness and contact with medical services is stressful for families. It tests parental resilience (Ramchandani and McConaghie 2005) and may exacerbate existing difficulties in family functioning (Johnson *et al.* 2005). As there is evidence that adjustment following illness is frequently related to family functioning (Johnson *et al.* 2005), supporting mothers and fathers and promoting effective family functioning can promote children's recovery.

Principles for practice

- The prevalence of the concept of involved fathering and changing parental responsibilities within families means that fathers are more likely to be present with their child in hospital than in earlier decades. Even if they are not present in hospital or normally resident with the child, their child's hospitalization has an impact on fathers.
- In order to support fathers, nurses need to understand their experiences and needs, yet the British literature on parents' involvement in their children's care in hospital reveals little of them.
- Without evidence from research, nurses have to depend on their personal knowledge and experience. The discussion in this chapter thus far has demonstrated that nurses need to be aware of their own assumptions and expectations in relation to fathers' roles, and guard against imposing these on families in practice.

In the remainder of this chapter, current knowledge from research in relation to fathers' experiences during their child's healthcare will be explored.

What is known about fathers' experiences and needs when their child is ill?

The needs and experiences of fathers of children in acute care have been largely overlooked by researchers, although research has been undertaken in relation to fathers in neonatal care and in relation to chronic illness.

Fathers in acute settings

No British research has been done which has focused on fathers' experiences in the acute inpatient setting. Although, initially, it was mothers who accompanied their children in hospital, the term parents has been commonly used since the 1980s, while research was actually being conducted with mothers. As society has changed, more fathers are likely to be present in hospital, and it has been assumed that what we know from research with parents (really mothers) is relevant to them. The oversight of fathers' needs appears to have resulted, at least in part, from a focus on understanding the perspectives of the parent who is resident in hospital, as in the past this has predominantly been mothers.

Some of the research examining parents' experiences in this area has touched on fathers' experiences, although samples in these studies are predominantly mothers. Darbyshire (1994) investigated the experiences of parents who were resident in hospital with their child. His research participants included 24 mothers and four fathers, reflecting the ratio of resident parents at the time. He suggests that fathers were marginalized by organizational policies which constructed 'parents' to mean mothers (e.g. the facility for resident parents was called the 'mothers unit'), and there is a suggestion that fathers were largely ignored by nurses (Darbyshire 1994). Callery (1995) also explored parental experiences, interviewing the member of the family most involved in the child's care, predominantly mothers but including a minority of fathers and a grandparent. He found that some fathers were involved in care but they were relegated to a secondary role, as substitutes for the real carers or an optional extra. Coyne (2003), in a study into nurses', parents' and children's views of parental participation, found fathers acting as supporters to mothers – by relieving them at the child's bedside and sharing duties at home. Nurses had clear but subconscious expectations of the roles that parents would play when in hospital with their child (Coyne 2007).

In Kristensson-Hallström's study (1999) into factors influencing levels of parental participation in care, Swedish fathers said they wanted to participate in only those aspects of care with which they were familiar more commonly than mothers, whereas mothers wanted to participate as much as possible provided they had guidance. This may suggest a lack of confidence in fathers or a reluctance to expose their competence to nurses' scrutiny.

Board (2004) explored sources of stress for fathers of children on the PICU and on a general ward: 70% of participants from the general ward reported symptoms of stress, including headaches, having unpleasant thoughts, being easily annoyed and worrying too much (Board 2004). Participants were also asked to identify the sources of their stress, with 90% of general ward fathers citing 'seeing their child have needles' and 80% 'not knowing how to help' (Board 2004). Children's nurses can use this information to help prepare fathers for how they might feel, and this might reduce the stress fathers experience.

Tourigny et al. (2004) videorecorded mothers' and fathers' presence and actions in the first hour after their child's surgery, rather than relying on self-reported behaviours. They found that, although mothers were present for longer at the child's bedside in the first hour postoperatively, mothers and fathers demonstrated a similar range of helpful behaviours, though fathers showed them with less frequency (Tourigny et al. 2004). These findings suggest that mothers and fathers adopted similar roles in relation to their child in hospital. Thompson et al. (2009) found higher agreement between fathers' preoperative predictions of their child's level of anxiety at anaesthetic induction and scores from a behaviour ratings scale completed by researchers than mothers' predictions. At face value this would suggest that fathers were better able to predict their child's anxiety than mothers, although the researchers argue that mothers' predictions may have been based more on their child's internal state than behavioural and that the children's anxiety cues were too subtle to be picked up by the assessment tool used, resulting in falsely low anxiety scores, so that in fact mothers' predictions were accurate (Thompson et al. 2009).

'Being there' is a recurring theme in relation to the parents of children in hospital, yet Kars et al. (2008) found differences in the meaning of 'being there' for mothers and fathers. Mothers focused on empathy, involvement and child and parent staying together, whereas, for fathers, 'being there' had a more active meaning, seeing it as advocating and supporting their children in a more practical way, i.e. 'doing something' (Kars et al. 2008). In light of this finding, nurses may interpret fathers' actions such as asking questions about treatment plans or questioning professionals' actions and decisions as their way of 'being there', not necessarily a criticism of care.

Fathers in neonatal units

The birth of a sick or preterm infant is always a shock for parents, with long-term consequences for both parents. Fathers whose babies are admitted to neonatal units face particular challenges in addition to the shock and stress of the birth of a sick or preterm infant which they have to confront in the very visible context of the neonatal unit. If they are first-time fathers, their transition to fatherhood takes place in the public setting of the unit, as does their bonding with their baby. There may be physical barriers which prevent or inhibit them from holding their child. If they have other children, they will be concerned about how to tell them that their anticipated sibling will not be coming straight home or may not survive. In addition to concern for their infant, they will be concerned for the welfare of their partner post-delivery, who may have undergone a caesarean section or may be ill, and may be in a different hospital to the child. Yet, the father is very frequently the parent who is able to be most present in the earliest hours of a child's stay in a neonatal unit. Fathers may have to negotiate with employers about rescheduling their planned paternity leave or they may continue to work normally, saving their paternity leave until after the child is discharged, but increasing their stress in the short term. Children's nurses have a crucial role to play in supporting both mother and father at this challenging time.

Johnson (2008) has argued that engaging fathers in the care of their infants in neonatal intensive care is much more challenging than involving mothers. Identification of family care needs is part of nursing assessment and contributes to developmental care (Johnson 2008), yet just as in the acute setting, most studies of parents' experiences in neonatal units focus on mothers (Deeney *et al.* 2009). Arockiasamy *et al.* (2008) suggests that existing parental support mechanisms are based on healthcare providers' perceptions of what parents might need rather than having been developed with parental input. There is clearly a need to understand fathers' perspectives on their experiences and needs.

Fegran and Helseth (2009) argue that the neonatal intensive care unit is an environment in which two worlds meet. Parents are experiencing an ontological change, i.e. their way of being in the world is changing forever, whereas nurses are doing an ordinary day's work. Furthermore, parents need privacy and individualized care while nurses need efficiency, visibility and access (Fegran and Helseth 2009). Approximately 40% of neonatal intensive care units in the UK allowed both parents to stay overnight whenever they chose (Greisen *et al.* 2009), suggesting that separation of mothers and fathers at this stressful time is common. Pöhlman (2009) found that the necessary precedence given to technological care of infants in neonatal intensive care left fathers feeling frustrated, afraid and alienated and that nurses were unaware of how fathers were feeling. Fathers wanted to be involved but felt there was little they could 'do' (Pöhlman 2003). Arockiasamy *et al.* (2008) interviewed fathers of extremely ill infants in neonatal intensive care, finding that there was a universal sense of lack of control. Specific activities identified by fathers as helping them regain control were relationships with the healthcare team, friends and family together with consistent information, including short, relevant written information (Arockiasamy *et al.* 2008). Fathers also reported taking on a protector role towards both their partner and child (Arockiasamy *et al.* 2008).

Sloan *et al.* (2008) found that fathers identified their partners and families as sources of emotional support. This research highlights the importance of parents' relationships with each other and with family members, and nurses need to consider how they can promote and support these. Although sibling and grandparent visiting is permitted in many units, this is often conditional on being accompanied by parents (Greisen *et al.* 2009). Thus, grandparents can be prevented from staying with the child to enable parents to take a break and support one another, and inhibited from developing their bond with the baby.

Information needs vary. Fathers in one study identified staff as sources of informational support, although less than half were satisfied with the information they received (Sloan *et al.* 2008). Some fathers actively sought information as a means of regaining some control whereas others wanted limited information (Arockiasamy *et al.* 2008). In the UK, only 40% of neonatal intensive care units were found to permit completely open 24 hour parental visits, including during ward rounds (Greisen *et al.* 2009). While this policy may be predicated on the need to protect confidentiality, given the confines of space on neonatal units, it may also exclude parents from important exchanges of information and decision-making.

The formation of attachment bonds between parents and child is a crucial process during the neonatal period, which is disrupted if the child is born preterm or sick. In a natural setting, proximity, reciprocity and commitment are central characteristics of the attachment process (Goulet *et al.* 1998, cited by Fegran *et al.* 2008). Again, most of the literature on this topic is focused on mothers (Fegran *et al.* 2008). Fegran *et al.* (2008) argue that touch and visual contact are the most powerful communication tools by which parents communicate with their infants. Fathers in their study described how touching and holding their child, even if they were reluctant to do so initially, transformed their relationship with their child from an impersonal one to one of belonging and protection, having a positive effect on fathers' self-esteem and coping (Fegran *et al.* 2008).

Here lies a challenge for the practitioner: how to gently encourage the overwhelmed, shocked, frightened father to hold his child, knowing that in the longer term it is beneficial for him to do so. Knowing how much and what sort of information to give – whether he needs a broad overview or specific details – is a further challenge. It is not surprising, therefore, that neonatal nurses experience interaction with parents as perhaps the most challenging part of their job (Fegran and Helseth 2009).

Case study

Sixteen year old Becky has given birth at 27 weeks to Mia, who is admitted to a neonatal unit (NNU). Becky and Jake, Mia's father, live with Becky's parents, Phil and Jan. Becky is ill postnatally and is unable to visit the NNU. Jake seems overwhelmed with the situation. He visits the unit for short periods only and is yet to touch or hold Mia and does not speak to the staff. Phil and Jan are keen to be involved in Mia's care. The staff are concerned about Jake's apparent lack of commitment to Mia. Jan tells a staff nurse that Jake feels like everyone is staring at and judging him. She asks staff to back off a bit and let her and Phil get Jake involved at his own pace.

Reflection points

★ How do you think nurses should react to Jan's request to 'back off a bit'?

★ How might nurses support young fathers without making them feel unde pressure or scrutiny?

Fathers of children with chronic illness

There is a significant body of research in relation to fathers of children with chronic illness which provides evidence of relationships with healthcare professionals and child health services, the social and emotional impacts of having a child with chronic illness on fathers, the coping strategies fathers use and fathers' role expectations.

Clarke *et al.* (2009) argue that father involvement in aspects of a child's chronic illness may positively influence marital, family and child psychological outcomes.

Some fathers have seen health services as being oriented towards women (Clarke 2005; Ware and Raval 2007) and reported that they, as men, felt they had been treated differently from women to the extent of feeling ignored or abandoned by healthcare professionals (Ware and Raval 2007; Hayes and Savage 2008). Dealing with healthcare professionals was seen as challenging by some (Chesler and Parry 2001; Clarke 2005; Waite-Jones and Madill 2008). Clarke (2005) discusses the barriers to fathers' greater involvement in medical care, such as outpatient appointment times within normal working hours. Similarly, ward round times may mean that working fathers are unable to be present. This can mean that fathers have to depend on second-hand medical information from the child's mother, adding to stress and anxiety and potentially causing conflict between the parents (Chesler and Parry 2001).

The social effects on fathers of having a child with a chronic illness include social isolation, with family, friends and others seen as not understanding (Katz and Krulik 1999; Goble 2004; McNeill 2004; Waite-Jones and Madill 2008) or not being as supportive as anticipated (Ware and Raval 2007). In some studies, fathers reported increased strain on the couple's relationship, but also increased closeness with their partner along with increased closeness to the ill child (McNeill 2004; Ware and Raval, 2007) or to the other well children in the family (Goble 2004). Some fathers felt that having a chronically ill child had led to increased division of labour within the family along gendered lines (Goble 2004; Waite-Jones and Madill 2008) with consequent greater pressure on fathers to provide financially.

In terms of the emotional effects of childhood chronic illness on fathers, a sense of chronic sadness is evident, for example among fathers of children with diabetes (Sullivan-Bolyai *et al.* 2006) and or of children with life-limiting illness (Ware and Raval 2007). Fathers have described multiple losses: of a 'normal' family life, of an ideal healthy child, of their role as a protector and provider and of opportunities for shared family and father–child activities (Waite-Jones and Madill 2008). Fathers also faced anxiety arising from uncertainty in relation to their child's condition from day to day (Cashin *et al.* 2008; Hayes and Savage 2008), and fears for the future in relation to either the effects or management of the illness or their child's position in society as an adult (McNeill 2004; Sullivan-Bolyai *et al.* 2006).

Fathers of children with chronic illness express reluctance to discuss or show their feelings with family members or professionals. This reluctance is identified by men as arising from a need to 'be strong' and support their partners (Chesler and Parry 2001; McNeill 2004; Sullivan-Bolyai *et al.* 2006; Ware and Raval 2007). In short, research with fathers reveals:

- a reluctance to burden partners with their feelings (McNeill 2004)
- a view that men generally do not and should not talk about or show their feelings (Ware and Raval 2007; Waite-Jones and Madill 2008; Hayes and Savage 2008)
- the attitude that it is better not to talk about issues in order to avoid painful emotions (Hayes and Savage 2008).

The range of coping strategies fathers of children identify include:

- denial (Waite-Jones and Madill 2008)
- distraction (McNeill 2004; Peck and Lillibridge 2005; Waite-Jones and Madill 2008)

- 'time out' (McGrath and Chesler 2004)
- focusing on the here and now (Peck and Lillibridge 2005; Hayes and Savage 2008)
- taking positive action (McNeill 2004; Sullivan-Bolyai *et al.* 2006; Ware and Raval 2007)
- maintaining a positive outlook (McNeill 2004).

Some fathers respond to their child's chronic illness by seeking information about it and its management (Ware and Raval 2007; Cashin *et al.* 2008), whereas others described avoiding finding out more because such knowledge could increase stress and cause powerful emotions (Peck and Lillibridge 2005; Hayes and Savage 2008).

Although Clarke *et al.* (2009) argue that gender roles predominate in relation to care-giving when a child is diagnosed with cancer, many fathers of children with chronic illness are direct care-givers, reflecting today's changing fatherhoods. Examples include commitment to a range of direct care-giving, including routine childcare for the affected child, becoming the main carer for siblings when a mother's time was consumed by the needs of an ill child, becoming the main carer for the ill child (Clarke 2005; Bonner *et al.* 2007), performing medical aspects of care (Clarke 2005; Sullivan-Bolyai *et al.* 2006) and providing emotional support for all family members (Chesler and Parry 2001). Yet fathers of neonates and chronically ill children experience mothers as the 'experts' in the child's care (Pelchat *et al.* 2003; Pohlman 2003), with the authority to include fathers or keep them on the periphery (Pohlman 2003). Mothers have acknowledged not leaving room for fathers to participate in care and feeling that fathers were not able to adequately care for the ill disabled child (Pelchat *et al.* 2003). Thus, there is evidence to support maternal gatekeeping. Healthcare professionals may unwittingly perform gatekeeping of their own if they assume that 'mother knows best'.

Fathers identified that the protector element of their father identity was challenged by their child's chronic illness, in relation to both the ill child and other family members (McGrath and Chesler 2004; McNeill 2004; Clarke 2005). One father in McGrath and Chesler's (2004) study spoke of how his role as a father was 'to fix things', and of the anger and frustration resulting from not being able to 'fix' his son's cancer. The protector role is also expressed in discussion of the need for advocacy for their ill child in healthcare situations (McNeill 2004; Clarke 2005). For fathers, such advocacy included asking awkward questions or monitoring the performance of hospital staff. One can see that there is potential for tension to arise between fathers and nurses when fathers behave in this way.

There are some positive aspects of being a father of a child with a chronic illness. A sense of gradual adjustment, acceptance over time and of personal growth is evident in some studies (e.g. Chesler and Parry 2001; McNeil 2004). Despite intra-family stresses and strain, mothers and fathers reported stronger marriages and closer families (Chesler and Parry 2001). Fathers described opportunities to become more involved in family life that they would not have had if their child were healthy (Hayes and Savage 2008) and heightened relationships with their partner, the ill child (McNeill 2004; Ware and Raval 2008) or their healthy children (Goble 2004).

In the past, fathers of children with disability have been evaluated by health professionals in terms of the support they gave to the mother (Pelchat *et al.* 2003), be that emotional, practical or financial, whereas health professionals need to recognize, value and support the father–child relationship in and of itself.

> ## Key points
>
> - Healthcare professionals are largely unaware of fathers' needs.
> - Fathers in acute care have been overlooked.
> - Researchers are beginning to investigate the experiences and needs of fathers of sick or preterm neonates.
> - Many fathers of chronically ill children are active givers of care who experience social and emotional consequences as a result of their child's condition.
> - These consequences challenge the fulfilment of the father role.
> - There is contradictory evidence in relation to fathers' information needs.

Conclusions

It has been beyond the scope of this chapter to address either the needs or contributions to care of siblings of the sick child, but they too should feature in the children's nurse's mindful planning and implementation of family-centred care.

Children's nurses' everyday practice involves working with families of all descriptions in which individual members undertake a wide range of roles. Roles and relationships within families cannot be assumed. Fathers are more involved in their children's lives than in previous generations and consequently are in contact with healthcare professionals more frequently. Fathering is both a role and relationship and the nurse needs to consider this child–father relationship independently of the child–mother and mother–father relationship, while respecting family functioning.

The use of the term *parents* rather than *mothers* in children's nursing literature has led nurses to apply understanding drawn from research with mothers to their work with fathers. This has been exacerbated by a tendency for researchers to examine the experiences of the parents of hospitalized children from the perspective of the resident parent only. Yet we know that the wider family is affected by the child's hospitalization and can support the parents. There is as yet very little research on the contributions that grandmothers, grandfathers and other family members make to the care of ill children.

In this chapter, some of the research evidence concerning fathers' experiences of their child's healthcare has been outlined. There is some evidence to support the notion that fathers' needs when their children are ill are different from those of mothers. Children's nurses need to be aware of this evidence and consider how they identify and meet fathers' needs, particularly given the evidence that some fathers feel the need to appear strong and may be reluctant to talk. Children's nurses need to learn to consider fathers in their own right and in relationship to the child, not just as support or a substitute for mothers.

There is a need for further research with fathers, particularly in the acute setting, to improve understanding of their needs. Yet researchers undertaking such work face challenges, such as some men's reluctance to talk about their feelings. Approaches such as peer research may prove fruitful in future.

There is also clearly a need for pre-registration and continuing professional development programmes to reflect the fact that parenting is in reality mothering and fathering and to prepare nurses to work effectively with mothers, fathers and other family members.

This chapter has identified that, even though fathers play a vital role in caring for their child in sickness and in health, this has often been overlooked or disregarded by health and social professionals, including children and young people's nurses. Family-centred care, if it is to be implemented in its truest sense, must take value from and respect the contribution made by fathers and consider their needs as active carers.

Summary of principles for practice

- Children and young people's nurses must consider fathers in their own right and in relationship to the child and not merely as a support or substitute for mothers.
- Children and young people's nurses must recognize, value and support the father–child relationship.
- Children and young people's nurses must consider how they may identify and meet fathers' needs with regard to information-giving and negotiation over care.
- Children and young people's nurses must consider the child–father relationship while at the same time recognize family functioning.

References

Ahmann E (2006) Supporting fathers' involvement in children's health care. *Pediatric Nursing* **32**: 88–90.

Allen SM, Hawkins AJ (1999) Maternal gatekeeping: mothers' beliefs and behaviors that inhibit greater father involvement in family work. *Journal of Marriage and the Family* **61**: 199–21.

Archard D (2003) *Children, family and the state.* Aldershot: Ashgate.

Arockiasamy V, Holsti L, Albersheim S (2008) Fathers' experiences in the neonatal intensive care unit: a search for control. *Pediatrics* **121**: e215–22.

Board R (2004) Father stress during a child's critical care hospitalization. *Journal of Pediatric Health Care* **18**: 244–9.

Bonner M, Hardy K, Willard V, Hutchinson K (2007) Brief report: psychosocial functioning of fathers as primary caregivers of pediatric oncology patients. *Journal of Pediatric Psychology* **32**: 851–6.

Bowlby J (1965) *Child care and the growth of love*, 2nd edn. Harmondsworth: Penguin.

Brain D, Maclay I (1968) Controlled study of mothers and children in hospital. *British Medical Journal* **1**: 278–80.

Burgess A (2008) *The costs and benefits of active fatherhood.* London: Fathers Direct. See www.fathersdirect.com

Burgess A, Ruxton S (1996) *Men and their children: proposals for public policy.* London: Institute for Public Policy Research.

Burghes L, Clarke L, Cronin N (1997) *Fathers and fatherhood in Britain.* London: Family Policy Studies Centre.

Cabinet Office and Department for Children, Schools and Families (2008) *Families in Britain: an Evidence Paper.* London: DCSF. See http://www.cabinetoffice.gov.uk/media/111945/families_in_britain.pdf

Callery P (1995) An investigation into the role of parents in hospital. PhD thesis, University of Liverpool, Liverpool.

Cannon E, Schoppe-Sullivan S, Mangelsdorf S, *et al.* (2008) Parent characteristics as antecedents of maternal gatekeeping and fathering behavior. *Family Process* **47**(4): 501–19.

Casey A (1988) A partnership with child and family. *Senior Nurse* **8**(4): 8–9.

Cashin G, Small S, Solberg S (2008) The lived experience of fathers who have children with asthma: a phenomenological study. *Journal of Pediatric Nursing* **23**(5): 372–84.

Central Health Services Council (1959) *The welfare of children in hospital.* The Platt Report. London: Ministry of Health.

Cheal D (2002) *Sociology of family life.* Basingstoke: Palgrave Macmillan.

Chesler M, Parry C (2001) Gender roles and/or styles in crisis: an integrative analysis of the experiences of fathers of children with cancer. *Qualitative Health Research* **11**: 363–84.

Children in Wales (2008) *Including fathers in early years services: positive practice for professionals.* Cardiff: Children in Wales.

Clarke J (2005) Fathers' home health care work when a child has cancer: I'm her Dad; I have to do it. *Men and Masculinities* **7**(4) 385–404.

Clarke N, McCarthy M, Downie P, *et al.* (2009) Gender differences in the psychosocial experience of parents of children with cancer: a review of the literature. *Psycho-oncology* **18**: 907–15.

Coleman V (2010) The evolving concept of child and family-centred healthcare. In: Smith L, Coleman V (eds) *Child and family centred-care: concept, theory and practice,* 2nd edn, pp. 1–26. Basingstoke: Palgrave.

Coyne I (2003) A grounded theory of disrupted lives. PhD Thesis, King's College London, London.

Coyne I (2007) Disruption of parent participation: nurses' strategies to manage parents on children's wards. *Journal of Clinical Nursing* **17**: 3150–8.

Craig J, McKay E (1958) Working of a mother and baby unit. *British Medical Journal* **1**: 275–7.

Cunningham-Burley S, Beckett-Millburn K, Kemmer D (2006) Constructing health and sickness in the context of motherhood and paid work. *Sociology of Health and Illness* **28**(4): 385–409.

Dallos R, Sapsford J (1997) Patterns of diversity and lived realities. In: Muncie J, Wetherell M, Langan M, *et al.* (eds) *Understanding the family,* 2nd edn, pp. 126–70. London: Sage.

Daniel B, Featherstone B, Hooper CA, Scourfield J (2005) Why gender matters for Every Child Matters. *British Journal of Social Work* **35**: 1343–55.

Darbyshire P (1994) *Living with a sick child in hospital: the experiences of parents and nurses.* London: Chapman and Hall.

Deeney K, Lohan M, Parkes J, Spence D (2009) Experiences of fathers of babies in intensive care. *Paediatric Nursing* **21**: 45–7.

Department for Children, Schools and Families (2009) *Common Assessment Framework: practitioners' and managers' guides.* Nottingham: DCSF. See http://www.dcsf.gov.uk/everychildmatters/strategy/deliveringservices1/caf/cafframework/

Department for Children, Schools and Families and Department of Health (2009) *Statutory guidance on promoting the health and well-being of looked after children.* Nottingham: DCSF.

Department for Education and Skills (2003) *Every child matters.* London: DfES.

Department for Education and Skills (2004) *Engaging fathers: involving parents, raising achievement.* London: DfES.

Department for Education and Skills (2007) *Every parent matters.* London: DfES.

Department of Health (2004) *The National Service Framework for children, young people and maternity services.* London: Department of Health.

Department of Health and Department for Children, Schools and Families (2009) *Healthy lives, brighter futures: the strategy for children and young people's health.* London: Department of Health.

Dex S (2003) *Families and work in the 21st century.* York: Joseph Rowntree Foundation. See www.jrf.org.uk/publications/ families-and-work-twenty-first century

Edwards J (1998) Screening out men or 'Has Mum changed her washing powder recently?'. In: Popay J, Hearn J, Edwards J (eds) *Men, gender and masculinities,* pp. 259–86. London: Routledge.

Ellison G, Barker A, Kulasuriya T (2009) *Work and care: a study of modern parents.* Manchester: Equality and Human Rights Commission. See www.equalityhumanrights.com

Equal Opportunities Commission (2007) *Fathers and the modern family.* Manchester: Equal Opportunities Commission.

Fairtlough A (2008) Growing up with a lesbian or gay parent: young people's perspectives. *Health and Social Care in the Community* **16**(5): 521–8.

Fathers Direct (2007) *Family friendly practice: including fathers.* London: Fathers Direct.

Featherstone B (2009) *Contemporary fathering: theory, policy and practice.* Bristol: The Policy Press.

Fegran L, Helseth S (2009) The parent-nurse relationship in the neonatal intensive care unit context-closeness and emotional involvement. *Scandinavian Journal of Caring Sciences* **23**: 667–73.

Fegran L, Helseth S, Fagermoen M (2008) A comparison of mothers and fathers' experiences of the attachment process in a neonatal intensive care unit. *Journal of Clinical Nursing* **17**: 810–16.

Ferri E, Smith K (1996) *Parenting in the 1990s*. London: Joseph Rowntree Foundation. See www.jrf.org.uk/publications/parenting-1990s

Ferri E, Smith K (1998) *Step-parenting in the 1990s*. York: Joseph Rowntree Foundation. See www.jrf.org.uk/findings

Flouri E (2005) *Fathering and child outcomes*. Oxford: Wiley Blackwell.

Franck L, Callery P (2004) Re-thinking family-centred care across the continuum of healthcare. *Child: Care, Health and Development* **30**(3) 265–77.

Gaunt R (2008) Maternal gatekeeping: antecedents and consequences. *Journal of Family Issues* **29**(3): 373–95.

Goble L (2004) The impact of a child's chronic illness on fathers. *Issues in Comprehensive Pediatric Nursing* **27**: 153–262.

Golden A (2007) Fathers' frames for childrearing: Evidence toward a masculine concept of care-giving. *Journal of Family Communication* **7**(4): 265–85.

Goulet C, Bell L, Tribble D, Lang A (1998) A concept analysis of parent-infant attachment. *Journal of Advanced Nursing* **28**: 1071–81.

Greisen G, Mirante M, Haumont D (2009) Parent, siblings, grandparents in the neonatal intensive care unit: a survey of policies in eight European countries. *Acta Paediatrica* **98**: 1744–50.

Griggs J, Tan J-P, Buchanan A, *et al.* (2009) 'They've always been there for me': grandparental involvement and child well-being. *Children and Society* **24**: 200–14.

Hatter W, Vinter L, Williams R (2002) *Dads on dads: needs and expectations at home and work*. Manchester: Equal Opportunities Commission.

Hayes C, Savage E (2008) Fathers' perspectives on the emotional impact of managing the care of their children with cystic fibrosis. *Journal of Pediatric Nursing* **23**(4): 250–6.

Hearn J (1998) *The welfare of men*. In: Popay J, Hearn J, Edwards J (eds) *Men, gender and masculinities*, pp. 11–36. London: Routledge.

Henwood K, Proctor J (2003) The 'good father': reading men's accounts of paternal involvement during the transition to first-time fatherhood. *British Journal of Social Psychology* **42**(3) 337–55.

Higham S (2009) Fathers are parents too: fathers' involvement in the care of their acutely ill children in hospital. Paper presented at the Royal College of Nursing Conference: Back to the future – a celebration of 25 years of children and young people's nursing, Liverpool 12th September 2009.

HM Treasury and Department for Education and Skills (2007) *Aiming high for children: supporting families*. London: The Stationery Office.

Hobson B, Morgan M (2002) Introduction. In: Hobson B (ed.) *Making men into fathers: men, masculinities and the social politics of fatherhood*, pp. 1–24. Cambridge: Cambridge University Press.

Hughes B (2006) *Minister calls for public services to think differently about fathers*. See www.fatherhoodinstitute.org.uk

Hutchfield K (1999) Family-centred care: a concept analysis. *Journal of Advanced Nursing* **29**(5) 1178–87.

Johnson A (2008) Engaging fathers in the NICU: taking down the barriers to the baby. *Journal of Perinatal and Neonatal Nursing* **22**(4) 302–6.

Johnson G, Kent G, Leather J (2005) Strengthening the parent-child relationship: a review of family interventions and their use in medical settings. *Child: Care, Health & Development* **31**(1): 25–32.

Jolley J (2007) Separation and psychological trauma: a paradox explained. *Paediatric Nursing* **19**(3): 22–5.

Kars M, Duinjnstree M, Pool A, *et al.* (2008) Being there: parenting the child with acute lymphoblastic leukaemia. *Journal of Clinical Nursing* **18**: 1553–62.

Katz S, Krulik T (1999) Fathers of children with chronic illness: do they differ from fathers of healthy children? *Journal of Family Nursing* **5**(3): 292–315.

Kerr M, McKee L (1981) The father's role in child health care: is Dad an expert too? *Health Visitor* **54**: 47–55.

Krampe E (2009) When is the father really there? A conceptual reformulation of father presence. *Journal of Family Issues* **30**(7): 875–97.

Kristensson-Hallström I (1999) Strategies for feeling secure influence parents' participation in care. *Journal of Clinical Nursing* **8**: 586–92.

Lamb M (2000) The history of research on father involvement: an overview. *Marriage and Family Review* **29**(2): 23–42.

Layard R, Dunn J (2008) *A good childhood: searching for values in a competitive age*. London: The Children's Society/Penguin.

Lewis C, O'Brien M (1987) Constraints on fathers: research, theory and clinical practice. In: Lewis C, O'Brien M (eds) *Reassessing fatherhood: new observations on fathers, mothers and the modern family*, pp. 1–22. London: Sage.

Mac an Ghaill M, Haywood C (2007) *Gender, culture and society: contemporary femininities and masculinities*. London: Palgrave Macmillan.

Marsiglio W, Cohan M (2000) Conceptualizing father involvement and paternal influence. *Marriage and Family Review* **29**(2): 75–95.

McGrath P, Chesler M (2004) Fathers' perspectives on the treatment for pediatric hematology: extending the findings. *Issues in Comprehensive Pediatric Nursing* **27**: 39–61.

McNeill T (2004) Fathers' experience of parenting a child with juvenile rheumatoid arthritis. *Qualitative Health Research* **14**(4): 256–545.

McNeill T (2007) Fathers of children with a chronic health condition: beyond gender stereotypes. *Men and Masculinities* **9**: 409–24.

Meadow SR (1964) No thanks; I'd rather stay at home. *British Medical Journal* **2**: 813–14.

Moncrieff A, Walton A (1952) Visiting children in hospital. *British Medical Journal* **1**: 43–4.

Morton S, Jamieson L, Highet G (2006) *Cool with change: young people and family change*. Research Briefing 23. Edinburgh: Centre for Research on Families and Relationships. See www.crcf.ac.uk

Muncie J, Sapsford J (1997) The concept of the family. In: Muncie J, Wetherell M, Langan M, *et al*. (eds) *Issues in the study of the family*, 2nd edn, pp. 7–39. London: Sage.

Ochieng B (2003) Minority ethnic families and family-centred care. *Journal of Child Health Care* **7**(2): 123–32.

Office for National Statistics (2004) *Census 2001: National reports for England and Wales*, part 2. London: ONS.

Office for National Statistics (2006) *Social trends 36*. Basingstoke: Palgrave Macmillan.

Office for National Statistics (2009) *Social trends 39*. Basingstoke: Palgrave Macmillan.

One Parent Families/Gingerbread (2007) *One parent families today: the facts*. See www.oneparentfamily.org.uk

Page J, Whitting G, McLean C (2008) *A review of how fathers can be better recognised and supported through DCSF policy*. London: Department for Children, Schools and Families.

Palkovitz R, Palm G (2009) Transitions in fathering. *Fathering* **7**(1): 3–22.

Parenting UK (2009) *National occupational standards for work with parents*. London: Parenting UK. See http://www. parentinguk.org/search/node/national+occupational+standards

Peck B, Lillibridge J (2005) Normalization behaviours of rural fathers living with chronically ill children: an Australian perspective. *Journal of Child Health Care* **9**: 31–45.

Pelchat D, Lefebre H, Perreault M (2003) Differences and similarities between mothers' and fathers' experiences of parenting a child with a disability. *Journal of Child Health Care* **7**(4): 231–47.

Pickford R (1999) *Fathers, marriage and the law*. London: Family Policy Studies Centre.

Pöhlman S (2003) When worlds collide: the meanings of work and fathering among fathers of premature infants. PhD thesis, St Louis University, St Louis, MO.

Pöhlman S (2009) Fathering premature infants and the technological imperative of the neonatal unit: an interpretive inquiry. *Advances in Nursing Science* **32**(3): e1–16.

Ramchandani P, McConaghie H (2005) Mothers, fathers and their children's heath. *Child: Care, Health and Development* **31**: 1, 5–6.

Röndahl G, Bruhner E, Lindhe J (2009) Heteronomative communication with lesbian families in antenatal care, childbirth and postnatal care. *Journal of Advanced Nursing* **65**: 2337–44.

Sainsbury C, Gray O, Cleary J, *et al.* (1986) Care by parents of their children in hospital. *Archives of Diseases in Childhood* **61**: 612–15.

Sloan K, Rowe J, Jones L (2008) Stress and coping in fathers following the birth of a preterm infant. *Journal of Neonatal Nursing* **14**: 108–15.

Smith L, Coleman V (eds) (2010) *Child and family centred-care: concept, theory and practice,* 2nd edn. Basingstoke: Palgrave.

Smith L, Coleman V, Bradshaw M (2002) Family-centred care: a practice continuum. In: Smith L, Coleman V, Bradshaw M (eds) *Family centred-care: concept, theory and practice,* pp. 19–43. Basingstoke: Palgrave.

Sullivan-Bolyai S, Rosenburg R, Bayard M (2006) Fathers' reflections on parenting young children with type 1 diabetes. *Maternal-Child Nursing* **31**: 24–31.

The Children's Society and Princess Royal's Trust for Carers (undated) *Making it work: good practice with young carers and their families.* London: The Children's Society and Princess Royal's Trust for Carers. See www.youngcarer.com

The Scottish Government (2009) *The experiences of children with lesbian and gay parents – an initial scoping review of evidence.* Edinburgh: The Scottish Government. See www.scotland.gov.uk/socialresearch

Think Fathers (2008) *The Think Fathers campaign.* Abergavenny: Think Fathers. See www.think-fathers.org

Thompson C, MacLaren J, Harris A, Kain Z (2009) Brief report: prediction of children's pre-operative anxiety by mothers and fathers. *Journal of Pediatric Psychology* **34**(7): 716–23.

Tourigny J, Ward V, Lepage T (2004) Fathers behaviour during their child's ambulatory surgery. *Issues in Comprehensive Pediatric Nursing* **27**: 69–81.

Utting D (2007) *Parenting and the different ways it can affect children's lives; research evidence.* York: Joseph Rowntree Foundation. See www.jrf.org.uk/publications

Videon T (2005) Parent-child relations and children's psychological well-being: do Dads matter? *Journal of Family Issues* **26**: 55–77.

Waite-Jones J, Madill A (2008) Concealed concern: fathers experiences of having a child with juvenile idiopathic arthritis. *Psychology and Health* **23**(5): 585–601.

Ware J, Raval H (2007) A qualitative investigation of fathers' experiences of looking after a child with a life-limiting illness, in process and retrospect. *Clinical Child Psychology and Psychiatry* **12**(4) 549–65.

Warin J, Solomon Y, Lewis C, Langford W (1999) *Fathers, work and family life.* York: Joseph Rowntree Foundation. See www.jrf.org.uk/publications

Webb N, Hull D, Madeley R (1985) Care by parents in hospital. *British Medical Journal* **291**: 176–7.

Williams F (1998) Troubled masculinities in social policy discourse: fatherhood. In: Popay J, Hearn J, Edwards J (eds) *Men, gender and masculinities,* pp. 63–97. London: Routledge.

Williams R (2009) Masculinities and fathering. *Community, Work and Family* **12**(1): 57–73.

Chapter 3

The need for a culturally sensitive approach to care

Vasso Vydelingum and Pat Colliety

Overview

This chapter will focus on contemporary issues of growing up as a member of a minority in a predominantly White majority culture for children and young people who may perceive themselves as not belonging to the mainstream culture. The chapter starts with an explanation of terms such as culture, 'race', ethnicity and whiteness, and a discussion of terminologies such as Black and Asian, as well as factors affecting child-rearing practice are considered. Using a rights-based approach, the chapter then addresses issues affecting caring for children and young people from ethnic minorities in community, school and healthcare settings. The chapter seeks to engage the reader with contemporary issues that affect the provision of culturally sensitive care such as safeguarding children, health problems such as sickle cell disease, thalassaemia and diabetes, health inequalities and talking to children about death and grieving. Within school settings, issues such as bullying, school uniforms, teenage pregnancy, obesity, mental health issues and arranged marriages are discussed. The last section of the chapter addresses the implications for practice through the development of cultural competence and the provision of antidiscriminatory practice.

Introduction

From the early age of 6 months children are able to differentiate colours and shapes, and by the age of 3 years children certainly can recognize differences, including skin colour differences, long before they go to school. They are clearly learning to recognize the colours of the objects around them. Ouseley and Lane (2008) argue that children are not born with attitudes that view colour necessarily in negative terms. They are reflecting the attitudes and values derived from their parents and significant others. This is particularly true of both Black and White children, although some Black children may also be carrying the burden of learning that they are the objects of racism or negative experiences. It must be noted that children do not live in a colour-blind environment.

How far children and young people 'participate' varies enormously within and between societies, and the ratification of the UN Convention on the Rights of the Child (1989) by many countries, including the UK, should demonstrate a change in the approaches that such countries have towards children's rights. This is particularly important in relation to children and young adults from minority ethnic groups.

Culture, ethnicity and race

The aim of exploring definitional aspects of current terms is to provide readers with a critical overview of terminology and discuss some of the theoretical concepts which affect the way children and young people from ethnic minorities are viewed. The following sections will explore definitions of culture, ethnicity and race.

Culture

CULTURE DIFFERENCES

i Thoughts
ii Beliefs
iii Diet
iv Dress
v Music
vi Art

Culture refers to habits of thought, beliefs, diet, dress, music and art and reflects ethnicity. Helman (1994) refers to culture as a set of guidelines which an individual inherits as a member of a particular society that tells him/her how to view the world and how to behave in relation to other people. It also provides him/her with a way of transmitting these guidelines to the next generation through the use of symbols, language, art and rituals.

It is important for community children's nurses and other practitioners to recognize the value of language and the socialization process in the way children and young people learn about culture as it is a way of life that is shared by all members of that particular group. There is a danger of viewing culture as static with frozen attributes about people, as culture is constantly evolving and people respond to the technological developments in a dynamic fashion. Box 3.1 summarizes the key characteristics of culture.

Key points

- Culture is learned both through language acquisition and socialization.
- The individual is fitted into the way of life.
- Culture is shared by all members of the group – it gives group identity.
- Culture responds to factors such as technology and the environment.
- Culture is dynamic and evolving.

Box 3.1	**Ethnicity classification in the 2001 UK census in England and Wales**

- White
  — British
  — Irish
  — Any other White background
- Mixed
  — White and Black Caribbean
  — White and Black African
  — White and Asian
  — Any other mixed background
- Asian or Asian British
  — Indian
  — Pakistani

- — Bangladeshi
  — Any other Asian background
- Black or Black British
  — Caribbean
  — African
  — Any other Black background
- Chinese or other ethnic group
  — Chinese
  — Any other ethnic group
- Not stated

(Office of Population, Censuses and Surveys 2001)

[handwritten: Ethnic]

Ethnicity *[handwritten: ⇒ IS NORMALLY ASSOCIATED WITH NON-WHITE!]*

Ethnicity, on the other hand, refers to social groups who often share a cultural heritage with a common language, values, religion, customs and attitudes. Members are aware of sharing a common past, possibly a homeland, and experience a sense of difference. An 'ethnic person' may be used to refer to a foreigner or member of an immigrant community, whereas an 'ethnic minority' is used to describe someone related to a group of people having common racial, national, religious or cultural origins, existing within a majority culture. Such a person may belong to an ethnic group that is a group of people whose members identify with each other, through a common heritage that is real or presumed.

The classification of ethnicity in the UK, as shown in Table 3.1, has attracted controversy in the past, particularly at the time of the 2001 Census, when the existence and nature of such classifications, which appeared on the Census form, became public. If one goes by the above definitions of ethnicity, the labels included in the census form were not really seeking ethnic identities of people as labels, such as White and Black, African, Caribbean, Asian, Indian and Chinese, will do very little to reveal the ethnic identities of people, as Africa and Asia are vast continents with such a diversity of people that to classify oneself as 'Asian' or 'African' might suggest no more than a desire, from the authorities, to count the number of non-White people in the UK rather than truly reflecting the ethnicity of the population. The self-defining nature of ethnicity, the basis for categorization in the UK, lacks objectivity as the classification is centred on the self-report of how subjectively meaningful the label is to that person, unlike the data for age and gender.

The use of the term ethnicity in common usage and in the academic literature is not without controversy, as the term is more often used to describe non-White groups, which assumes that there is no ethnicity in the White population, when there clearly is. In addition, ethnicity may be inaccurately used to describe other objects such as 'ethnic' food, 'ethnic' décor or 'ethnic' vegetables, which can mean nothing more than foreign or non-European. Such an approach often ignores ethnicity in

Table 3.1 Key points for practitioners on the current terminology to use

Acceptable usage	Not acceptable as likely to cause offence
African: often used as a prefix, e.g. African Caribbean and African American, to denote the origins. Some early literature still refers to West Indian for people from the Caribbean	Afro-Caribbean Nigger Negro Negroid Wog Coloured Half-caste Paki Coolie Ethnics Ethnic minorities
Black: a political category to denote all non-Whites; children and young people may wish to be identified as *Black British*	
Mixed race: children and young people with mixed parentage such as a Black father and a White mother or vice versa	
South Asian: people who hail from or who descend from people from the Indian subcontinent such as India, Pakistan, Sri Lanka and Bangladesh. Some may prefer to be called Hindu, Muslim or Sikh. Children and young people may wish to be identified as *British Muslim, British Hindu* or *Sikh*	
White: a political category to denote people from a European origin	
Minority ethnic groups: to denote people who are minorities, but also indicates that there is a majority ethnic group	

White majority groups. McKenzie and Crowcroft (1996) argue that the term ethnicity may be used as a euphemism for race in health research and this can lead to spurious results owing to the lack of specificity about the term ethnicity.

'Race'

Use of the term 'race' has been controversial as the term is a social construct to refer to the genetic or biological differences (usually skin colour), without scientific basis. The idea of 'race' has developed from evolutionary theories and also physical differences, based on geography, such as skin colour or hair colour and type, but no other corresponding variation in other human characteristics (Appiah 1996). While it is recognized in academic circles that 'race' *per se* does not exist, as there is only one human race, Appiah (1996) also suggests that it is important to understand how people think about race and how such concepts, ideas and definitions of the term vary in time and place. Biological definitions have been discredited by scientists as there are greater differences within than between what is called 'races'; consequently, the term is used with inverted commas in social science literature (Pfeiffer 1998).

Mixed 'race' children and young people

Children and young people with mixed parentage, however, often seem to be excluded in any discourse about categorization, and in both the UK and the USA a major factor of differentiation is based upon Whites in an epicentre of swirling colours. In effect, to be 'mixed' is a function of coloured realities, not White ones, as some people of mixed race may feel that the blanket use of the term 'Black' often robs them of the pride of their mixed parentage (Gordon 1995).

Iyabo (1999) suggests that the relationship between racial and ethnic identity remains unclear in the literature. Research with British teenagers of mixed parentage (one Black and one White) revealed that about 39% regarded themselves as 'Black'; 49% did not regard themselves as 'Black' and instead referred to themselves as 'Brown' or 'half and half' or 'mixed'; with 10% saying that they too sometimes felt 'White' or 'felt more White than Black'; but none said that they would call themselves White (Tizard and Phoenix 1993).

Whiteness → Think they are highly privileged than the rest!

While 'White' is always in the list of categories for ethnicity classification, there is a dearth of definitions about what it is. It is assumed to be a neutral category against which all other classifications are measured. However, Puzan (2003) argues that 'White' is about White privilege, conferring certain indelible and undeniable advantages to those who fit that category. Such a view is supported by Marx and Pennington (2003), who suggest that whiteness is a highly privileged social construction rather than a neutral racial category. Puzan (2003) further adds that the inherent power assumed in 'acting White' has been underestimated and explains that acting White means adhering to the behaviours, values, beliefs and practices of the dominant culture. Community children's nurses and other health and social care practitioners should be aware of this assumption when dealing with children and young people from ethnic minorities as this inherent power difference may be the cause of friction and resentment.

of course!

What's in a name? (A note on terminology)

Vydelingum (1998) suggested that, whatever label or name is used for members of the diverse minority ethnic population in Britain, it is problematic and it changes over time. Often, practitioners can be reluctant to use terms which might cause offence, whereas other people might quite rightly reject terms used to describe them, especially when such terms are no more than euphemisms for inferiority. Some terms may do no more than emphasize a minority ethnic's differentness, which, in turn, may lead to the legitimation of discrimination against them.

Permissible nomenclature is transitory and writers are often guilty of using currently in-vogue words which may in later years invite criticism. For example, just over three decades ago, 'coloured' was polite common currency in describing 'non-Whites' in the UK and the USA, except for 'Orientals' and 'American Indians', notes Gaine (1987). 'Coloured', until the dismantling of apartheid, remained a legal category, though a controversial one, in South Africa. The Black is Beautiful movement by people of African origins in the USA assisted them tremendously in ridding themselves of the negative connotations of the word 'Black', and for African Americans, which now seems to be the currently preferred term in the USA, the term 'coloured' is a euphemism – an apology for a skin colour socially defined as undesirable. 'Black' has gained new meaning, suggestive of political identity and ethnic pride.

Objections to the 'Black' label

In Britain, young 'South Asians' may object to the term 'Black' to describe them as this may appear to conflate a variety of ethnic groups which should be treated separately, e.g. African Caribbeans, Bangladeshis, Indians, Pakistanis, Sikhs, Hindus and Muslims, and which may relate to their parents' country of origin. Within the sociology of race, Modood (1994) argues that the term 'Black' and its concept are harmful to British Asians. The reason why many young South Asians continue to reject the label 'Black' lies in the attempts to impose it on them by the advocates of 'Black' rather than being actively sought by them. 'Black' has limited applicability as it has to do with socially defining a group of people not by themselves but by the majority (White, dominant) group.

Modood (1994) suggests that 'Black' evokes a false essentialism: that all 'non-White' groups have something in common other than how others treat them. 'Black', being evocative of people of African origins, understates the size, needs and specific concerns of Asian communities. However, Modood fails to recognize that 'Black' also treats people of African origins as a homogeneous group, which they are not, with the resultant underemphasizing of the multiplicity of cultures and the diversity of languages among the African Caribbean too (Figueroa 1991). Modood (1994) further argues that while African Caribbeans can use the concept for the purposes of ethnic pride, for South Asians it can be no more than 'a political colour', leading to a politicized identity, consequently resulting in a smothering of Asian ethnic pride. The 'smothering of ethnic pride' created by the use of the blanket term 'Black' is also true of people of African Caribbean origins whose identities as Shonas or Endebeles (Zimbabwean tribes), Tanzanians, Zambians, Zulus, Jamaicans or Barbadians are denied.

What is an Asian child or young person?

The term 'Asian' is misleading as it was a colonial invention used to describe people of Indian descent who had either been transported as indentured labourers or encouraged to settle as traders in the British colonies, suggest Westwood and Bachu (1988). Few young Asians in Britain identify with the term or attach great meaning to it. 'Asian' refers to people who were either born in or whose forebears originated from the Indian subcontinent, often living as ethnic minorities in Britain, excluding the Japanese, Chinese or 'Southeast Asians'. Just like the use of the term 'Black' discussed earlier, utilization of the catch-all 'Asian' term also suppresses cultural diversity and tends to mask the many types of family structures, specific religions, culture and migratory patterns of the 'Asian' people.

Under some circumstances, there may be objections to bracketing together a wide variety of cultural ethnic groups often with different positions within British society argues Vydelingum (1998). Young 'Asians' would prefer to be seen as people of Indian, Pakistani, Bangladeshi or Sri Lankan origins. However, some young people may prefer to be identified as Black British: this has the advantage of stressing the fact that the people are referred to first as British; other young people might prefer use of the term British Asians or British Hindu, Muslim or Sikh.

Cultural conflicts

Community children's nurses and other health and social care practitioners must note that the contemporary issue here is that children and young people from minorities may not always assign the same ethnic identities as their parents to themselves. Such children growing up in the UK may be experiencing conflict about straddling two or more cultures and also speaking more than one language. For example, a child born to Asian Bangladeshi parents may speak Sylheti or Bengali. Children born of Bangladeshi parents will probably enter the school with a degree of fluency in Sylheti, but with a very limited knowledge of Bengali and, often, with little exposure to the written word. Through exposure to the British schools system and meeting children from other cultures and backgrounds the child will learn English and may later wish to self-identify as both Bangladeshi and British or a British Bangladeshi.

Ethnocentrism and racism

Far too many practitioners are unsure when dealing with cultural aspects of care as a high level of confusion exists about ethnocentrism and racism. Ethnocentrism is the tendency to use one's own group as the basis for all comparison, and to view

What's in a name? (A note on terminology)   Page 63

PART I

one's own group as the norm. Herberg (1995, p. 38) defines ethnocentrism as the 'unconscious' tendency to look at others through the lens of one's own cultural norms and customs and take for granted that one's own values are the only objective reality'.

Racism is more about discriminating and providing a less favourable service to someone on the basis of 'race' or racial features and can prevail as part of the ethos or culture of the organization. It is a corrosive disease, suggests Macpherson (1999), who believes that institutional racism can be the most difficult organizational process to tackle. Concluding from the Stephen Lawrence Inquiry, MacPherson (1999) suggested that institutional racism is the collective failure of an organization to provide an appropriate and professional service to people because of their colour, culture or ethnic origin. It can be seen or detected in processes, attitudes and behaviour, which amount to discrimination through the unwitting prejudice, ignorance, thoughtlessness and racist stereotyping which disadvantages ethnic minority people.

In the following case study we will illustrate the meaning of ethnocentrism, and we believe that this is far more common in practice, especially when dealing with children and young people from ethnic minorities.

Case study

In the early 1980s, a nurse was training to be a health visitor in the West Midlands, UK. During the practice placement, the nurse was placed in a very middle class area and saw mainly White families. The nurse asked the health visiting practice teacher if she could spend some time in an alternative placement to enable her to gain experience of health visiting with minority ethnic families. The teacher arranged for the trainee to spend some time with a health visitor in Birmingham. The trainee visited daily with the health visitor and went from one house to another, calling in on young Asian women and their babies. As far as communication was concerned, it was a rather difficult situation as the health visitor did not speak Hindi or Bengali and the mothers did not speak English. Most of the communication was done using sign language. One day after a visit, the health visitor asked the trainee if she had noted that Mrs Begum was a good mother. The trainee thought that she had missed something rather important, and asked the health visitor to explain why she thought that Mrs Begum was a good mother. She said, 'Did you not see how Mrs Begum had started to give her baby, now 4 months old, Cow and Gate weaning food from the jars, instead of Indian food?'

This was not racism but ethnocentrism as the health visitor's judgement was based on her dominant values, making these the only objective reality. Community children's nurses and other healthcare practitioners should be aware of their own stereotypical views and the impact such views might have on the care for sick children.

Reflection points

★ Can you recall times in practice when obvious ethnocentric views have been expressed?

★ Describe what happened?

★ Were the views of individuals challenged in any way?

★ How do you handle people who hold strong stereotypes?

Stereotyping

Ethnocentric approaches in care provision can be the result of stereotyping, which assumes that cultures are static, homogeneous and have a biological basis. Ahmad (1993) suggests that such stereotyping can be based on the notion of exotica – studying exotic diseases, exotic customs and exotic people. This leads to a pathologizing of culture, meaning the locating of people's health problems in terms of their pathological culture; for example, children from South Asian parents tend to be submissive because of the oppressive patriarchal family relationships, and children from West Indian families tend to lack discipline as they come from single-parent families with matriarchal relationships. Furthermore, *Asian rickets* in children; *Asian tuberculosis*; *self-harm* in young female Asians, etc. Rickets is a disease of calcium deficiency, which can occur in any child who has calcium deficiency, and low calcium serum levels do not have an Asian marker; similarly, the tubercle bacillus that infects Asians does not have a specific biological marker and is the bacillus that would infect anyone (Black or White) who was malnourished and living in overcrowded conditions. The use of such terms would lead practitioners to believe that these were new diseases. Such an approach, argues (Ahmad 1993), not only pathologizes minority cultures but also ignores issues of power, deprivation and racism and distracts from putting more resources into exploring such diseases; the end result is a Black family pathology, i.e. problems with children and illnesses are due to the nature of Black families. Further examples of stereotyping and ethnocentric approaches in care can be found in Vydelingum (2006).

Cultural diversity and transcultural nursing

In a critical review of concepts and definitions, Kroeber *et al.* (1952) explained that cultural diversity in nursing practice derives its conceptual base from nursing, other cross-cultural health disciplines and the social sciences such as anthropology, sociology and psychology. Culture is conceptualized broadly to encompass the belief systems of a variety of groups. Cultural diversity refers to the differences between people based on a shared ideology and valued set of beliefs, norms, customs and meanings, evidenced in a way of life. However, the term 'transcultural nursing', coined by Dr Madeleine M. Leininger in the mid-1950s, began to attract more widespread interest and concept development in the 1970s and 1980s. A comparatively new and marginal discipline in the UK, transcultural nursing refers to a specialty

What's in a name? (A note on terminology)   **Page 65**

PART I

within nursing focused on the comparative study of different cultures and subcultures (Papadopoulos 2006).

What is important when dealing with children and young people from minority ethnic groups is that the values and beliefs of the practitioner, more often White middle class, may not be convergent. For example, the values of nursing in the USA or the UK are embedded in the values of a Western culture placing stress on self-reliance and individualism – beliefs that 'individuals have the ability to pull themselves up by their bootstraps' and that an individual's rights are more important than a society's. However, many cultures, especially Asian and African cultures, do not share the primacy of the value of individualism. With individualism, importance is placed on individual inputs, rights and rewards (Andrews and Boyle 1999). It is worth noting that the majority of cultures around the world are in essence collectivistic, meaning that the loyalties of a person to a group exceed the rights of the individual, rather than individualistic, in which the rights of the individual supersede those of the group. In many cultures, health decisions are not made by an individual but by a group – family, community and/or society – and this is a very important point to remember when dealing with sick children.

Factors affecting child rearing

The immigration process is a change agent in family life and affects people's roles, expectations and obligations; however, children born to immigrants are UK citizens and are as entitled to all rights and entitlements as any other child. It should be noted that the worst affected are asylum seekers and refugee families, because of government dispersal policies.

The relationship between family and society is dynamic, and rapid changes in family structure, values, customs and systems of obligations are major catalysts for social change, as noted way back by Wilmot and Young (1957). Family reproduces culture, through ideological, structural and personal factors, but what is important is that the rate of social change for immigrants may be faster than for 'natives', and differences between generations may be greater at the level of both assumptions and behaviour. The contemporary issue here is that external social, economic and legal constraints may exert greater pressure for change in children born to minority ethnic families (Ahmad 1996).

The role of the family

The family reproduces values and behaviours, e.g. honour, shame, identity, religion, obligations and expectations, and these are often seen as the prime responsibility of parents. Religious and cultural institutions assist the family in cultural retention.

Concerns about the values and institutions of the wider society and external hostility may reinforce encapsulation. Hence, in addition to going to a British school, some children may attend afternoon or evening classes at their local religious centres, such as Madrassahs (for Muslims) or Gudwarahs (for Sikhs), to learn about their language, religion or culture. Here, gender differences in childhood upbringing, as seen by that particular culture, may also be reinforced. This may be a cause for conflict in children and young people growing up in the UK, particularly if such differences are in conflict with the wider values of British society.

For example, if some girls are brought up in such a way that they are not able to participate as equal citizens, they may resent such gender stereotypes, leading to generational conflicts. Such demands on young people about roles, obligations, honour and respect may set some of them on a collision course with their parents, when taking the 'personal choices' route can lead to personal rejection by family and local community.

Cultural influences on child-rearing practices

Most Southeast Asian groups (Vietnamese, Cambodian and Laotian) share cultural values that influence parental socialization practices. Confucian principles of filial piety, ancestral unity and lineage are the most crucial of these, according to Morrow (1989), Vernon (1982) and Yamamoto and Kubota (1983). A central principle – 'pride and shame', in which an individual's action reflects either positively or negatively on the entire family – is inherent within each culture. Right from an early age, children are taught to respect their parents, older siblings and other adults in positions of authority, and individual family members are made aware of their place in the vertical hierarchy. The fostering of mutual interdependence is started from an early age, such that obligation to parents and family is expected to outweigh personal desires or needs (Morrow 1989). Such an upbringing may be in stark contrast to Western values of assertiveness and independence and raises questions about children's rights in the context of childhood. Morrow (1999, p. 157) illustrates these from research on children's perspectives on their rights and decision-making, and quotes from young children of Pakistani origin, as follows:

My mum and my dad make all the decisions and my sisters.

Me and my mum decide.

I listen to my mum and dad, children should listen to parents, that's good manners.

Community children's nurses and other practitioners should be cognizant of the fact that, although such practices may infringe the rights of the young people, the wider role of the family should be acknowledged, especially in relation to the education of children and young people from minority ethnic groups.

Practice

Safeguarding children from minority ethnic groups

The common core set of knowledge and skills required to practise at a basic level in six areas when dealing with safeguarding children is shown in Box 3.2.

The Children Act 1989 (s.22 (5)) (Office of Public Sector Information 1989) states that local authorities have a duty to give due consideration 'to the child's religious persuasion, racial origin and cultural and linguistic background' in decision-making, and under the United Nations (UN) Convention (UN Convention on the Rights of the Child 1989), all children have the right to be protected from harm. Boushel (2000) suggests that there are only a small number of studies that incorporate

Box 3.2	Core knowledge and skills

- Effective communication and engagement
- Child and young person development
- Safeguarding and promoting the welfare of the child and young person
- Supporting transitions
- Multiagency working
- Sharing information

'race' and 'ethnicity' in social welfare research and children from minority ethnic groups are disproportionately represented both in child protection registrations and in the looked after population (Barn *et al.* 1997). The Social Services Inspectorate (2000) has noted that disparities have been found to be particularly pronounced in local authorities that have a small proportion of ethnic minority families. Stereotyping, colour blindness, cultural deficit and inadequate training of professionals lead to failures in the statutory processes designed to protect children, according to Webb *et al.* (2002). More children from minority ethnic groups were permanently placed away from their birth parents than their White peers, although they were more likely to be placed with relatives. Such placements may reflect stereotypical views concerning the family support available to minority ethnic groups. Hunt *et al.* (1999) found that court proceedings were instigated faster when children came from minority ethnic groups, although the families displayed fewer pathological profiles.

Research evidence (Jones and McCurdy 1992; Chamba *et al.* 1999; Ghate and Hazel 2002) indicates that the perception that minority ethnic groups receive additional support from their extended family is an oversimplification, and that there is considerable diversity across minority communities. Many parents from minority ethnic groups have restricted informal social networks, less practical and emotional support from family or friends and are less likely to use community-based services. Basing decisions upon erroneous assumptions about different cultures can have grave consequences.

Using such an uncritical approach may lead to dire consequences, as seen in the Victoria Climbié case. Professionals' perceptions of respect and obedience in African Caribbean families were cited as reasons why they failed to note or act upon signs of ill-treatment in the case of Victoria Climbié (Laming 2003, p. 16). The report states 'cultural norms and models of behaviour can vary considerably between communities and even families' (Laming 2003, p. 345).

Large numbers of children and young people arrive into this country from overseas every day. Many of these children do so legally in the care of their parents. However, many children are arriving into the UK who may be in the care of adults who, although they may be their carers, have no parental responsibility for them, and some may be in the care of adults who have no documents to demonstrate a relationship with the child. Evidence from the Inter-Agency Protocol on Safeguarding Children From Abroad shows that unaccompanied children or those accompanied by someone who is not their parent are particularly vulnerable. The children and many of their carers will need assistance to ensure that the child receives adequate care and accesses health and education services. A small number of these children may be exposed to the additional risk of commercial, sexual or domestic exploitation.

PART I

Assessment for safeguarding children and young people from minority ethnic groups

Harran (2002, p. 413) emphasizes the importance of recognizing 'that professionals and clients are not culturally neutral but a product of their own cultural conditioning and life experiences'. Practitioners do not necessarily have sufficient understanding of cultural diversity (Farmer and Owen 1998), which may lead to a failure to conduct 'culturally competent assessment and intervention'. It may also undermine the emphasis placed upon the child's or young person's rights and needs and cause delays in the decision-making process.

The Social Services Inspectorate (2000) report on services for minority ethnic children and families, *Excellence Not Excuses*, expressed concerns about assessment and care planning and identified cases where children's safety was compromised because physical and sexual abuse had not been identified or properly dealt with.

They found that, although it was generally acknowledged that meeting the holistic needs of the child was important, in practice, this was problematic, and particularly when dealing with children with mixed ethnicities.

Reflection points

★ What are the developmental needs of Black children and their families?

★ In what ways are these similar to, and in what ways do they differ from, the developmental needs of White children and families?

★ How can these developmental needs be responded to in work with Black children and families?

Dutt and Phillips (2000, p. 38) point out that 'both black and white children require their parents or carers to respond to their same fundamental care needs' and state that 'the base lines for assessing parenting capacity and the child's developmental needs should be the same irrespective of whether a black child or a white child is being assessed'. Webb *et al.* (2002) raise additional issues that may influence the recognition of abuse in children from minority ethnic groups (Box 3.3).

Box 3.3	Assessment of abuse in children from minority ethnic groups

- Dark skin complexions may mask evidence of bruising
- Some children from minority ethnic groups may show dark patches on their lower back 'Mongolian blue'; this is normal
- Female genital mutilation may be seen as normal practice in some cultures though illegal in the UK
- Language barriers may prevent children and young people from expressing their wishes and views or disclosing abuse
- Some children and young people may not view corporal punishment as abuse if it is perceived as endemic in the household, and such practice may be viewed as 'normal' child-rearing practices
- Professionals may be reluctant to express concerns for fear of being viewed as racist

When is abuse not abuse?

Cultural differences in the way families rear their children should be respected, but when child abuse does occur it should be understood that this particular family has gone beyond what is acceptable not only in their own and British culture (Chand 2000, cited in Harran 2002, p. 411) but also in the law of the land. In the USA, statutes specify exemptions regarding abuse thresholds, most commonly in relation to religious belief (e.g. concerning withholding medical treatment on religious grounds) or cultural practice; such considerations do not operate in the UK. As Chand points out, extensive recruitment from overseas into the health and welfare services may increase the diversity of cultural norms and expectations. Health and social care practitioners need to be aware that their beliefs may affect the decisions they make. Furthermore, Welbourne (2002, p. 353) emphasizes the importance of taking into account the fact that 'tensions exist between different cultural norms and values within the UK, not only between ethnically and culturally distinct groups of people'.

Female genital mutilation is one of the troubling issues relating to culture and ethics, argues Gallagher (2006). She cites the British Medical Association's (2001) definition of female genital mutilation as

> *a collective term used for a range of practices involving the removal of parts of healthy female genitalia, from the removal of the head of the clitoris to the total amputation of the clitoris and labia minora and part of the labia majora, the remainder of which is stitched together leaving a matchstick-sized opening for the passage of urine and menstrual blood.*

Female genital mutilation is still a widely used traditional practice in Northern Africa, and the World Health Organization (2010) estimates that over 2 million girls have this operation every year.

Reasons for such social, cultural and religious practices are put forward as the preservation of chastity and the restoration of family honour in that the woman remains a virgin until she has intercourse with her husband. However, Lindroos and Luukkainen (2004), in a study in Nigeria, found that this practice was more a matter of male domination and a convenient way of controlling sexual behaviour in women. They also found that female genital mutilation was a significant factor in maintaining high numbers of maternal mortality because of the associated pain, infections and haemorrhage during labour. Practitioners should keep in mind that female genital mutilation is illegal in the UK, whatever the cultural reasons behind it.

Other health issues for children and young people

Infant mortality

There are large differences in the infant mortality rates of ethnic groups in England and Wales, according to new statistics published by the Office for National Statistics (2008). Data reveal that, for babies born in 2005, infant mortality in both the Pakistani and Caribbean groups was twice that of the White British group. Asian and Black ethnic groups accounted for over 11% of live births in England and Wales in 2005, and 17% of infant deaths. Babies in the Pakistani and Caribbean groups had particularly high infant mortality rates: 9.6 and 9.8 deaths per 1000 live births, respectively, which is double the rate in the White British group (4.5 deaths per 1000 live births). Mortality in the Pakistani group was high throughout the first year of life whereas mortality in the Caribbean group was especially high in the first month of life. One-half of all infant deaths in the Pakistani group were due to congenital anomalies compared with only one-quarter of deaths in the White British group (Office for National Statistics 2008).

Sickle cell disease and thalassaemia

In England, sickle cell disease (SCD) is as common as cystic fibrosis. Sickle cell disease affects an estimated 12 500 people, with a further 240 000 thought to be carriers. Modell *et al.* (2007) estimate that there are approximately 214 000 carriers of thalassaemia, with around 700 people suffering from thalassaemia major, the most severe form of the disease. SCD presently affects more than 1 in every 2400 births in the UK. Sickle cell and thalassaemia are both increasingly common in countries of Northern and Western Europe and this is likely to increase further with greater population movement. SCD is found to be highest among people of Black Caribbean and Black African descent, with a high risk of sudden death in the early years of life. SCD is the commonest cause of stroke in childhood in the UK; the peak incidence is between the ages of 2 and 7 years, and by the age of 10 about 6% of children have suffered clinical strokes.

Thomas *et al.* (2001) have noted that thalassaemias are less common than SCD, with the highest prevalence found among Cypriots, Indians, Pakistanis, Bangladeshis, Chinese and other Asian groups. Because both conditions can restrict a child's or an adult's ability to conduct normal daily activities, they can also have profound psychosocial effects on individuals and their families. Implications for practice involve adequate screening programmes such as the NHS Sickle Cell and Thalassaemia Screening Programme, which was set up in England in 2001. Early detection and adequate management of the condition can improve quality of life. For SCD, this enables parents/guardians to learn to recognize certain risk factors in their child, to avoid those that can trigger painful 'crisis' attacks and to administer antibiotics each day to prevent infections. Children with thalassaemia major will require blood transfusions every 4–6 weeks and can suffer from chronic diseases (such as diabetes) and growth or puberty failure.

Diabetes

Rates of obesity are significantly higher for Asian/Asian British children in the UK (Saxena *et al.* 2004; Department of Health 2008a) than for White British children. Children who are overweight/obese are at higher risk of insulin resistance, type 2 diabetes, metabolic syndrome, coronary artery disease, some cancers, breathing problems, arthritis and psychological problems, according to Zimmet *et al.* (2007). Recent research points to lifestyle issues within the minority ethnic families.

Hanif (2008) summarized the evidence concerning the relationships between traditional South Asian diets, physical inactivity and central adiposity in adults. In children, familial perceptions of a 'healthy' weight, activity levels and food choices have an impact upon childhood obesity. Khunti *et al.* (2007) have shown that children from ethnic minorities have lower levels of physical activity than White European contemporaries, although activity levels were poor in general. They also found that dietary habits were generally unhealthy in children of all ethnicities. Moreover, 'normal' weight may be perceived differently within cultures, families or generations. In a multiethnic UK sample of 14–15 year olds, boys and children from ethnic minorities were most likely to underestimate their level of obesity (Standley *et al.* 2009).

Health inequalities within Black and minority ethnic communities

Disadvantage and discrimination characterize the experiences of many people from Black and minority ethnic communities, especially in the area of health and healthcare, in that they experience poorer health, generally have reduced life expectancy and, in certain areas of the UK, experience greater problems accessing health services than the majority White population.

Cooper *et al.* (1998) reported that South Asian children and young people used GP services more than any other ethnic group after controlling for socioeconomic background and perceived health status, but the use of hospital outpatient and inpatient services was significantly lower for children and young people from all minority ethnic groups compared with the White population. Key findings from the survey are illustrated in Box 3.4.

In Britain, minority ethnic groups lead a parallel existence to that of the population as a whole, through greater rates of poverty and deprivation. Platt (2002) identified the ways in which past discrimination and disadvantage has affected the current welfare of minority groups. The report evaluates the extent to which current structures and policies perpetuate or mitigate deprivation.

A Barnardo's (2007) report, *It Doesn't Happen Here: The Reality of Child Poverty in the UK*, revealed that, within Black or Black British households, 48% of children were living in poverty. This rose to 67% in Pakistani and Bangladeshi households compared with 27% of White children. Worklessness was one of the key drivers for higher poverty rates for some ethnic minority groups. Educational achievement was

---

Box 3.4	Key points for practitioners

- The use of GP, outpatient and inpatient services by children and young people does not vary significantly according to their socioeconomic status
- Indian children and young people are more likely to consult a GP than any other ethnic group
- Black Caribbean, Indian, and Pakistani or Bangladeshi children and young people are less likely to use hospital inpatient and outpatient services than White children and young people
- These ethnic differences have important implications for the quality of healthcare received by children and young people

(adapted from Cooper et al. 1998)

an important factor in poverty rates among ethnic minority groups. The achievement gap between White pupils and their Pakistani and African Caribbean classmates has almost doubled since the late 1980s. The report also found that 54% of Pakistani and Bangladeshi children in working households were in poverty, compared with 12% of White children.

Talking to children about death

Children and young people from minority ethnic groups are more likely to know someone who has died or been involved in honour killings, which are becoming a major problem in the UK. Honour killing is the murder of a woman accused of bringing shame upon her family. In recent years, more and more cases have reached the UK courts, but many crimes remain unresolved or even undetected. The UN Population Fund (UNFPA 2000) estimates that the annual worldwide total of killings might be as high as 5000 women (BBC News 2003).

The BBC report indicates that, in the UK, murders have sometimes taken place after a family has reacted violently to their son or daughter taking on the trappings of Western culture. Killings are often disguised as suicide, fire or an accident. Police believe that there may be as many as 12 honour killings in the UK every year. They will typically occur within Asian and Middle Eastern families when a person is believed to have 'dishonoured' their loved ones. In 2003, the Metropolitan Police set up a strategic task force to tackle the issue. A specialist unit was given the task of researching honour crimes, and 100 murder files spanning the last decade were reopened in an effort to find common links.

In a multicultural society, each culture has it own way of dealing with death and dying, and aligned with this are rituals and practices that may be very dear to the people concerned. While today's diversity adds to the richness of British culture, misunderstandings by health and social care practitioners may lead to accusations of insensitivity and ethnocentric approaches. Grief and bereavement are emotions that are experienced by all people, but these are expressed differently in different communities.

Box 3.5	Understanding rituals

- Ask the family if there are specific things in their culture that they do when someone is dying
- Ask whether there are specific rituals/customs that they use to recognize death
- Do they have certain traditions surrounding the disposal of the body?
- Ask about their beliefs about what happens after death
- Explore what their feelings are about mourning after death
- Ask whether there are any social stigmas associated with certain types of deaths
- Ask how important a transition death of a child or young person is
- What are their views on post-mortem and tissue donation?

When children and young people from such communities are dying, their parents often want certain religious rituals and practices to be carried out properly. Although it is not expected that health and social practitioners will be aware of all the rituals, parents of children and young people would expect a degree of sensitivity. In such circumstances, it is better to ask rather than show ignorance; respect should be shown for the body as it is almost a universal practice to treat the dead body with reverence, rather than just a dead body. Some guidelines for practitioners are summarized in Box 3.5.

Helping children and young people cope with loss and grief

While grieving processes may appear to be generic, the way children and young people from minority ethnic groups may cope will be shaped by the religious upbringing and socialization and acculturation into their own cultures. Children's coping with grief may be affected by the way they are brought up, and is influenced by the values and beliefs enshrined in their culture, such as respect, honour, responsibility and caring for others. Sandra Fox, from the Boston Medical Center (Fox 1985), has developed a framework outlining four psychological tasks that children and adolescents must accomplish if their grief is to be 'good grief', i.e. a 'grief' that promotes coping skills and prevents future mental health problems. They are understanding, grieving, commemorating and going on.

Understanding

Children and young people need honest age-appropriate information to make sense of death, and need to know what happened and why and that the person is no longer alive and will never be part of their lives in the way he or she used to be. Children go through 'magical thinking', which is especially true when death occurs because it is so hard to make sense out of death. Therefore, children often feel that the death must be the result of something they did or said or failed to do or say. Magical thinking must be challenged, so as not to leave them with life-long guilt.

Grieving

While the style of grieving will differ depending on the age of the child, the relationship with the person who died, and perhaps the suddenness of the death, may involve many feelings such as sadness, anger, abandonment and ambivalence. There is no one way or right way to grieve. All feelings must be validated as children grieve in spurts. They will re-grieve through adolescence. It is important to be aware of the anniversary date of the death and other significant dates to the bereaved child.

Commemorating

Commemorating is done both formally or informally, remembering the person who died and confirming the reality of the death and the value of human life. In this stage, friends, fellow students and teachers may be involved in the planning of the commemoration.

Going on

During this phase children and young people are expected to be returning comfortably to regular activities. This process becomes easier and healthier after the tasks of understanding, grieving and commemorating have been gone through, although all tasks are spiral not linear. Pain should be anticipated at anniversaries, and special times of remembering as 'going on' is not about forgetting or loving that person any less but about the reality of moving on in life.

Steps nurses and other practitioners can take to help bereaved children

The ways that nurses can help bereaved children according to the four steps suggested by Fox are outlined below.

Share the fact of the death with children and parents

Explain to children what has happened in an age-appropriate way, but share only the information that is public knowledge. Explain to younger children that a person dies when his or her body stops working totally. Communicate to parents or send a letter home telling them what has happened, what you have discussed at the clinic, ward or nursery and encourage them to listen to their children's reactions to the death and to talk with them about it.

Recognize your own feelings

Particular events or anniversaries of losses in our own lives can make it difficult to talk with children about death. It is all right to tell children how hard it is for you to talk about what has happened, and it is all right to cry. If your own grief makes it impossible for you to talk to children or young people, find someone who can. Stay in the room during the discussion, however, so you will know which children still have questions or concerns. Be authentic!

Watch particularly vulnerable children carefully

Be aware of children who may be 'at risk' for later emotional problems as a result of the death. For example, close friends or enemies of a child who died or children whose parents or siblings have illnesses similar to the one that caused the recent death. When someone's parent dies, all children worry about the mortality of their own parents. The death of a friend or classmate raises similar fears, particularly if one has the same symptoms or has done the same things as the child who died. Remind children that most people live very long.

Address the children's fears and fantasies

Children's active imaginations sometimes lead them to think something they have done or have not done has caused a death. Give them accurate information about the cause of the death. The following case study raises questions about the standards of care for a young Muslim man.

Case study

A young male Asian patient (teenager) had died in a ward in a general hospital. His mother was called in to see the body. She had been horrified to find him in a smelly side room, on a bed lying in a pool of vomit. She was very distressed as the picture of her son, in such a disgusting state in that bed, had been haunting her ever since. She complained to the hospital authorities and said that, in her mind's eye, the only picture she could see of her son was the last time she saw him lying in that bed. The nursing staff's comments were that, as he was a Muslim, they did not think they were allowed to touch the body: 'We usually let the family deal with the body'. The staff nurse said that the nurses were just following the guidelines.

Reflection points

★ What about the rights of the teenager whose body was left in a pool of vomit?

★ Were nurses providing culturally sensitive care?

★ Could the nurses have used gloves to wash the body to make it presentable to the mother?

★ What were the nurses' responsibilities under their professional code of conduct?

★ Is it right to follow guidelines to the letter even if these could lead to insensitive and poor practice?

Issues facing school nurses and community children's nurses

All children within the UK are required by law to be in full-time education between the ages of 5 and 16. There is, however, a huge range of settings within which this education can occur, including state schools, both selective and comprehensive entry, and those that are private (fee paying), single sex, mixed and affiliated to a religious group. Being at school is a central part of a child or young person's life as they spend a large proportion of their time there. As well as the more obvious learning that occurs in school, such as literacy, numeracy and science, more subtle learning occurs; for example, secondary socialization, which imparts the morals of the school and the society within which it is located, and peer learning, which involves the child or young person in discovering the culture of their peer group and deciding to accept it or reject it.

Reflection points

★ What was the ethnic mix in your school?

★ Was one ethnic group in the majority?

★ Did this have an influence on the culture of the school?

★ How did it affect those from other ethnic groups?

Bullying

Schools are also communities that, as with any community, can be either nurturing or destructive. Bullying, both face to face and cyber bullying, is a worldwide phenomenon that is gaining an increasing amount of attention (Ybarra and Mitchell 2004; Cowie and Jennifer 2007; Byron 2008). Much of the literature on bullying suggests that one of the factors involved is a perception of being different (Kowalski and Limber 2007; Williams and Guerra 2007; Wolak *et al* 2007; Ybarra *et al.* 2007). The UK has a very diverse ethnic mix, which suggests that bullying is an issue that needs to be considered in relation to children and young people from diverse backgrounds.

The ethnically diverse population in the UK is increasing: in 2004 an estimated 8.9% of the population was born outside the UK; in 2007, the figure was 10.6 (Office for National Statistics 2009). In 2004, the five most common non-UK countries of birth were India, Republic of Ireland, Pakistan, Germany and Bangladesh. In 2007, this had changed to India, Republic of Ireland, Poland, Pakistan and Germany (Office for National Statistics 2009).

Country of birth does not necessarily correlate to ethnicity; for example, the high numbers born in Germany can be attributed to the UK military bases in the country. However, for the other groups, the country of birth tends to correlate with ethnicity.

There also tends to be clusters of people from different ethnic groupings in the UK. For example, those of Polish origin tend to settle in the east of England and Scotland; those of Pakistani origin in the northwest of England, Yorkshire and Humberside; those of Indian origin in the Midlands and the southeast of England (Office for National Statistics 2009). London and other UK cities have large numbers of ethnic groups, with 2.3 million (32%) of Londoners being born outside the UK compared with 7% of the rest of the population. Outside London, the southeast and West Midlands have the highest migrant populations (Spence 2008).

In London, the largest migrant populations are from India, Bangladesh, Ireland, Jamaica, Nigeria, Poland, Kenya, Sri Lanka, South Africa and Ghana, making up 42% of the migrant population in London. Another 27% are from the EU, USA, Australia, New Zealand, Hong Kong and Japan (Spence 2008).

One consequence of this ethnic mix in London is that it is estimated that over 300 languages are spoken by children in London schools, and for more than one-third of children English is not the language that is used in their homes (National Literacy Trust 2006).

The internet is an integral part of young people's lives and it is an excellent means of communication. As Huesmann (2007) suggests, it has the potential to offer varied experiences, broadening horizons and helping children to become effective in adult life. It has been estimated that over 80% of adolescents own at least one of the following: computer with internet access, personal data assistant or cell phone (David-Ferdon and Hertz 2007). The majority of young people report that the internet is a valuable resource and enables them to engage socially with others (David-Ferdon and Hertz 2007).

It does, however, have a negative side, which is that the ease of access to communication means that young people may be vulnerable to bullying and harassment through these media. As Huesmann (2007) argues, this has not led to new psychological threats and bullying behaviours, but it is now more difficult to protect children from them. Huesmann (2007, p. S6) points out that 'It is now not just kids in bad neighbourhoods or with "bad" friends who are likely to be exposed to bad things when they go out on the streets. A "virtual" bad street is easily available to most youth now'. Ybarra and Mitchell (2004) argue that, for some young people who are bullied face to face at school, the internet simply means that the bullying continues into the evening and the night in places that might previously have been considered 'safe', e.g. at home with parents and family.

Reflection points

★ Think about your own educational experience. Did you or anyone you knew experience bullying?

★ What form did this bullying take?

★ What was done about it? By whom?

★ Can you identify any factors that led to this bullying?

★ What would you do about it now?

School uniforms and rights of minority ethnic children

Eason (2005), a BBC Education editor, reported on the Court of Appeal ruling that a Muslim girl's human rights were violated by a school's insistence on its dress code. The Court called on the Department for Education and Skills (DfES) to give schools more guidance on how to meet their obligations under the Human Rights Act 1998 (Office for Public Sector Information 1998).

He outlined the case of Shabina Begum, aged 15, who had accused Denbigh High School in Luton, Bedfordshire, of denying her the 'right to education and to manifest her religious beliefs' over her wish to wear a full-length jilbab gown.

The school, where most pupils were Muslim, had consulted Islamic scholars for advice, and had argued that Ms Begum had chosen a school with a uniform policy and, if she did not like it, could move to another school. However, Lord Justice Brooke, Vice President of the Civil Division of the Court of Appeal, ruled that her exclusion was unlawful and that the school had unlawfully denied her 'the right to manifest her religion'.

A representative for the DfES had reported that school uniform guidance states that governors should bear in mind their responsibilities under sex and race discrimination legislation and the Human Rights Act; be sensitive to pupils' cultural and religious needs and differences; and give high priority to cost considerations.

Eason reports that, currently in the UK, there is no legislation that deals specifically with school uniforms, and that individual schools, their governing bodies and the head teacher enforce the policy as part of day-to-day discipline. However, the DfES 'does not consider that exclusion from school would normally be appropriate where a pupil fails to comply with the school's rules on uniform'. The guidelines say schools must be 'sensitive to the needs of different cultures, races and religions' and accommodate those needs within their general uniform policy, such as allowing Muslim girls to wear appropriate dress and Sikh boys to wear traditional headdress'.

Reflection points

★ Consider whether members of other religious groups might wish to wear clothing not permitted by a school's uniform policy, and the effect this might have on its inclusiveness.

★ Is it appropriate to override the beliefs of very strict Muslims, when liberal Muslims had been permitted the dress code of their choice?

★ Is it appropriate to take into account concerns about such things as other pupils feeling intimidated or coerced by the presence of very strict Muslim garb?

★ Could schools do more to reconcile their wish to retain a uniform policy with the beliefs of those who considered it exposed too much of their bodies?

★ Could schools apply a policy without considering the individual child or young person?

Principles for practice

- The culture within the family, the school and the peer group may not be compatible.
- Practitioners need to be aware that any child or young person may be being bullied and that any child or young person who may be perceived as different is particularly vulnerable.
- Many people from the same ethnic groups live in the same area. This may result in cultural and social isolation for those who live in other areas.
- For some children and young people, English may not be the language that is used at home.

Public health priorities

The UK government has put public health high on the policy agenda, and a number of reports have been published on the state of the nation's health and identifying the public health priorities arising from it (Department of Health 2003, 2004, 2008b, 2009).

In relation to children and young people the priorities are focused around obesity, mental health, sexual health and teenage pregnancy. Here, we will consider teenage pregnancy and obesity.

Teenage pregnancy

The UK has one of the highest teenage pregnancy rates in the world and the highest rate in Europe (Fig. 3.1).

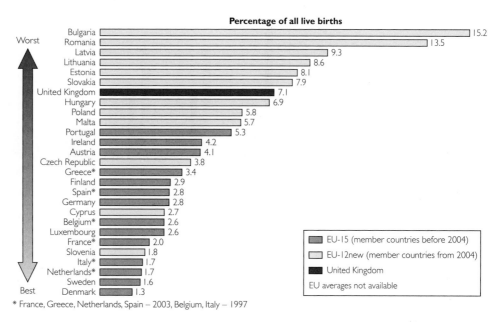

* France, Greece, Netherlands, Spain – 2003, Belgium, Italy – 1997

Figure 3.1 Percentage of all live births to mothers aged under 20 years. Reproduced from Health Profile of England 2007. Department of Health

Reflection points

★ Why do you think that the UK has one of the highest rates of teenage pregnancy in the world?

★ Why do you think that it matters?

In the UK, reducing the number of teenage pregnancies (those ending in a live birth or a termination) is a priority (Department of Health 2009). There is a link between social deprivation and the rates of teenage pregnancy, with girls from socially deprived backgrounds being more likely to become pregnant than others (Office for National Statistics 2009). There is also a link between the age of the mother at the time of conception and the socioeconomic outcomes for the mother and the child (Department of Health 2009), which tend to be worse for mothers and children when the mother was younger at the time of conception.

It is difficult to disentangle official statistics relating to the ethnic origin of teenage mothers, but as can be seen from Figs 3.2 and 3.3, there is a clear link between the age of the mother and her socioeconomic group. These statistics are for premaritally conceived first live births in England and Wales; Fig. 3.2 shows the socioeconomic status of the mother for all ages of mother, and Fig. 3.3 shows the socioeconomic status of the mother for those who gave birth aged 20 or younger.

It can be seen from Figs 3.2 and 3.3 that women from the more socially deprived groups are more likely to have a live birth before the age of 20 than those from the higher socioeconomic groups. However, Figs 3.2 and 3.3 show only the births to married women, rather than all women under the age of 20. Figure 3.4 shows the rates per thousand for women under the age of 16.

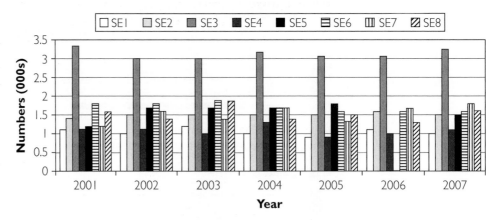

Figure 3.2 Premaritally conceived first live births to married women; estimated distribution by socioeconomic classification of father, 2001–2007 (all ages) (thousands). SE, socioeconomic group. Reproduced from Office for National Statistics (2009).

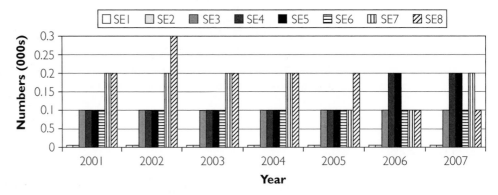

Figure 3.3 Premaritally conceived live births to married women under the age of 20, by socioeconomic classification. Reproduced from Office for National Statistics (2009).

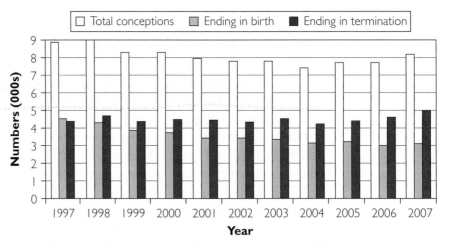

Figure 3.4 Reproduced from Office for National Statistics (2009).

It can be seen, therefore, that the chances of a young woman becoming pregnant before the age of 20 is much greater for those in the lower socioeconomic groups. There is also a link between country of origin and conception and births below the age of 20, as can be seen in Table 3.2. The UK, therefore, has a high rate of conception among young women aged 20 and under, many of which end in abortion.

Table 3.2 Age of mother and country of birth, 2007 (live births)

Country of birth of mother	Age of mother at birth		
	All ages	Under 20	20–24
Total	690 013	44 805	130 784
UK	529 655	40 766	103 142
Total outside the UK	160 340	4036	27 637
Irish Republic	3232	59	290
Australia, Canada and New Zealand	4707	30	161
New Commonwealth	68 678	1375	12 276
India	12 012	115	1727
Pakistan	17 648	382	4451
Bangladesh	8775	216	2586
East Africa	4197	84	422
Southern Africa	4657	78	476
Rest of Africa	12 700	254	1428
Caribbean	3578	200	625
Far East	1329	3	55
Rest of New Commonwealth	3782	43	506
Other European Union	34 117	1142	6834
Rest of Europe	7715	199	1433
USA	3111	48	328
Rest of the world	38 780	1183	6315

Reproduced from Office for National Statistics (2009).

There appears to be a higher rate of births to women under the age of 20 among some groups than among others; for example, women whose country of origin is India, Pakistan and Bangladesh. What the statistics do not explain, however, is the possible cultural influences on these rates. For example, within some cultures it is the norm for women to marry and have babies much younger than in other cultures. In addition, the statistics do not differentiate the ethnic groups which make up the UK as their country of origin. As has been discussed, the UK is an ethnically diverse population with many people from different ethnic groups describing themselves as 'British', and they, their parents, grandparents and previous generations were born here.

Reflection points

★ What does Table 3.2 tell you about the link between country of origin and rates of birth to mothers below the age of 20?

★ What important information is missing from Table 3.2?

A contemporary issue is sexual health. In 2008, the UK government began immunizing girls against the human papilloma virus, which has been linked to the development of cervical cancer. It has been estimated that this immunization campaign will save thousands of deaths from cervical cancer per year. As with any immunization, parental consent is sought. Some parents have refused consent as they believe that their daughters are not sexually active and therefore their daughters do not need it; others believe that having the immunization may encourage promiscuity.

Some Hindu and Muslim parents may find the suggestion very offensive that their teenage schoolchildren might be considered sexually active and that they need to be protected against what could be considered a sexually transmitted disease.

Reflection points

★ If you were the parent of a teenage girl who was offered the human papilloma virus vaccine, what might your concerns be?

★ What cultural or religious issues do you think there might be in relation to this?

Obesity

Obesity is another public health priority for the government, and it has initiated a number of strategies to try to halt the year-on-year increase in the incidence of obesity. The National Child Measurement Programme (Department of Health 2006) involves all children in reception and year 6 having their height and weight recorded. The exercise will take place in schools every year. Primary care trusts coordinate the exercise with the support and cooperation of schools, and the exercise allows collection and monitoring of information about children's health to inform local planning and targeting of resources and to enable tracking of local progress against government targets on childhood obesity.

Figures 3.5 and 3.6 show the changes in the proportion of children of normal weight, those who are overweight and those who are obese in reception and year 6 over a 2 year period; these are the only statistics currently available.

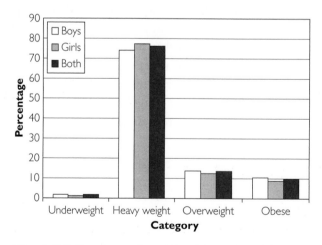

Figure 3.5 Prevalence of normal weight, underweight, overweight and obese children, 2007–8, reception year.

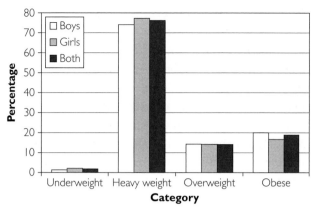

Figure 3.6 Prevalence of normal weight, underweight, overweight and obese children, 2007–8, year 6.

Case study

A health visitor in an ethnically varied area of London visited a family who had had their first baby 6 months previously. At the time, the advice was to begin weaning between the ages of 4 and 5 months. Both parents had been born in India and the father had lived in the UK from the age of 10 and spoke good English. His wife, however, had only recently come to the UK and spoke very little English. The health visitor took a range of leaflets giving information about weaning and initiated a discussion with both parents, with the father acting as interpreter. It was soon obvious that there were few common reference points about food and food preparation and the health visitor and the parents had to start from basics to build this common understanding.

Reflection points

★ Think about your own diet. Try to explain the nutritional value (or otherwise!) of the food that you eat to someone who has no experience of your culture or lifestyle.

★ What resources would you like to help you to do this?

★ When you are in practice, try to find information leaflets in different languages for different topics, e.g. immunization, feeding, health advice. Are they easily available? Which topics do they cover?

Mental health issues

Self-harm

The term self-harm is now used to replace terms such as 'attempted suicide' or 'parasuicide' because the range of motives or reasons for this behaviour includes several non-suicidal intentions (Mental Health Foundation 2006). Although young people who self-harm may claim that they want to die, the motivation in many is more to do with an expression of distress and desire for escape from troubling situations. Even when death is the outcome of self-harming behaviour, this may not have been intended (Mental Health Foundation 2006). Hawton and James (2005) found that young South Asian females in the UK seem to have a raised risk of self-harm. Intercultural stresses and consequent family conflicts may be relevant factors. Hicks *et al.* (2003), in a study on perceived causes of suicide attempts in 180 ethnic South Asian women living in the London area, found three factors which were endorsed most frequently and strongly as causes of suicide attempts: violence by the husband, being trapped in an unhappy family situation and depression.

The evidence for conflicts between teenage girls and their families is provided by the Asian Family Counselling Service's (2005) annual report, which highlights not only intergenerational conflict but also issues surrounding forced marriages.

Arranged and forced marriages

Children and young people's nurses and other practitioners must not confuse an arranged marriage and a forced marriage. Arranged marriages have been common practice in the UK, especially among the nobility. Casciani (2009) highlights findings from a report for the Department for Children, Schools and Families (2009), which details criticisms of some schools and education authorities.

Critics say some schools are 'non-responsive' and failing to intervene as they dismiss forced marriage as a 'cultural issue' or fear a backlash from powerful figures in minority communities: 'One respondent talked about how it was precisely those cases of children [going missing from education] that showed the signs of forced marriage that were less likely to be followed up in schools as this was seen as an issue specific to the culture of the child' (Department for Children, Schools and Families 2009, p. 43)

Casciani (2009) comments on the new guidance urging schools to identify signs of forced marriages ahead of the holidays. The guidance comes as an official report, *Forced Marriage: Prevalence and Service Response* (Department for Children, Schools and Families 2009), and raises questions about how some schools and councils have failed to act on suspicions or evidence of abuse. The report calls on schools to play a greater preventative role, saying some are clearly reluctant to get involved.

The government's Forced Marriage Unit (FMU) says it has received 770 calls for help this year, an increase of 16% compared with 2008. There is growing evidence that abusive families use the school summer holidays to coerce daughters and sons to marry abroad (Department for Children, Schools and Families 2009). Guidance published by the FMU (Forced Marriage Unit 2008) urges those who work in schools to be aware of signs of a possible forced marriage because school or college is often the only place where the potential victim can speak freely.

Forced marriages are not something that practitioners must be culturally sensitive about as such an act could be seen as a child abuse issue, and practitioners must treat it in that way and follow child protection procedures. The FMU, run jointly by the Home Office and Foreign Office, received 1600 reports last year and intervened in 420 actual cases, reports Casciani (2009); overall, there are estimated to be at least 5000 cases of forced marriage, but it is impossible to know for certain.

Principles for practice

- Be aware of links between social deprivation and rates of teenage pregnancy.
- The statistics for higher rates of teenage pregnancy among some ethnic groups do not account for the cultural trends of younger age of marriage in such ethnic groups.
- Human papilloma virus vaccination may be an emotive and/or inappropriate topic for discussion in some ethnic and cultural groups.
- Levels of obesity are increasing, but the data are not detailed enough to make links to socioeconomic status, ethnic origins or culture.

Implications for practitioners

Health and social care practitioners should respond to ethnic diversity by recognizing and acknowledging the continuing and contextual nature of culture and ethnicity. There is a need to critically reflect on personal values and beliefs, relating these to professional understanding within the wider ideological and policy contexts. More importantly, practitioners must develop cultural competence. According to Campinha-Bacote (1999) the process of cultural competence is divided into five interdependent constructs: cultural awareness, cultural knowledge, cultural skill, cultural encounters and cultural desire.

Cultural awareness

This domain is about appreciating and accepting differences, and the ability of health and social care providers to appreciate and understand their clients' values, beliefs, practices and problem-solving strategies. Self-awareness is also a vital part of this construct. This allows practitioners to analyse their own beliefs to avoid bias and prejudice when working with clients. On cultural awareness of the 'other', Duffy (2001) argues that there are more similarities than differences between cultures; therefore, it is important to celebrate the similarities and acknowledge the differences.

Cultural knowledge

Knowledge can help promote understanding between cultures, and practitioners must deliberately seek out various world views and explanatory models of disease. Although it is essential to gather cultural knowledge, it is an equally important, but sometimes neglected, culturally competent skill to be humble enough to let go of the security of stereotypes and ethnocentric views and remain open to the individuality of each client or patient. Central to the development of cultural knowledge lies the ability for health and social care providers to have an educated knowledge base about various cultures to better understand children and young people who may come from a culture different from their own.

Cultural skill

The need for practitioners to carry out an adequate effective assessment, whether this be for educational or for health and social care intervention, rests on the centrality of effective communication. Far too often practitioners complain of language barriers as obstacles to their ability to conduct an accurate and culturally competent history-taking and physical examination. Most children or young people from a minority ethnic group may be able to speak English and may be either bilingual or even trilingual. In the event that a child or young person does not speak English, unless you are thoroughly effective and fluent in the target language, always use a professional interpreter, preferably of the same sex. Plan what needs to be said ahead, and always address the client/patient directly when talking. Putsch (1995) suggests using simple language, avoiding technical jargon and using a list format for instructions to reinforce understanding.

Cultural encounters

Meeting and working with people of a different culture will help dispel myths and stereotypes and may contradict academic knowledge. However, sometimes, when cultural encounters are set up as part of an educational visit, this can, if not done sensitively, re-establish and reinforce negative stereotypes of people from different cultures.

Cultural desire

Achievement of all the above domains will be dependent on the desire of practitioners to possess a drive to achieve cultural competence and to provide antidiscriminatory practice.

Antidiscriminatory practice

Antidiscriminatory practice is an approach to working with people that promotes diversity and self-esteem, positive group identity, fulfilment of the individual and the full participation of all groups in society. Practitioners need to explore their own work setting to consider whether it values people for their individuality and ensures a sense of belonging that promotes self-esteem. Does the setting respect where people come from, what they achieve and what they bring to the learning situation?

There is so much discrimination and inequality that seemingly go unchallenged by our institutions, despite legislation to the contrary.

Reflection points

★ Should a disabled child who is not ready to be toilet trained be prevented from attending a local playgroup because there is a shortage of staff and no convenient changing area?

★ Should a traveller child never get to go to a nursery because he or she is always at the bottom of the waiting list because of first come, first served admission policies?

Conclusion

This chapter has provided an overview and explanation of the various terminologies about culture, 'race' and ethnicity, and discussed the problematic nature of using such labels and definitions uncritically. Contemporary issues such as obesity, bullying, sexual health, human papilloma virus vaccination, the contentious issue of wearing uniforms and arranged marriages have been considered.

Issues around practice have engaged the reader on aspects that affect the provision of culturally sensitive care, such as safeguarding children, as well as health issues, such as sickle cell disease, thalassaemia and diabetes, health inequalities, talking to children about death, grieving and developing cultural competence. Finally, the chapter addressed the implications for children and young people's nurses and other health and social care practitioners using a cultural competency framework.

Children and young people are entitled to culturally sensitive care and children and young people's nurses have a moral, ethical and professional duty to ensure this is respected in practice.

Summary of principles for practice

- Children and young people's nurses must ensure that children and young people from ethnic minorities receive the culturally sensitive care they are entitled to.
- Children and young people's nurses must take into account cultural diversity and develop cultural competence.
- Children and young people's nurses must meet their moral, ethical and professional obligations to provide care that is culturally sensitive for every child and young person.

References

Ahmad WIU (1993) *'Race' and health in contemporary Britain*. Milton Keynes: Open University Press.

Ahmad WIU (1996) Family obligations and social change among Asian communities. In: Ahmad WIU, Atkin K (eds) *'Race' and community care*. Milton Keynes: Open University Press.

Andrews MM, Boyle JS (1999) *Transcultural concepts in nursing care*, 3rd edn. Philadelphia: Lippincott, Williams & Wilkins.

Appiah KA (1996) Race, culture and identity: misunderstood connections. In: Appiah KA, Gutman A (eds) *Color conscious, the political morality of race*. Princeton, NJ: Princeton University Press.

Asian Family Counselling Service (2005) *Annual report*. See www.asianfamilycounselling.org.uk/AFCSAnnualReport05.pdf

Barn R, Sinclair R, Ferdinand D (1997) *Acting on principle: an examination of race and ethnicity in social service provision for children and families*. Batsford: British Agency for Adoption and Fostering.

Barnardo's (2007) *It doesn't happen here: the reality of child poverty in the UK*. London: Barnardo's.

BBC News (2003) *Honour killings*. See news.bbc.co.uk/1/hi/england/London/3149030.stm

Boushel M (2000) Childrearing across cultures. In: Boushel M, Fawcett M, Selwyn J (eds) *Focus on early childhood: principles and realities*, pp. 65–77. Oxford: Blackwell Science.

British Medical Association (2001) *The medical profession and human rights: handbook for a changing agenda*. London: Zed books in association with the BMA.

Byron T (2008) *Safer children in a digital world: the report of the Byron Review.* See http://www.dcsf.gov.uk/byronreview/

Campinha-Bacote J (1999) *The process of cultural competence in the delivery of healthcare services: a culturally competent model of care*, 3rd edn. Thousand Oaks, CA: Sage.

Casciani D (2009) Forced marriage plea to schools. *BBC News Online* 2 July 2009.

Chamba R, Ahmad W, Hirst M, *et al.* (1999) *On the edge: minority ethnic families caring for a disabled child.* Bristol: The Policy Press.

Cooper H, Smaje C, Arber S (1998) Use of health services by children and young people according to ethnicity and social class: secondary analysis of a national survey. *British Medical Journal* **317**: 1047–51

Cowie H, Jennifer D (2007) *Managing violence in schools: a whole school approach to best practice.* London: Sage.

David-Ferdon C, Hertz M (2007) Electronic media, violence, and adolescents: an emerging public health problem. *Journal of Adolescent Health* **41**(6): S1–5.

Department for Children, Schools and Families (2009) *Forced marriage: prevalence and service response.* Research report DCSF-RR128. National Centre for Social Research. See http://www.natcen.ac.uk/study/forced-marriage

Department of Health (2003) *Tackling health inequalities: a programme for action.* London: DH.

Department of Health (2004) *Race equality action plan.* See www.dh.gov.uk/en/Publicationsandstatistics/Publications/ PublicationsPolicyAndGuidance/DH_116731

Department of Health (2006) *National child measurement programme 2006/07.* See www.dh.gov.uk/en/Publichealth/Obesity/ DH_083093

Department of Health (2008a) *Healthy weight, healthy lives: a cross-government strategy for England.* London: Stationery Office.

Department of Health (2008b) *Health profile for England 2008.* London: DH.

Department of Health (2009) Abortion Statistics, England and Wales: 2008. See http://www.dh.gov.uk/en/ Publicationsandstatistics/Publications/PublicationsStatistics/DH_099285

Duffy E (2001) A critique of cultural education in nursing. *Journal of Advanced Nursing* **36**(4): 487–95.

Dutt R, Phillips M (2000) *Assessing black children in need and their families.* London: HMSO.

Eason G (2005) School uniforms needs a review. *BBC News Online* 2 March 2005.

Farmer E, Owen M (1998) *Child protection practice: private risks and public remedies.* London: HMSO.

Figueroa P (1991) *Education and the social construction of 'race'.* London: Routledge.

Forced Marriage Unit (2008) *The right to choose: multi-agency statutory guidance for dealing with forced marriage.* London: FMU.

Fox S (1985) *Boston Medical Center: good grief program.* See www.wayland.k12.ma.us/claypit_hill/GoodGriefHandout.pdf

Gaine C (1987) *No problem here: a practical approach to education and 'race' in white schools.* London: Hutchinson Radius.

Gallagher A (2006) The ethics of culturally competent health and social care. In: Papadopoulos I (ed.) *Transcultural health and social care.* Edinburgh: Churchill Livingstone.

Ghate D, Hazel N (2002) *Parenting in poor environments: stress, support and coping.* London: Jessica Kingsley.

Gordon LR (1995) Critical 'mixed race'? *Social Identities* **1**(2): 281–396.

Hanif W (2008) *Type 2 diabetes and obesity in the south Asian population.* NHS Evidence: Diabetes. See http://www.library.nhs. uk/ethnicity/viewResource.aspx?resid=296344&code=a650e11a04575c761e6a1bb48671f39d

Harran E (2002) Fragile: handle with care – protecting babies from harm. *Child Abuse Review* **11**(1): 65–79.

Hawton K, James A (2005) Suicide and deliberate self harm in young people. *British Medical Journal* **330:** 891–4.

Helman C (1994) *Culture, health and illness*, 3rd edn, p. 2. Oxford: Butterworth-Heinemann.

Herberg P (1995) Theoretical foundations of transcultural nursing. In: Andrews MM, Boyle JS (eds) *Transcultural concepts in nursing care*, 2nd edn. Philadelphia: J.B. Lippincott & Co.

Hicks M, Hsiao-Rei M, Bhugra D (2003) Perceived causes of suicide attempts by U.K. South Asian women. *American Journal of Orthopsychiatry* **73**(4): 455–62.

Huesmann LR (2007) The impact of electronic media violence: scientific theory and research. *Journal of Adolescent Health* **41**(6): S6–13.

Hunt J, Macleod A, Thomas C (1999) *The last resort: child protection, the Courts and the 1989 Children Act.* London: Department of Health.

Iyabo FA (1999) Of jewel heritage: racial socialization and racial identity attitudes amongst adolescents of mixed African-Caribbean/white parentage. *Journal of Adolescence* **22**: 303–18.

Jones E, McCurdy K (1992) The links between types of maltreatment and demographic characteristics of children. *Child Abuse and Neglect* **16**(2): 201–15.

Khunti K, Stone MA, Bankart J, *et al.* (2007) Physical activity and sedentary behaviours of South Asian and white European children in inner city secondary schools in the UK. *Family Practice* **24**(3): 237–44.

Kowalski RM, Limber SP (2007) Electronic bullying among middle school students. *Journal of Adolescent Health* **41**(6): S22–30.

Kroeber AL, Kluckhohn C, Untereiner W, Meyer AG (1952) *A critical review of concepts and definitions.* New York: Vintage Books.

Laming W (2003) *The Victoria Climbié Inquiry: summary report of an inquiry by Lord Laming.* London: HMSO.

Lindroos A, Luukkainen A-R (2004) *Antenatal care and maternal mortality in Nigeria.* See www.uku.fi/kansy/eng/antenal_care_nigeria.pdf

Macpherson W (1999) *The Stephen Lawrence Inquiry*, p. 28, para. 6.34. London: Home Office.

Marx S, Pennington J (2003) Pedagogies of critical race theory: experimentation with white pre-service teachers. *International Journal of Qualitative Studies in Education* **16**(1): 91–110.

McKenzie KJ, Crowcroft NS (1996) Ethnicity, race and culture: guidelines for research. *British Medical Journal* **312**: 1094–6.

Mental Health Foundation (2006) *The Truth Hurts.* Report of the National Inquiry into Self Harm Among Young People. London: MHF.

Modell B, Darlison M, Birgens H, *et al.* (2007) Epidemiology of haemoglobin disorders in Europe: an overview. *Scandinavian Journal of Clinical and Laboratory Investigation* **67**(1): 39–69.

Modood T (1994) Political Blackness and British Asians. *Sociology* **28**(4): 859–76.

Morrow R (1989) Southeast Asian parent involvement: can it be a reality? *Elementary School Guidance and Counseling* **23**, 289–97.

Morrow V (1999) 'We are people too': children's and young people's perspectives on children's rights and decision making in England. *The International Journal of Children's Rights* **7**: 149–70.

National Literacy Trust (2006) *Literacy and education levels by ethnic group and populations.* See http://www.literacytrust.org.uk/Database/STATS/EALstats.html#20languages

Office for National Statistics (2008) *Infant mortality statistics.* See www.statistics.gov.uk

Office for National Statistics (2009) *Population estimates for UK, England and Wales, Scotland and Northern Ireland: current datasets.* See http://www.statistics.gov.uk/statbase/Product.asp?vlnk=15106

Office of Population, Censuses and Surveys (2001) Census. Newport: ONS. See http://www.ons.gov.uk/search/index.html?newquery=census+2001

Office of Public Sector Information (1989) *The Children Act 1989.* London: OPSI. See http://www.opsi.gov.uk/acts/acts1989/ukpga_19890041_en_1

Office of Public Sector Information (1998) *Human Rights Act 1998.* London: OPSI. See http://www.opsi.gov.uk/acts/acts1998/ukpga_19980042_en_1

Ouseley H, Lane J (2008) Nipping prejudice in the bud. See www.guardian.co.uk, 7 August 2008.

Papadopoulos I (ed.) (2006) *Transcultural health and social care.* Edinburgh: Churchill Livingstone.

Pfeiffer N (1998) Theories of 'race', ethnicity and culture. *British Medical Journal* **317**: 1381–4.

Platt L (2002) *Parallel lives? Poverty among ethnic minority groups in Britain.* London: Child Poverty Action Group.

Putsch R (1995) Cross-cultural communication – the special case of interpreters in health care. *Journal of the American Medical Association* **254**(23), 3344–8.

Puzan E (2003) The unbearable whiteness of being (in nursing). *Nursing Inquiry* **10**(3): 193–200.

Saxena S, Ambler G, Cole TJ, Majeed A (2004) Ethnic group differences in overweight and obese children and young people in England: cross sectional survey. *Archives of Disease in Childhood* **89**: 30–6.

Social Services Inspectorate (2000) *Excellence not excuses: inspection of services for ethnic minority children and families.* See www.doh.gov.uk/scg/social.htm

Spence L (2008) *A profile of Londoners by country of birth estimates from the 2006 Annual Population Survey.* DMAG Briefing February 2008. London: Greater London Authority. See http://www.legacy.london.gov.uk/gla/publications/factsandfigures/dmag-briefing-2008-05.rtf

Standley R, Sullivan V, Wardle J (2009) Self-perceived weight in adolescents: over-estimation or under-estimation? *Body Image* **6**(1): 56–9.

Thomas VJ, Hambleton I, Serjeant G (2001) Psychological distress and coping in sickle cell disease: comparison of British and Jamaican attitudes. *Ethnic Health* **6**(2): 129–36.

Tizard B, Phoenix A (1993) *Black, white, or mixed race? Race and racism in the lives of young people of mixed parentage.* London: Routledge.

United Nations (1989) *Convention on the Rights of the Child.* Adopted under General Assembly Resolution 44/25. Geneva: UN.

Vernon P (1982) *The abilities and achievements of Orientals in North America.* Calgary: Academic Press.

Vydelingum V (1998) 'We treat them all the same'. Nurses' and South Asian patients' experiences of care. Unpublished PhD thesis, University of Southampton, Southampton.

Vydelingum V (2006) Nurses' experiences of caring for South Asian minority ethnic patients in a general hospital in England. *Nursing Inquiry* **13**(1): 23–32.

Webb E, Maddocks A, Bonglli J (2002) Effectively protecting black and minority ethnic children from harm: overcoming barriers to the child protection process. *Child Abuse Review* **11**: 394–411.

Welbourne P (2002) Adoption and the rights of children in the UK. *The International Journal of Children's Rights* **10**(3): 269–89.

Westwood S, Bachu P (1988) *Images and realities*, 6th edn. Gabriola Island, BC: New Society.

Williams KR, Guerra NG (2007) Prevalence and predictors of internet bullying. *Journal of Adolescent Health* **41**(6) (suppl.): S14–21.

Wilmot P, Young M (1957) *Family and kinship in East London.* London: Routledge & Kegan Paul.

Wolak J, Kimberley JD, Mitchell J, Finkelhor D (2007) Does online harassment constitute bullying? An exploration of online harassment by known peers and online-only contacts. *Journal of Adolescent Health* **41**(6): S51–8.

World Health Organization (2010) Female genital mutilation. Geneva: WHO. See http://www.who.int/mediacentre/factsheets/fs241/en/

Yamamoto J, Kubota M (1983) The Japanese-American family. In: Powell GJ (ed.) *The psychosocial development of minority group children.* New York: Brunner/Mazel, Inc.

Ybarra M, Mitchell K (2004) Online aggressor/targets, aggressors, and targets: a comparison of associated youth characteristics. *Journal of Child Psychology and Psychiatry* **45**(7): 1308–16.

Ybarra M, Diener-West M, Leaf P (2007) Examining the overlap in internet harassment and school bullying: implications for school intervention. *Journal of Adolescent Health* **41**(6): S42–50.

UNFPA (2000) *The state of the world population.* UNFPA. See http://www.unfpa.org/swp/2000/english/

Zimmet P, Alberti KG, Kaufman F, *et al.* (2007) The metabolic syndrome in children and adolescents: an IDF consensus report. *Pediatric Diabetes* **8**(5): 299–306.

PART 2
A rights-based approach to care

Chapter 4

The right for children and young people to participate in their own healthcare

Jill John and Richard Griffith

Overview

This chapter will examine the evidence for children and young people's right to participate in their own healthcare. It will begin with an historical overview of children's rights and legislation and will then examine the evidence by exploring:

- How far have we come?

- Where are we now?
- What more can we do?

The chapter will examine case law examples and evidence-based research and will give examples of frameworks and excellent practice from healthcare and associated allied professions.

Introduction

There is a growing acceptance in the UK and elsewhere that children and young people should participate more in making decisions about issues that affect them. Increased children and young people's participation has been fuelled by a convergence of new and developing ideas from quite different perspectives, such as the growing children's rights agenda and the new sociology of childhood.

The key benchmark for children's rights is the 1989 United Nations Convention on the Rights of the Child (UNCRC) that the UK ratified in 1991. It is the most extensively ratified human rights treaty in history and was the culmination of six decades of work. Somalia and North America are the only UN member countries to opt out of the charter.

The UNCRC provides a framework for the development of national policies and laws to protect the rights of children and young people throughout the world, and is considered by many as being instrumental in the development of more child-friendly policies in Britain (O'Halloran 1999). The main weakness of the Convention, however, is that there is no direct method of formal enforcement and governments are merely directed to undertake all appropriate methods available to them to implement the rights. Member states do have to report back to the UN initially 2 years after ratification and implementation and then every 5 years.

Until recently, it has been difficult to reconcile differences between historically held beliefs about children and young people's inability to make decisions and findings from research that contradict these assumptions (Alderson and Montgomery 1996). Children and young people's participation in healthcare decisions is heavily influenced by such assumptions, in particular an identified need for adult guidance and the need to reduce attempts to reason and/or listen to their views (Flatman 2002). The notion of working with children, young people and families in the involvement of their care (physical and otherwise), let alone the decision-making process, would have been seen as totally inappropriate as little as 30 years ago, when parents and other family members were seen as amateurs who frequently got in the way of professionals trying to do their job (Darbyshire 1994).

Historical overview of childhood and children's rights

Until the nineteenth century and the increase of industrialization it could be argued that the notion of childhood was largely an invention (Boyden 1991, cited in James *et al.* 1999). Rates of fertility and mortality were high owing to the spread of deadly and untreatable infectious disease, including typhoid and cholera. Families therefore had many children because a high percentage of children died under the age of 1 and many more did not live beyond 5 years. It is difficult for historians and others to calculate infant mortality rates as births were not registered until 1837; however, church records before this time showed that funerals always exceeded baptisms. Aries (1962) identified that medieval European children were not segregated from adults and, therefore, were not thought to require any special needs and frequently were dressed in adult clothing. The further back in history one goes, the more evidence there is of a lower level of child care, including an increased likelihood of children not only being killed but also abandoned, beaten, terrorized and sexually abused (deMause 1974, cited in Mayall 1994). Aries (1962, p. 48) continues by describing childhood as 'A nightmare from which we have only recently begun to awaken'.

The status of children and childhood as it evolved was marked by the absence of practically all civil rights, with no philosophical or legal recognition to self-determination; this rendered children virtually powerless, having little or no control over their own lives, which many consider a marked characteristic of slavery (Verhellen 1996).

Early Roman law allowed a father to literally have the power of life or death over a child. The overwhelming power a father had was gradually removed during the nineteenth century by Talfourd's Act, the Custody of Infants Act 1839 and the Matrimonial Causes Act 1857. Yet, children were still seen to be in the custody of their parents, who retained considerable power over them. For example, parents could demand that a child in care be handed back when he or she was old enough to earn a wage (*Barnardo v McHugh* [1891]).

However, the twentieth century brought changes in family life associated with both industrial and urban expansion; childhood was gradually seen as a separate period of human life and children became central figures within the family (Boyden 1991, cited in James *et al.* 1999). Hygiene and public health were a defining feature of 'modern childhood', alongside the development of compulsory schooling. Impressive improvements were made in both the UK and other developed countries in the areas of health and physical development of children owing to higher standards of living and advances in sanitation and nutrition. Because of this, children have been attributed with certain qualities and/or disabilities and interest in them has grown considerably. However, socioeconomic inequalities in health still exist in developed societies today, including the UK, and sadly these have changed little in recent years (Van de Mheen *et al.* 1998).

Key point

- It has taken centuries to recognize children as important beings in their own right.

Reflection point

★ Why do you think that it has taken centuries to recognize children as important beings in their own right? Take a few moments to think of two reasons why children held little importance within the family before the twentieth century.

How far have we come?

Some consider that current-day perception of childhood has changed little and is essentially a preparation for 'adulthood', with a particular onus on guiding, educating, developing and sustaining the physical and moral well-being of children and young people through social institutions that include the family, school, health and welfare agencies. All too frequently, however, these agencies speak for children and young people on the basis that they are incapable of thinking 'like adults' until a certain developmental age is reached (Mayall 1996).

This view of regarding children and young people as 'future adults' instead of 'current or present persons' leads to the knowledge and beliefs of children and young people being either disregarded as irrelevant or totally ignored as a means of understanding their actions, concerns and needs (James and Prout 1990; Mayall 1998). There is an unquestionably growing counterview to this among both academics and professionals, in that children and young people are social actors in themselves and not just subjects of social processes and structures (James and Prout 1990). The emerging sociology of childhood indicates the importance of children and young people actively constructing their own lives by, for example, participating in and negotiating their own healthcare, education and social welfare by utilizing skills that often go unrecognized (Mayall 1998). However, the approaches adopted to children's rights and adults' beliefs about this concept in the UK undoubtedly have their origins in the evolution of the child and childhood with an indication that this history continues to influence current attitudes towards children and young people in society and contemporary healthcare practice (Lowden 2002).

Overall, the 54 Articles in the Convention can be broadly divided into three types of rights:

- provision
- protection
- participation.

Provision

Article 24 of the UN Convention indicates that children and young people have the right to the:

> *Highest attainable standard of health and to the facilities for the treatment of illness and rehabilitation of health.*

The first named concern within the Article is:

> *to diminish infant and child mortality.*

Children and young people's right to good healthcare is enshrined in various policy and public documents, including, most importantly, the UNCRC and the 1989 Children Act. Alderson (2002) indicates that Article 24 of the Convention balances local with global attainment and indicates how inspirational some children's rights are. She argues that children and young people's right to be healthy is often unrealistic and unattainable, although the Convention clearly indicates the right to every type of healthcare available to them within their own culture.

Area of concern in the UK

Inequalities in health in the UK have been identified for over 30 years in both research and policy. They are linked to social exclusion and poverty, which can include unemployment, homelessness and family breakdown, which are significant factors to poor health and premature death. Infant mortality figures (deaths per 1000 infants under 1 year), which are an acknowledged robust indicator of public health, are also a major statistic for comparing child health from one nation with that of another. In most parts of the UK, the figures are falling and are roughly half of what they were in the 1950s; however, despite this, there are currently 5.2 deaths per 1000 infants in comparison with 2.8 in Sweden (US Census Bureau 2006). One reason for the difference is that the poor are getting poorer in the UK, keeping the overall figure higher than most EU countries (Department of Health 2007).

Protection

Article 19 clearly identifies the need for:

> *legislative, administrative, social and educational actions to protect children from all types of violence including neglect and abuse.*

Theories of child development and in particular Bowlby's work in the 1950s identified that a lack of attachment in early life to main carers could lead to poor parenting in the next generation. His work attracted and influenced the medical professions' interest in child abuse, with Kempe's (1962) writings on the 'battered baby' syndrome over 40 years ago opening a long and continuous debate on the subject. The decades since have seen a gradual increase in knowledge and expertise in child abuse as well, of course, in both the public's and government's increasing concern. Protection in law came eventually in the form of the 1989 Children Act after a period of considerable debate, activity and consultation with a range of groups except children and young people. It brought together for the first time both public and private law and sought to establish a new basis for intervention in family life in cases of child abuse, with one of the key principles underpinning the legislation being that the 'child's welfare should be paramount'. It opens with a 'Welfare Check List' (Section 1.1) and in Part 3 defines the 'child in need'.

Area of concern in the UK

The UK is repeatedly criticized by the UN Inspection Committee for not legislating against the hitting of children and young people by their parents/guardians, and is the only country that was a member of the EU prior to 1997 not to do so. The judgment in *A v United Kingdom* [1998] contained a promise from the UK government to change its legislation as the defence of reasonable chastisement was unclear and allowed the severe beating of a child in UK law. However, the government has consistently refused to completely prohibit parental use of physical punishment as the government sees it as an unwarranted intrusion in family life.

Participation

The principle of the child's right to participate in decision-making is indicated in Article 12 of the Convention in that the child who is capable of forming his or her own views has the right to:

> *Express those views freely in all matters affecting the child, the views of the child being given due weight in accordance with the age and maturity of the child.*

This has been identified by the Committee on the Rights of the Child as a central underlying principle which must be considered with regard to all other rights (Lansdown 2001). The Article is one of the most far-reaching rights of the UNCRC, but it is also the provision most widely violated and disregarded in almost every sphere of children and young people's lives.

Principle for practice

- Participation is the keystone of the arch which is the UNCRC. Without the active participation of children and young people in the promotion of their rights to a good childhood, none will be achieved effectively (Badham 2002, cited in Willow 2002).

Acceptance of this principle is beginning to be seen through an increase in participation in activities involving children and young people; however, participation is currently still viewed very much as the younger sibling to both provision and protection.

Why is participation important?

This has been expressed in several ways, often grouped into legal, political or social reasons (Children and Young People's Unit 2001; Willow 2002; see Box 4.1).

For many, a child's or young person's participation is a value or rights-based principle much like democracy and is not something that has to be justified by either

Box 4.1	Rationale for children's participation in decision-making

- To uphold children and young people's rights
- To fulfil legal responsibilities (UNCRC; Children Act 1989)
- To improve services
- To improve decision-making
- To enhance democratic processes

- To promote children and young people's protection
- To enhance children and young people's skills
- To empower and enhance self-esteem

(Sinclair and Franklin 2000)

evidence or proof that it works (Sinclair 2004). This should not diminish, however, the need to monitor or evaluate to ensure the widest representation of children and young people in a variety of settings and circumstances.

Legal rights

The United Nations (1989) Convention on the Rights of the Child is a universally agreed set of standards that set minimum entitlements and freedoms that should be respected by governments. It is founded on respect for the dignity and worth of each child, regardless of race, colour, gender, language, religion, opinions, origins, wealth, birth status or ability.

Although the UK ratified the Convention some 20 years ago, its 54 Articles do not have direct effect in domestic law and children and young people cannot take action in court against them. The Convention's Articles act only as a yardstick against which the government's treatment of children and young people is audited on a 5 yearly basis by the UN.

Unless incorporated into UK domestic law the rights set out in the Convention do not have the weight of law, they are not legal rights and children and young people cannot rely on them to insist that they be allowed to participate in their healthcare.

A legal right is defined as an interest recognized and protected by law (Kennedy and Grubb 2002). All other rights, argues Bentham, are 'merely nonsense upon stilts' as once these worthy values are held up to scrutiny by the law they are quickly found to have no legal remedy attached to them (Tait 1883).

In the UK, legal rights are bestowed on people by placing obligations, called legal duties, on others. Under the Human Rights Act 1998 the state has a legal duty to ensure that it has laws and policies in place to ensure that one person does not violate the human rights of another.

Legal right to participate in healthcare

Consent

Consent to examination and treatment is an area of law that relies on a child/young person's ability to decide rather than an arbitrary age limit. It is an essential element of the lawfulness of treatment and upholds the ethical principle of autonomy or self-determination by allowing a person to decide whether to have an examination or treatment. For the nurse it provides a defence to criminal assault and the tort or civil wrong of trespass to the person (*F v West Berkshire HA* [1990]).

The nature of consent

Consent is a state of mind in which a person agrees to the touching of his or her body as part of an examination or treatment (*Sidaway v Bethlem Royal Hospital* [1985]). It has both a clinical and legal purpose:

- the clinical purpose recognizes that the success of treatment depends very often on the cooperation of the child/young person
- the legal purpose is to underpin the propriety of the treatment and furnish a defence to the crime and tort of trespass.

For capable adults the law recognizes the right to self-determination that includes the right to consent to or refuse medical treatment even if this would lead to their death.

Children reach the age of majority or adulthood at 18. Although the courts acknowledge that no child under 18 is wholly autonomous they do recognize the right of children/young people to decide whether they wish to participate in their healthcare by allowing them to consent to examination and treatment as they develop and mature with age.

Consent and children

Kennedy and Grubb (2000) argue that children pass through three developmental stages on their journey to becoming a fully autonomous adult:

1 the child of tender years
2 the Gillick-competent child
3 children aged 16–17 years.

Consent to treatment for a child of tender years is provided by a person with parental responsibility for the child, usually a parent. However, the decision of the parent must be in the best interests of the welfare of the child and can be overridden by a court exercising its inherent jurisdiction to act in the child's best interests.

Children of tender years and parental responsibility

The concept of parental responsibility replaced the notion of parental rights.

Parental responsibility is defined as all the rights, duties, powers, responsibility and authority which by law a parent of a child has in relation to the child and its property (Children Act 1989, Section 2). These are not defined or specified in the Act. In essence it empowers a person to make most decisions in a child's life including consenting to medical treatment on the child's behalf. A child of tender years must rely on a person with parental responsibility to make decisions about his or her healthcare (Box 4.2).

Box 4.2   Who has parental responsibility for a child?

Parental responsibility

- Parental responsibility is defined as the rights, duties, powers, and responsibility and authority, which by law a parent has in relation to a child (Children Act 1989, Section 3; Office of Public Sector Information 1989)
- Mother
  - Mother has automatic parental responsibility on the birth of the child (Children Act 1989, Sections 2(1) and (2); Office of Public Sector Information 1989)
- Father
  - Father has parental responsibility if he was married to the child's mother at the time of the birth (Children Act 1989, Section 2(1)) **OR**
  - If he subsequently married the mother of his child (Children Act 1989, Section 2(3) and Family Law Reform Act 1987, Section 1 (Office of Public Sector Information 1987)) **OR**
  - If he became registered as the father of the child after December 2003 (Children Act 1989, Section 4(1)(a)) **OR**
  - He and the child's mother make a parental responsibility agreement (Children Act 1989, Section 4 (1) (b)) that is made and recorded in the form prescribed by the Lord Chancellor **OR**
  - The Court on his application orders that he shall have parental responsibility (Children Act 1989, Section 4(1)(c) **OR**
  - He obtains a residence order (Children Act 1989, Section 12, read with Section 4) **OR**

- He is appointed as the child's guardian and the appointment takes effect (Children Act 1989, Section 5)
- Acquired Parental Responsibility can be removed only by a Court

Others who can acquire parental responsibility

- A person in possession of a residence order which could include the father of the child (Children Act 1989, Section 12)
- A person appointed as the child's guardian; once the appointment takes effect this could include the father of the child (Children Act 1989, Section 5)
- A person, other than a police officer, who is in possession of an emergency protection order (Children Act 1989, Section 44(4)(c))
- A person who has adopted a child (Adoption Act 1976, Section 12 or Adoption and Children Act 2002, Section 46) (Office of Public Sector Information 1976, 2002)
- A step-parent with the agreement of the parent(s) with parental responsibility or by order of the court (Children Act 1989, Section 4A)

A local authority may additionally acquire parental responsibility

- By obtaining a care order (Children Act 1989, Section 31)
- By obtaining a freeing for adoption order (Adoption Act 1976, Section 18) or a placement order (Adoption and Children Act 2002, Section 21; Office of Public Sector Information 2002)

Delegation of parental responsibility

The Children Act 1989, Section 2(9) (Office of Public Sector Information 1989) allows a person with parental responsibility to arrange for someone else to exercise it on their behalf. This delegation need not be in writing and allows carers such as schools, nannies and childminders to make delegated decisions on behalf of a person with parental responsibility for the child or young person.

For example, a nurse may visit a young child to find her in the care of her grandmother. As long as the nurse is satisfied that the grandmother is acting with the authority of a person with parental responsibility such as the child's mother then she may accept the grandmother's consent as permission to treat the child.

Carers

The Children Act 1989 (Office of Public Sector Information 1989) allows those who have care for a child/young person but not parental responsibility to do what is reasonable in all the circumstances to promote or safeguard the child's welfare (Children Act 1989, Section 3(5); Office of Public Sector Information 1989). In terms of medical treatment, what is reasonable would generally require the consent of a person with parental responsibility unless it was an emergency or the treatment was trivial. In a medical emergency situation, abandonment of the child or child protection cases, medical staff can proceed without the consent of the child or parent if it is deemed in the child's 'best interests', although others named as *de facto* carers, e.g. teachers, can assume all duties, powers and responsibilities of a parent if required under these circumstances.

The extent of parental responsibility

Although the Children Act 1989 (Office of Public Sector Information 1989) does not describe the duties placed on parents, the courts have outlined what parental responsibility means in practice. Parents have a duty to care for their children. It is an offence under the Children and Young Persons Act 1933, Section 1 (Office of Public Sector Information 1933) to assault, ill-treat, neglect or abandon a child under the age of 16. It is one of the rare situations in law where the offence may be committed by omission as well as by action. That is, what a parent fails to do for his or her child is as relevant as what he or she does to the child if it results in neglect or ill treatment. This duty is not restricted to parents. Those who have responsibility for the care of a child are also bound by the same duty. It can be seen that parents are bound by a duty of care to their child and can be prosecuted if they fail to exercise that duty properly.

Although a person with parental responsibility can generally make decisions independently, the freedom of each to act alone is not unfettered.

Case law example

The Court held in *Re J* [2000] that there are a small group of important decisions made on behalf of a child that should not be carried out or arranged by one parent alone, although they have parental responsibility under the Children Act 1989. These include (*Re B (A Child)* [2003]):

- sterilization of a child
- the change of a child's surname
- circumcision of a child
- a hotly disputed immunization.

Best interests of the child

The parent's right to make healthcare decisions about his or her child is not absolute. Parents' rights exist only for the benefit of the child and must be exercised in the child's best interests. The courts exercise a supervisory role over parental decision-making and can overrule a decision that they consider as not being in the best interests of the welfare of the child (Children Act 1989, Section 1).

Under the private law provisions of the Children Act 1989, Section 8, the courts also have the power to settle disputes between two or more people with parental responsibility.

Private law is not a question of child protection and so the threshold criterion of significant harm does not have to be engaged for the court to have jurisdiction.

As long as there is a dispute between people regarding an issue of parental responsibility for a child the court can intervene to settle the issue.

The orders available to the court are:

- a Residence Order, which settles with whom a child should live and bestows parental responsibility on that person when necessary
- a Contact Order, which settles contact arrangements with a child; contact can be as widely interpreted as the court sees fit and ranges from telephone and email contact to visits and holidays
- a Prohibited Steps Order, which prohibits an action without the permission of the court
- a Specific Issues Order, which allows the court to settle a specific issue in relation to the parental responsibility of a child.

Prohibited Steps and Specific Issues Orders are also used by the courts to settle issues concerning a child's healthcare.

Principle for practice

- Children and young people are not the property of their parents/carers. Parents/carers have a responsibility for them that continues until such time as the children/young people reach 18 years or are adopted.

Case law example

In *J (A Minor) (Prohibited Steps Order: Circumcision)* [2000] the English mother of a 5 year old boy was granted a Prohibited Steps Order preventing his Muslim father from making arrangements to have him circumcised without a court order because ritual circumcision was an irreversible operation which was not medically necessary, had physical and psychological risks and in such cases the consent of both parents was essential.

Authorizing treatment against the wishes of a child's parents is reserved for the most serious cases. In *A&D v B&E* [2003] the High Court accepted that, in general, there is wide scope for parental objection to medical intervention. The court considers medical interventions as existing on a scale. At one end are obvious cases where parental objection would have no value in child welfare terms, e.g. urgent life-saving treatment such as a blood transfusion.

Case law example

In *Camden LBC v R (A Minor) (Blood Transfusion)* [1993] a child's parents refused to allow him to have a blood transfusion for the treatment of B-cell lymphoblastic leukaemia owing to their religious beliefs. The court found that, where the life of a child was at risk and it was essential to act urgently, the private law requirements of the Children Act 1989 Section 8 could be used to seek a Specific Issue Order. This procedure allows the matter to be brought before a High Court judge who could order the treatment without delay and without transferring parental responsibility.

At the other end of the scale are cases where there is genuine scope for debate and the views of the parents are important. These would not raise questions of neglect or abuse that would trigger child protection proceedings. Although a National Health Service (NHS) trust can obtain leave to apply for a Specific Issues Order (Children Act 1989, Section 8) it is unlikely that leave would be granted in the face of unified parental opposition to this type of treatment.

In *Re B (A Child)* [2003] the Court of Appeal held that, although it was prepared to settle a dispute between two parents on the issue of childhood immunizations, it would not do so when the dispute was between a parent and the health authorities.

The best interests test

The test for determining the best interests of a child has developed over a period of time as new cases have been brought to court for judgment. In one of the earliest cases the court limited its consideration of a best interest to the life expectancy of the child.

Case law example

In *Re B (A Minor) (Wardship: Medical Treatment)* [1981] a child born with Down's syndrome needed urgent surgery for an intestinal blockage. The parents took the view that it would be kinder to let the child die than to allow her to grow up as a physically and mentally handicapped person. The judge held that the surgery was straightforward and that, as the child was expected to live 20–30 years, surgery was in her best interests.

Some 10 years later the court refined the determination of a best interest to include pain and suffering. In *J (A Minor) (Child in Care: Medical Treatment)* [1993] a profoundly brain-damaged child with a very short life expectancy was not thought to be benefiting from treatment and both the parents and medical team sought an order allowing them to curtail treatment.

In the child's interest the Official Solicitor argued that an absolutist test applied that, in the case of a child, everything should be done to preserve the child's life right to the bitter end and a court was never justified in denying consent to treatment to save life.

The court held that the absolutist test never applied. The denial of treatment to prolong life could only be sanctioned when it was in the best interests of the patient and the test applicable was that of the child's best interests in those circumstances and that was based on an assessment of the child's quality of life and his or her future pain and suffering in relation to the life-saving treatment.

When those with parental responsibility strongly oppose the giving or withholding of treatment by a health professional to a child then the matter will need to be referred to the court for a decision unless it is an emergency (*Glass v United Kingdom* [2004]). Failing to seek the court's approval for a plan of care in these circumstances would be a breach of the child's right to respect for a private and family life under Article 8 of the European Convention on Human Rights (Council of Europe 1950).

Autonomy and children and young people

The Gillick-competent child

The argument that a child/young person should have the right to make decisions about his or her healthcare becomes more compelling as the child matures towards adulthood. The matter of whether a child under 16 has the decision-making capacity to consent to examination and treatment was decided by the House of Lords in *Gillick v West Norfolk and Wisbech AHA* [1986]. In this case a mother objected to Department of Health advice that doctors could give contraceptive advice and treatment to children under 16 without parental consent. The court held that a child under 16 had the legal capacity to consent to examination and treatment if they had 'sufficient maturity and intelligence to understand the nature and implications of that treatment'.

Test for Gillick competence

Nurses must apply the rule in *Gillick* when determining whether a child/young person under 16 has capacity to consent to examination and treatment.

When determining whether a child has sufficient maturity and intelligence to make a decision nurses will need to take account of:

> *the understanding and intelligence of the child/young person, their chronological, emotional and mental age, their intellectual development and their ability to reach a decision by appraising the advice about treatment in considering the nature, consequences and implications of that treatment.*

> (Gillick v West Norfolk and Wisbech AHA [1986] *per Lord Scarman*)

The aim of the rule in *Gillick* is to reflect the transition of a child to adulthood. Legal capacity to make decisions is conditional on the child gradually acquiring the maturity and intelligence to be able to make treatment decisions. The degree of maturity and intelligence needed depends on the gravity of the decision. A relatively young child would have sufficient maturity and intelligence to be capable of consenting to a plaster on a small cut.

Equally, a child who had the capacity to consent to dental treatment or the repair of broken bones may lack capacity to consent to more serious treatment (*Re R (A Minor) (Wardship Consent to Treatment)* [1992]).

Case law example

In *Re L (Medical Treatment: Gillick Competence)* [1998] a critically injured 14 year old Jehovah's Witness had refused to consent to life-saving medical treatment because it would involve blood transfusions. The court found that, despite her maturity, L was still a child and her beliefs had been developed through her sheltered upbringing within the Jehovah's Witness community. She knew that she would die without treatment but had not been informed of the likely nature of her death. She was not Gillick competent and it was in her best interests for the treatment to be carried out.

Indeed, to date, the courts have never found a child under 16 who wished to refuse life-saving treatment to be Gillick competent. Decision-making capacity therefore does not simply arrive with puberty; it depends on the maturity and intelligence of the child and the seriousness of the treatment decision to be made.

For example, a nurse giving contraceptive advice and treatment to a child will realize that there is much to be understood by the child if he or she is to have capacity to consent. The nurse would need to be satisfied that not only was the advice understood but that the child had sufficient maturity to understand what was involved.

This would include:

- moral and family questions such as the future relationship with parents
- longer term problems associated with the emotion of pregnancy or its termination
- the health risks associated with sexual intercourse at a young age.

> **Key point** 🔑
>
> Assessing Gillick competence of children and young people is complex and not just chronologically age related.

A nurse must be satisfied that a child/young person has fully understood the nature and consequences of treatment before he or she can accept their consent or refusal of treatment. It is for the nurse to decide whether or not a child is Gillick competent and able to consent to treatment. However, the power to decide must not be used as a licence to disregard the wishes of parents whenever the nurse finds it convenient to do so. Those who behave in such a way would be failing to discharge their professional responsibilities and could expect to be disciplined by their professional body (*Gillick v West Norfolk and Wisbech AHA* [1986]).

When a child or young person is considered Gillick competent then the consent is as effective as that of an adult. This consent cannot be overruled by a parent.

Fraser guidelines

Giving contraceptive advice and treatment to a child under 16 years gives rise to a concern that a practitioner may be accused of procuring sexual intercourse with a child under 16 years, a criminal offence under the Sexual Offences Act (Office of Public Sector Information 2003). To protect nurses from such accusations Lord

Fraser in *Gillick* issued guidance to ensure that contraceptive advice and treatment was given only on clinical grounds. There might be exceptional cases when in the interests of the child's welfare a nurse might give contraceptive advice and treatment without the permission or even knowledge of the parents. You must be satisfied:

1   that the girl understood the advice
2   that you could not persuade her to tell or allow you to tell her parents
3   that she was likely to have sexual intercourse with or without contraceptive treatment
4   that unless she received such advice or treatment her physical or mental health was likely to suffer and
5   her best interests required such advice or treatment without the knowledge or consent of her parents.

It is essential that this guidance is followed in practice to avoid any possibility of criminal conduct.

The defence offered by Lord Fraser's guidance has been extended by the Sexual Offences Act 2003, Section 13 (Office for Public Sector Information 2003). This provides a defence against aiding, abetting or counselling a sexual offence if the purpose is to:

- protect the child/young person from sexually transmitted infection
- protect the physical safety of the child/young person
- protect the child from becoming pregnant
- promote the child/young person's emotional well-being by the giving of advice unless the purpose is to obtain sexual gratification or to cause or encourage the relevant sexual act.

In *R (Axon) v Secretary Of State For Health* [2006] the court held that there was no reason why the rule in *Gillick* should not apply to other proposed treatment and advice.

The approach of a health professional to a young person seeking advice and treatment on sexual issues without notifying his or her parents should be in accordance with Lord Fraser's guidelines. There was no infringement of the rights of a young person's parents if a health professional was permitted to withhold information relating to the advice or treatment of the young person on sexual matters.

Legal issues in relation to protection and sexual activity

It has long been public policy to protect children/young people from being subjected to sexual activity while they are in what is considered to be a vulnerable stage of their development.

The age of consent for all sexual activity was amended by the Sexual Offences Act 2003. Both boys and girls over 16 can now engage in heterosexual and homosexual activity with persons over 16. It is an offence to engage in sexual activity with a person under this age regardless of the age of the offender. Such activity can range from kissing to sexual intercourse.

However, a person over 18 in a position of trust commits an offence if they engage in sexual activity with a person below that age. The Sexual Offences Act 2003 defines a position of trust as including people who normally have power or authority in a child/young person's life. These include:

- education staff
- staff in young offender institutions
- staff in accommodation provided by local authorities and voluntary organizations
- staff in hospitals, independent clinics, care homes, residential care homes and private hospitals.

It also includes people providing individual services such as court welfare officers and care or supervision order supervisors.

Children 16 and 17 years old

The assessment of the capacity of a 16 or 17 year old child to consent to treatment would be in accordance with the provisions of the Mental Capacity Act 2005 and its code of practice. Children and young people who have attained the age of 16 years have a right to consent to examination and treatment under the Family Law Reform Act 1969, Section 8 (Office of Public Sector Information 1969). It provides that:

(1) The consent of a minor who has attained the age of sixteen years to any surgical, medical or dental treatment which, in the absence of consent, would constitute a trespass to his person, shall be as effective as it would be if he were of full age; and where a minor has by virtue of this section given an effective consent to any treatment it shall not be necessary to obtain any consent for it from his parent or guardian.

(2) In this section 'surgical, medical or dental treatment' includes any procedure undertaken for the purposes of diagnosis, and this section applies to any procedure (including, in particular, the administration of an anaesthetic) which is ancillary to any treatment as it applies to that treatment.

This allows a child of 16 or 17 years to consent to examination and treatment as if they were of full age, that is, an adult. When such consent is given it is as effective as that of an adult. It cannot be overruled by the child's parent or guardian.

The courts have adopted a very narrow construction of the provisions of Section 8 of the 1969 Act. A child to whom the provisions apply can consent only to treatment or examinations which are therapeutic or diagnostic (*Re W (A Minor) (Medical Treatment Court's Jurisdiction)* [1992]). It does not allow consent for the donation of organs or blood. Even the giving of blood samples is excluded (separate provision is made for these under Section 21(2) of the Family Law Reform Act 1969).

Contraceptive advice and treatment is considered a legitimate and beneficial treatment under Section 5 of the National Health Service Act 1977 (Office of Public Sector Information 1977) and Section 41 of the National Health Service (Scotland) Act 1978 (Office of Public Sector Information 1978). Children who have attained 16 years can consent to contraceptive advice and treatment including termination of pregnancy.

Key point

Refusal of medical treatment for all children and young people under 18 will be overturned in the courts.

So where are we now?

The process so far has been painfully slow, although several authors identify that there have been some isolated efforts to enable children and young people to participate in decision-making over many years (Neill 1962; Holt 1975; Hoyles 1989). It has in fact been the UK's ratification of the UN Convention that has provided a powerful stimulus to discussion of the issue, creating not only an unprecedented high profile but also a growing body of literature devoted to the topic (Shier 2001).

Children and young people are one of the most governed groups by both the state and society and are also some of the highest users of state services including health, education and social services; thus, they are a primary focus for state intervention. This leads to them being frequently viewed as the entry route into social change with no exception when New Labour came into power in the UK and introduced major policy initiatives to tackle 'social exclusion'. Under this banner considerable government funds and commitments have been expended on children and young people in recent years. They may have been central to policy agendas but their views have not always been! Most initiatives were and are designed, delivered and evaluated by adults. Although intended to be protective towards children and young people, they frequently leave the adult–child power relations untouched. Yet participation is arguably central to policy agendas, in particular social exclusion, and with children and young people traditionally having limited input to local and national policies the need for greater social participation in ways that meet their wishes and felt need is crucial to their enhanced participation in decision-making (Hill *et al.* 2004).

Participation in practice has undoubtedly been given great impetus in recent years; in particular, with the commitment to children and young people's participation by the constituent governments of the British Isles (Sinclair 2004). However, the government's contribution has to be seen in light of the UN Committee reviewing the UK government's implementation of the UNCRC; although the Committee has recognized the increased encouragement by the government for consultation and participation by children and young people, the indication is that there is still more to do especially in ensuring that participation leads to change.

Youth parliaments: an example of good practice

This is one example of the implementation of children's rights at government level, consisting of democratically elected members between 11 and 18 years old. Formed in 2000 it now consists of 600 members who are elected to represent the views of young people in their area to government and service providers. Endorsed by the three main political parties, over half a million young people vote in the elections each year, which are held in 90% of constituencies. Members meet regularly to hold debates and plan campaigns at venues that include the House of Lords, House of Commons and the British Museum and have recently included topics such as:

- youth crime
- free transport for young people
- lowering the voting age to 16.

Evidence of participation policy in the UK

- Department of Health (2001) – *Seeking consent: working with children*
- Children and Young People's Unit (2001) – *Learning to listen: core principles for the involvement of children and young people*
- Children and Young People's Unit (2003) – *Action plan for children and young people's participation*
- Department of Education and Skills (2002) – *Listening to learn: an action plan for the involvement of children and young people*
- Department of Health (2002) – *Listening, hearing and responding: Department of Health action plan – core principles for the involvement of children and young people*
- Department of Health (2004) – *The national service framework for children, young people and maternity services*
- Welsh Assembly Government (2005a) – *The national service framework for children, young people and maternity services*

From policy to practice

Until recent years there had been no systematic monitoring of health processes for 'looked after children' and evidence from localized studies indicated the neglect of routine immunizations and screening, lack of appropriate care for acute and chronic health conditions and failure to diagnose other health (particularly mental) problems (Hall and Elliman 2003). The comparative controlled study carried out by Williams *et al.* (2001) aimed to assess the health needs and provision of healthcare to school-age children in local authority care. Health needs in the context of this study included mental, emotional and physical health, health education and health promotion. A total of 142 children aged 5–16 in local authority care and 119 control children matched by sex and age were studied. The results showed clearly that 'looked after children' were more likely to:

- experience frequent changes in their general practitioner
- have incomplete immunization status
- have inadequate dental care
- suffer from anxieties and difficulties in relationships with others
- wet the bed
- smoke
- use illegal drugs
- receive less health education.

However, the overall conclusion of the findings of this study were not dissimilar to those of the aforementioned uncontrolled observational studies in that, although there was no clear evidence that the physical health of these children and young people suffered significantly, the overall healthcare of children and young people who had been established in care for more than 6 months was significantly worse than for children and young people living in their own homes, particularly in regard to emotional and behavioural health and health promotion.

Examples of policy: social exclusion

The Department of Health (2002) identified eight key priorities for tackling social exclusion and poverty as being the need to improve the life chances of 'looked after children' through expenditure and education. Both England (Quality Protects) and Wales (Children First) had provided considerable monies since 1999 to improve the health, education and welfare of 'looked after children' and they were identified within the National Service Frameworks (Department of Health 2004; Welsh Assembly Government 2005a) as 'children and young people with special circumstances'.

Legislative changes

Children Act 2004

The legislation that emerged from the Children's Bill was the end result of the government green paper 'Every Child Matters' (HM Government 2004) published alongside the Victoria Climbié Inquiry (Laming Report) (Department of Health and the Home Office 2003), which summed up the findings of the very public enquiry into the tragic death of Victoria Climbié at the hands of her paternal aunt and her aunt's lover. It proposed changes in legislation to minimize risk for all children and young people and a legislative spine for improving children's lives. It identified five outcomes of 'well-being':

1 be healthy
2 be safe
3 enjoy and achieve
4 make a positive contribution
5 achieve economic well-being.

The main aims included:

- integrated services – the need to encourage integrated planning, commissioning and delivery of services
- safeguarding – the need for a radical overhaul of child protection procedures to protect vulnerable children
- information sharing – the promotion of interagency cooperation by the facilitation of legislation that will support information sharing
- workforce reform – the need for suitable trained staff and the need for multidisciplinary teams with lead professionals.

Changes in policy in Wales

The Welsh Assembly Government has established participation as a core value of devolved government in Wales in that 'children and young people are to be treated as valued members of the community whose voices are heard and needs considered across the range of policy making'. It established seven core aims for all its activities for children and young people in its *Framework for Partnership* (Welsh Assembly Government 2000).

Seven core aims

- Flying start in life
- Comprehensive range of education and learning opportunities
- Enjoy the best possible health and free from abuse, victimization and exploitation

- Have access to play, leisure, sporting and cultural activities
- Listened to and treated with respect
- Have a safe home and a community that supports emotional and physical well-being
- Are not disadvantaged by poverty

Example of good practice: Funky Dragon interactive website

To facilitate participation, the Welsh Assembly Government helped to set up, and funds, the Children and Young People's Assembly for Wales (known as the Funky Dragon). The Funky Dragon is a peer-led organization made up of a Grand Council of representatives from local children and young people's fora and national and local peer-led groups. It ensures that the views of children and young people aged 0–25 are heard and taken into account in the decision-making process, particularly by the Welsh Assembly Government.

Evidence of participation policy in Wales

- Welsh Assembly Government (2000) – *Framework for partnership with children and young people*; seven core aims identified
- House of Commons (2001) – Children's Commissioner for Wales Bill; first in UK
- Welsh Assembly Government (2002) – participation of children via an interactive website (www.funkydragon.org)

- Welsh Assembly Government (2004) – *Children and young people: rights to action*
- Welsh Assembly Government (2008a) – *Rights in action*
- Welsh Assembly Government (2009) – *Getting it right*

Children's commissioners

Norway was the first country to appoint a children's commissioner, called an 'ombudsman', in 1981 to safeguard children and young people's rights. Following the agreement of the UN on the UNCRC, other countries began to follow suit; first Sweden, then others in Europe and the rest of the world.

Frequently described as 'watchdogs' and 'champions' for children and young people they are high-profile independent bodies established to monitor, promote and safeguard children and young people's human rights (Children's Rights Alliance for England 2004). Within the UK, the campaign began in the early 1990s and, gradually, over 130 organizations in the UK supported the campaign for children's commissioners urged on by the fact that when, in 1995, the UK Government presented its initial report to the UN Committee it was highly criticized for failing to support children and young people's human rights through an independent mechanism.

Devolved countries encouraged progress and, in 2001, Peter Clarke took up the post of Children's Commissioner, the first appointment of such a post in the UK. This came sooner in Wales than in the rest of the UK because of the results of the inquiry by Waterhouse *et al.* (1999) into child abuse in children's homes in North Wales. The Care Standards Act 2000 (Office of Public Sector Information 2000) created a children's commissioner post for Wales following a key recommendation of Waterhouse *et al.* The report indicated findings that when the children and young people in care had complained about being abused and ill-treated they had not been listened to. Initially, the post was there to mainly protect children and young people in care, but this was amended by the Children's Commissioner for Wales Bill in late 2000 to give the post holder more powers to protect the rights of all children and young people. Appointments of other children's commissioners in the UK followed soon afterwards, with Northern Ireland in 2003, Scotland in 2004 (also the Irish Republic) and eventually England in 2005, although this post is still not as independent as the others but has responsibilities over policies that affect children and young people in England and Wales such as youth crime and asylum.

These posts not only significantly raise the profile of children and young people but also have a critical role in raising children's awareness about their rights. The success of these posts to some degree relies upon their independence from government.

Example of participation: evaluation of the commissioner's role

This took place over a 3 year period and was published in December 2008. It involved children and young people from the start. They were on the initial panel to appoint a researcher prior to forming a steering group to look at planning and designing the research methods; in year 2, they were involved with data collection; and in year 3 in the analysis and writing up. The adults were facilitators and the report is full of individual pages of their experience through the research journey (Swansea University/ University of Central Lancashire/Save the Children 2008).

One of the 13 recommendations was to:

ensure that all organisations providing services for children and young people consider that staff are well informed about the role of the commissioner.

(Towler in Swansea University/University of Central Lancashire/Save the Children 2008)

Key point

- Children's commissioners are frequently described as 'watchdogs or champions' for children and young people and are independent from any government organization.

From policy to practice

Children's rights is a curriculum topic in the undergraduate programme in children and young people's nursing in Welsh universities to clearly identify the UNCRC (UN 1989); also included are three main areas of rights – provision, protection and participation – in relation to children and young people's health and how they apply to the holistic nursing of children, young people and their families

National service framework for children, young people and maternity services

This blueprint (Department of Health 2004; Welsh Assembly Government 2005a) clearly sets out and defines standards for the universal services (in England and Wales) which all children and young people should receive including not only optimum health and well-being but also a programme for sustained improvement in children's health. It is a joint policy initiative across both the NHS and local government and supports the Welsh Assembly Government's seven core aims for children and young people and includes them from conception to the age of 18. The National Service Framework was already in the early stages of development when Wanless (2003) was released, but it recommends the proposed extensions to other areas of the NHS. Undeniably there has been involvement of both children and families in the development of the framework (especially in Wales), reflecting the intent shown in the second report to the UN Committee on the Rights of the Child (Department for Children, Schools and Families 1999) to 'Promote the voice of the child'.

Example of implementing policy in practice: self-assessment audit tool

The Welsh Assembly Government (2004) published *Children and Young People: Rights to Action*, which set out that all government policies would deliver children's rights based on the UNCRC; however, the framework used to help make this happen is the National Service Framework through the planning processes of local children and young people's partnerships. Those responsible for the key actions will use a self-assessment audit tool (SAAT) to measure their own progress and this information is used along with other statistics to write their children and young people's plan (CYPP). There are already systems in place to check how well those responsible for the key actions are doing and to make sure that what is entered into the SAAT is correct. The Welsh Assembly Government will then look at the results for the SAAT to identify whether they correspond with the local authority CYPP.

Nursing practice

Within healthcare, however, the Convention represents a shift from a 'highly paternalistic' and medically dominated view to a children's rights-based approach that endorses the child and young person's right to express his or her views and opinions in all matters that affect them. To enable them to do this, however, they require the appropriate information to be given by the appropriately trained professionals. Effective training for healthcare professionals would address common attitudes and prejudices about children's rights and would promote greater respect for the autonomy of children and young people (Lowden 2002). The planning of children's services was made mandatory in 1996 and the second report to the UN Committee (Department for Children, Schools and Families 1999) by the UK did at long last include the importance of this as a critical mechanism for improving a broad range of services for children in need and their families.

All health professionals should understand the imperative to work for child- and family-friendly services as an integral part of the philosophy of 'family-centred care' (Casey 1988, cited in Muir and Sidey 2000). This phrase has become the touchstone for children and young people's nursing practice in the UK, where the needs of the child and young person are considered within the context of the family unit and effective care depends upon negotiation and partnership. Although family-centred care gives a welcome emphasis to the nursing relationship in practice, it has its shortcomings, none the least because it gives little consideration to the very difficult professional, ethical, political and rights-based issues that occur in the nursing of children and young people (Samwell 2000, cited in Muir and Sidey 2000).

A qualitative study by Noyes (2000) goes some way to demonstrate this. A sample of 18 young 'ventilator-dependent' people was purposely selected to reflect age, gender, ethnicity, level of need and location with the aim of describing young people's views (and those of their parents) of their health, social care and education by conducting in-depth interviews. The findings (which are impossible to discuss at great length) are summarized under the relevant Articles of the UNCRC and commence with a clear breach of Articles 4 and 42 in failing both to implement the Convention effectively and to inform the young people and their parents of their rights. It continues with the failure to uphold Articles 12 and 13 following the identification that some of these young people did not have access to an adequate communication system (if non-verbal); when they did have access, they frequently did not have contact with the people who understood it, so their ability to freely express their views was particularly restricted. In addition, there was evidence of them not always being offered the full protection of both the Children Act (1989) and the Patient's Charter (Department of Health 1991, 1996). A particular finding on analysis of the in-depth interviews with these young people was an overwhelming agreement of the need for them to be placed at the centre of decision-making and subsequently allowed to be in charge of their own lives. This led the researcher to seriously question the appropriateness and effectiveness of the health services offered to these young people who had (when enabled) been highly critical of some of the aspects of their care.

What more can we do?

Children, as minors in law, have neither autonomy nor the right to make choices or decisions on their own behalf, and only too frequently responsibility for such decisions and for their welfare has traditionally been vested with those adults who care for them (Lansdown 2001). Children's rights activists Shakespeare and Watson

(1998), in agreement, indicate that the different perspectives on children's rights can result in services being developed, for example, for a child or young person that are determined by other people, particularly professionals and especially for very young and disabled children (cited in Noyes 2000). The need to allow children and young people to participate in matters that affect them is in recognition that they are individuals who not only have opinions and views of their own but that these cannot always be represented necessarily by parents or professionals (Sinclair 1996). Payne (1995) also adds with caution that professions such as nursing can be dangerous and restricted places, giving an example of how children who are disabled are frequently treated as an 'object' of concern or care and not, unfortunately, as a citizen with rights.

Consumer participation is now a major component of contemporary health and nursing policy, with the importance emphasized of partnership working with nurses, midwives and health visitors. The NHS Plan (Department of Health 2000) clearly identified for the first time that patients should have a real say in the NHS, and subsequent documents indicated that this included consumers becoming empowered participants. However, there was limited mention of children and young people's services in the initial plan. It could be argued that consumer participation at the individual level is familiar territory to children and young people's nurses because of the long history of practising family-centred care (Coleman *et al.* 2002). However, it is considered by many that, to date, healthcare staff and parents may have been overcautious in their assessment of children and young people's ability to understand and contribute their opinions and feelings around healthcare decisions (Foley *et al.* 2001). Although parents may have realistic expectations of their child's ability, children and young people need to know that nurses and doctors will respect their views and opinions as well (Alderson and Montgomery 1996). In fact, overall, they consider that there should be no need for young people's rights to conflict with the values of the healthcare professional, but that health professionals need in fact their own code of ethics, to incorporate respect for these rights. Bricher (2000) identifies the importance of reflection and rights and indicates that it is imperative that nurses on both an individual and organizational level reflect on their practice to identify just where children and young people's nursing practice is addressing a rights-based approach.

The education of children and young people's nurses to a minimum of degree level (since 2002 in Wales and from 2013 in England) indeed is a step in the right direction for them to examine and understand what is required to enable a rights-based approach to the nursing of children, young people and their families. Advanced Nurse Practitioners and Consultant Nurse posts that require education to at least Masters level are still in their infancy in children and young people's nursing; however, these highly educated nurses should be able to push the boundaries forward both strategically and in nursing practice and challenge the paternalistic attitudes that persist within healthcare.

Principle for practice

- Children and young people need to know that their views will be respected by nurses and doctors.

Autonomy, consent and the need for children's nurses to be advocates

Although both the courts and parliament allow children and young people to make treatment decisions for themselves as they mature, no child/young person under 18 years is a wholly autonomous being (*Re M (A Child) (Refusal of Medical Treatment)* [1999]). There is nothing compelling a nurse to take consent from an obviously Gillick-competent child. The nurse may, if he or she so chooses, take the consent from a person with parental responsibility. Similarly, if a child/young person under 18 refuses medical examination or treatment then the law does allow others to consent even if the child/young person has capacity. Lord Donaldson summed up the position thus:

> *I now prefer the analogy of the legal 'flak jacket' which protects you from claims by the litigious whether you acquire it from your patient, who may be a minor over the age of 16 or a 'Gillick competent' child under that age, or from another person having parental responsibilities which include a right to consent to treatment of the minor.*
>
> *Anyone who gives you a flak jacket (i.e. consent) may take it back, but you only need one and so long as you continue to have one you have the legal right to proceed.*
>
> (Re W (A Minor) (Medical Treatment Court's Jurisdiction) *[1992]*
> (Lord Donaldson MR at 641)

When a child/young person with capacity consents to medical examination or treatment it cannot be overruled by a parent. However, when the same child/young person refuses to consent then you can obtain it from another person with parental responsibility who has the right to consent to treatment on the child's or young person's behalf.

Key point

- An exception to this rule exists under the Mental Health Act 1983, Section 131 (Department of Health 1983), in which a child aged 16 or over can consent or refuse informal admission to a psychiatric hospital.

However, to grant autonomy to children and young people to consent to treatment without that of their parents (for whatever reason) and not grant the same autonomy to refuse treatment is a blatant disregard for the concept and of course for children's rights (Bijesterveld 2000). This is clearly indicated in the case of *Re M (A Child) (Refusal of Medical Treatment)* [1999], when a 15½ year old had her decision to refuse a heart transplant overruled by the High Court, failing to make any commitment to children's right to 'autonomy' and limited itself to allowing her views to be heard. A lack of respect for autonomy of the child serves to undermine not only their self-esteem and confidence but also their capacity to develop decision-making skills and the opportunity to actually make them (Foley *et al.* 2001; Flatman 2002).

This strong tendency towards judicial paternalism emerged and manifested itself in the 1990s and still (according to many children's rights promoters) continues despite clear standards within the UNCRC to the contrary (Flatman 2002). The trouble with consent law is that it appears to be 'all or nothing' and, although we have discussed the rights of competent children, it fails to address the rights of non-competent children and/or adults (Alderson and Morrow 2004).

So what is the way forward to allow children and young people to participate in the decision-making process of their care, and when relevant to give informed consent? The answers are manifold and are currently being addressed by policy-makers, educationalists and children's charities alike. One example is the Department of Health (2001) in its publication *Seeking consent: working with children*, which clearly indicates the increasing need for children and young people's nurses to ensure that they have evidence in their plans of care of actual involvement of children, young people and their families.

The regulatory body for nursing, midwifery and health visiting (Nursing and Midwifery Council 2008a) clearly indicates the importance of consent and advocacy in its Code of Professional Conduct. This includes (Nursing and Midwifery Council 2008a,b):

- You must ensure that you gain consent before you begin any treatment or care.
- You must respect and support people's rights to accept or decline treatment and care.
- You must uphold people's rights to be fully involved in decisions about their care.
- You must act as an advocate for those in your care, helping them to access relevant health and social care, information and support.

This clearly demonstrates to qualified nurses that, once they are on the professional register, they are responsible and accountable for implementing human rights by adopting their professional body's code of conduct.

Advocacy in the promotion of participation in healthcare

The requirement, therefore, for children's nurses to act as advocates for the child, young person and his or her family is imperative. It is described by many as ensuring that patients and their families are informed of all rights and subsequently have all the necessary information to make informed decisions, and then supporting them in those decisions while also safeguarding their 'best interests'. Bennett (1999) indicates that true advocacy in nursing practice represents an expressed need by the patient and not a perceived need by the nurse. However, there are broadly three types of advocacy, none of which is necessarily dependent on health professionals:

1 Independent advocacy-increased services are now available through government schemes and local councils.
2 Collective advocacy – this comes in the form of groups and charities that represent children and young people, including the National Society for the Prevention of Cruelty to Children, Barnardo's and Action for Sick Children.
3 Self advocacy – promoting the child/young person's ability to make his or her views known.

Example of implementing policy in practice: increased collective and independent advocacy services in Wales

A task force examined advocacy services for children and young people in Wales and delivered its recommendations in 2005 (Welsh Assembly Government 2005b). This included a tiered model of advocacy delivery across health, education and social care settings. This was intended to streamline processes and encourage greater collaboration among providers, in line with the aims of the Children Act 2004 (Office of Public Sector Information 2004); to improve outcomes for vulnerable children and young people; and to ensure more effective use of resources. The task force proposed a collaborative regional model for delivery of children and young people's advocacy services, which should allow greater independence for advocacy providers from service commissioners.

Funding of over £1.2 million has been given to key children's advocacy providers in Wales: Barnardo's, Tros Gynnal, Voices from Care, and the National Youth Advocacy Service. Funding has also been given to local authorities through the Children First programme, to extend advocacy services to children in need.

The Welsh Assembly Government is reviewing arrangements for children and young people to complain about any health service as currently a complaint can only be made against treatment given in a hospital. However, development of advocacy services for children and young people offers considerable support for them as discussed below.

Further advocacy development in Wales: the New Service Framework for the Future Provision of Advocacy Services for Children in Wales (Welsh Assembly Government 2008b)

This will provide a locally/regionally commissioned service covering health, social care services and education with a particular focus on providing support to assist vulnerable children and young people and is currently being rolled out.

But what more can children and young people's nurses do to advocate for children and young people in healthcare? Critics of the UNCRC suggest that, in fact, it is inherently paternalistic and is closely related to upholding 'positive rights', which generally impose a duty that requires another to do something for you and are founded on the ethical principle of beneficence – 'doing good to another'. Charles-Edwards (2000) identified that advocacy in healthcare should be about promoting negative rights as well as positive, which, for example, would be the child's right to contribute his or her viewpoint and participate in decisions even if the healthcare professionals think that the child is wrong, thus highlighting the difference between advocacy and acting in the child's 'best interests'. So nurses and other healthcare workers need to work towards:

- ensuring that families are aware of all available health services
- ensuring that families are informed adequately regarding treatments and procedures
- encouraging and/or supporting existing healthcare practices
- ensuring all rights are protected.

Example of good practice

Community children's nurses who are educated to degree level and hold a specialist practice award frequently work closely with children with severe and life-threatening disabilities and are aware of these children's qualities of life (as small as they may be) and frequently act as advocates for the child and family in helping others to understand this perspective.

Principle for practice

- Advocacy in children's nursing should be about promoting negative rights as well as positive rights.

However, the UNCRC (UN 1989) clearly sets out three levels that respect all children in regard to participation rights and include the right

1 to be informed
2 to form and express views
3 to influence a decision.

The fourth level goes beyond the UNCRC and includes the sharing of power and responsibility for decision-making. This is actually what is addressed in Gillick, although most children and many adults prefer to stop at stage 3 and to share the decision-making with people close to them (Alderson and Montgomery 1996; Royal College of Paediatrics and Child Health 2000; British Medical Association 2001). In regard to other models of participation, one has been uniquely influential: Roger Hart's 'ladder of participation', which first appeared in 1992 (cited in Shier 2001) and has been reproduced many times since (Fig. 4.1). It was adapted from Arnstein's (1969) 'ladder of citizen participation', and Arnstein originally suggested that different levels of control and participation could be compared with rungs on a ladder. However, the influence of Hart's model was confirmed by research conducted by Save the Children in 1995 when Barn and Franklin (1996) carried out a survey of organizations throughout the UK that included questions on what models and theories had been the most helpful in regard to participation; Hart's was one of the two most frequently mentioned, the other being the theories of Paulo Freire (cited in Shier 2001). Their work is based on general principles such as empowerment and respect for young people rather than specific models and theories. The steps on Hart's ladder describe the degree to which children are in control of the process, up to the eighth level where children initiate the process and invite adults to join them in the decision-making.

However, there are many criticisms of Hart, including that the ladder is too idealistic and hierarchical with the objective in striving for the top rung. But what this and other models do is highlight the need to understand and distinguish different levels of empowerment afforded to children and young people. This is somewhat controversial for many people working with and around young people. Essentially, the debate is which of these levels of participation is actually the most meaningful?

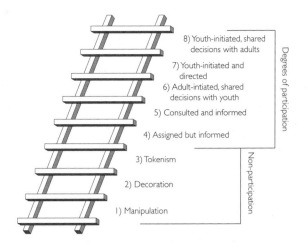

Figure 4.1 Hart's ladder of participation. Adapted from Hart RA (1992) *Children's participation: from tokenism to citizenship*. Innocenti Essays No. 4. Florence: UNICEF International Child Development Centre.

Hart's ladder was not constructed to be utilized in a healthcare context and was developed initially for use with 'common children' in society. The Royal College of Paediatrics and Child Health (1997) has now distinguished four levels of participation:

1 informing children
2 listening to them
3 taking account of their views so they can influence decisions
4 respecting the competent child as the main decider about proposed healthcare interventions.

Many believe that shared decision-making is most beneficial to both young people and adults. Others believe that young people are most empowered when they are making decisions without the influence of adults. Most often, this does not exclude adults but reduces their role to that of support.

Case study

Members of the young people's executive at Oxford Radcliffe (known as YiPpEe for short) are children and young people who either have been in hospital themselves or have a sibling who has. They meet and work with adults, giving them ideas about what children and young people want and need in hospital. Some recent projects that they have been involved in include:

- reviewing food quality and developing menus
- creating an information booklet for children and young people in hospital
- making children's rights clearer and more obvious to adults and young people
- discussing the importance of privacy and dignity for children and young people.

Best interests

Disabled children

When the issue of consent for a disabled child/young person reaches the court, it is nearly always in regard to life-saving treatment and the judge has to rule on the basis of what is in the best interests of the child/young person. Parental consent might be valid if it does not go against the child's or young person's rights as, for a disabled child/young person, it is less likely that their views will be sought, although the principle of an expert to represent them is explicit in the UN Convention. It is commonly assumed that a disabled child does not have quality of life and decisions are often influenced by this perception in terms of the best interests of the child (Campbell 2002). The child and young person's welfare is of paramount consideration and historically doctors were judged to know best; however, the courts now take a much more holistic approach to best interests that goes beyond the clinical needs of the child/young person.

Case law example

In *An NHS Trust v MB and Mr & Mrs B* [2006] an NHS trust sought a declaration that it should be lawful in M's best interests to withdraw all forms of ventilation from a seriously ill young boy but his parents objected. M had not been able to breathe unaided since before his first birthday and required positive pressure ventilation. The trust considered that his quality of life was so low and the burdens of living so great that it was unethical to continue artificially to keep him alive.

The court said that M's welfare was its paramount consideration under the Children Act 1989, Section 1. In considering his best interests the court had to take account of wider welfare issues.

It was probable and had to be assumed that M continued to:

- see
- hear
- feel touch
- have an awareness of his surroundings, in particular of the people who were closest to him, namely his family
- have the normal thoughts and thought processes of a small child of 18 months, with the proviso that because he had never left hospital he had not experienced the same range of stimuli and experiences as a more normal 18 month old
- have age-appropriate cognition, a relationship of value with his family, and other pleasures from sight, touch and sound. Those benefits were precious and real and the routine discomfort, distress and pain that M suffered did not outweigh those benefits.

It was therefore not in M's best interests to discontinue ventilation with the inevitable result that he would die. However, it would not be in M's best interests to undergo procedures that went beyond maintaining ventilation such as cardiopulmonary resuscitation or the administration of intravenous antibiotics.

How does the UN Committee think we are faring?   Page 121

PART 2

The law appears at times to be contradictory where disabled children are concerned, with an absence of clear guidance (Rowse 2007). Unfortunately, the Convention is not widely used in making healthcare decisions, but gradually the Human Rights Act 1998 (from October 2000 in the UK; Office of Public Sector Information 1998) has changed the position of children and young people in being involved in their own healthcare decisions, and health professionals such as children's nurses can act to ensure that this happens.

Law that allows treatment to be forced upon non-competent children and young people appears to assume that they have no understanding worth considering and in fact is at times in conflict with the 'best interests' of the child/young person. It needs work towards providing clearer frameworks comprehensible to professionals, parents, children and young people alike, with the focus of responsibility being on adults to demonstrate that the child/young person is incompetent rather than the child/young person needing to pass a test of competence that many adults would fail (Lowden 2002).

How does the UN Committee think we are faring?

Concluding Observations of the Committee on the Rights of the Child: United Kingdom of Great Britain and Northern Ireland (UN 2008)

The UN Committee on the Rights of the Child examined the UK government in September 2008 to see how well it was protecting children's human rights since the last reporting period, and information was provided by the four UK governments. Since considering this evidence, and in some cases visiting the country concerned, the Committee has made 124 concluding observations (recommendations) of where the government must do more to put the UNCRC fully into practice in the UK. The four countries, however, are at different points of development and have different priorities. All four have dedicated departments for children and young people and Ministers with special responsibilities for policies affecting them as well as their own Commissioners. Although all four recognize the challenge ahead of them and have their own plans, there has been a move forward in some areas:

- Article 22: refugee children and young people will now enjoy the same status as others in the UK.
- Article 37c: young people in custody will no longer be detained with adults under any circumstances.

The recognition is that, although it is important to take forward their own policies to meet local needs that achieve the goals set out, collaborative working is essential, as is having clearly defined joint targets to tackle child poverty and plans to enable children and young people to participate in decision-making on issues that affect their lives. Therefore, a joint commitment from all four nations of the UK has been made to take action in response to the UN Committee and has been clearly laid out in the document *Working Together, Achieving More* (Department for Children, Schools and Families 2009a); some examples follow.

Responsive policy in the UK

England

- Department for Children, Schools and Families (2007) – *The Children's Plan*
- Department for Children, Schools and Families (2009b) – *The Children's Plan Two Years On: A Progress Report*
- Department for Children, Schools and Families (2009c) – *UNCRC: Priorities For Action*

In October 2009 England published an update to the Children's Plan (Department for Children, Schools and Families 2009b) which sets out priorities for taking forward the UN Committee's recommendations. The English plan *UNCRC: Priorities for Action* (Department for Children, Schools and Families 2009c) was published alongside the above document.

Wales

- Welsh Assembly Government (2009) – *Getting It Right*

A 5 year rolling Action Plan for Wales setting out key priorities and actions to be undertaken by the Welsh Assembly Government in response to the Concluding Observations of the UN Committee on the Rights of the Child (UN 2008). It has 16 priorities that will be focused on, and will be a living document. It will be subject to regular review and updating to ensure that it keeps abreast of new developments in policy and strategy and remains relevant and timely. Two examples of these include:

- No. 1. Tackle poverty for children and young people in Wales – new legislation to address this major issue and local plans will be stronger and give more support.
- No. 8. To increase opportunities for all children and young people in Wales to participate in decision-making on issues that affect them.

There has been a good start to this in Wales, but work must continue and more must be done to ensure that the chance to take part is available to all children and young people. This may be in regard to their own healthcare at both a local and a national level.

Scotland

- Scottish Government (2009) – *Do the Right Thing*

Launched in September the Scottish Government's response to the Concluding Observations of the UN Committee sets out 21 priority areas of action.

Northern Ireland

As of 2009, Northern Ireland is still developing additional actions for inclusion in its existing children and young people's strategy action plan which are yet to be identified.

Conclusion

The UNCRC has made great progress in promoting children and young people's rights by providing a benchmark for the implementation of these rights throughout the world. The Convention's value, however, has been limited by the failure of many countries, including the UK, to incorporate its provisions into domestic law. Children and young people cannot enforce the rights guaranteed by the convention in a British court, and the UK government does not regard the criticisms of its performance by the UN Committee on the Rights of the Child as a reason to make the convention legally enforceable. Despite this, there is no doubt that the UNCRC has influenced governments towards increased participation by children and young people in policy planning and giving them a voice through the children's commissioners.

Participation in their own healthcare by children and young people remains little changed since the seminal case of *Gillick* in the late 1980s. Children and young people's nurses always work in a climate of consent with their young patients to encourage participation by taking the time to explain procedures and the reasons for treatment. This clinical function of consent is every bit as important as its legal function. Healthcare delivery is far more efficient and effective with the cooperation of the child and young person, and this is more likely to occur when the child/young person knows what the procedure is and why it needs to be performed. We have seen that a child and young person's legal right to express his or her autonomy has developed through a protective common law structure that always has someone available to step in should a child's or young person's refusal of treatment be contrary to their best interests. This paternalistic approach effectively restricts a child's or young person's participation in making choices about their healthcare; either the child/young person agrees to treatment or someone else makes the decision for them. Competence is the key to autonomy, so a competent child or young person should be free to make choices about his or her healthcare regardless of what others consider to be in their best interests. Until the licensed paternalism of health professionals is curtailed and the UK enshrines the Articles of the UNCRC in law, children and young people will not be free to fully participate in their healthcare.

Summary of principles for practice

- Children and young people's nurses must ensure that the rights of children and young people are upheld in all areas of practice.
- Children and young people's nurses must ensure that children and young people are given the opportunity to express their views and opinions and wherever possible participate in their own care.
- Children and young people's nurses must be knowledgeable about present-day law in relation to issues such as informed consent.
- Children and young people's nurses must be knowledgeable about policy in their own country in relation to participation by children and young people in all aspects of their own lives, including healthcare.

References

A v United Kingdom [1998] 2 FLR 959.

A&D v B&E [2003] EWHC 1376 ((FAM)).

Alderson P (2002) Young children's health care rights and consent. In: Franklin B (ed.) *The new handbook of children's rights: comparative policy and practice*. London: Routledge.

Alderson P, Montgomery J (1996) *Health care choices: making decisions with children*. London: Institute for Public Policy and Research.

Alderson P, Morrow V (2004) *Ethics, social research and consulting with children and young people*. London: Barnardo's.

An NHS Trust v MB and Mr & Mrs B [2006] EWHC 507.

Aries P (1962) *Centuries of childhood*. London: Jonathan Cape.

Arnstein S (1969) A ladder of citizen participation. *Journal of the American Planning Association* **35**:216–24.

Barn G, Franklin A (1996) Article 12: Issues in developing children's participation rights. In: Verhellen E. (ed.) *Monitoring children's rights*. Leiden: Martinus Nijhoff.

Barnardo v McHugh [1891] AC 388 ((CA)).

Bennett O (1999) Advocacy in nursing. *Nursing Standard* **14**(11): 40–1.

Bijesterveld P (2000) Competent to refuse. *Paediatric Nursing* **12**: 33–5.

Bricher G (2000) Children in the hospital: issues of power and vulnerability. *Pediatric Nursing* **26**(3): 277–81.

British Medical Association (2001) *Consent, rights, and choices in healthcare, children and young people*. London: BMA Publishing.

Camden LBC v R (A Minor) (Blood Transfusion) [1993] 2 FLR 757.

Campbell A (2002) Informed choice for adolescents. *Paediatric Nursing* **13**(10): 41–2.

Charles-Edwards I (2000) Children's nursing and advocacy: are we in a muddle? *Paediatric Nursing* **13**(2): 12–16.

Children and Young People's Unit (2001) *Learning to listen: core principles for the involvement of children and young people*. London: CYPU.

Children and Young People's Unit (2003) Action plan for children's and young people's participation. See www.allchildrenni.gov.uk

Children's Rights Alliance for England (2004) *The case for a children's rights commissioner for England*. London: CRAE.

Coleman V, Smith L, Bradshaw M (2002) *Family centred care: concept, theory and practice*. Basingstoke: Palgrave.

Council of Europe (1950) *European Convention on Fundamental Human Rights and Freedoms*. Rome: Council of Europe. See http://conventions.coe.int/treaty/Commun/QueVoulezVous.asp?NT=005&CL=ENG

Darbyshire P (1994) *Living with a sick child in hospital*. London: Chapman and Hall.

Department for Children, Schools and Families (1999) *UK 2nd report*. Report to the UN Committee on the Rights of the Child. London: HMSO. See http://www.dcsf.gov.uk/everychildmatters/strategy/strategyandgovernance/uncrc/unitednationsreportingprocess/uncrcreportingprocess/

Department for Children, Schools and Families (2007) *The children's plan*. London: DCSF. See http://publications.dcsf.gov.uk/default.aspx?PageFunction=productdetails&PageMode=publications&ProductId=DCSF-01099-2009

Department for Children, Schools and Families (2009a) *Working together, achieving more*. London: DCSF.

Department for Children, Schools and Families (2009b) *The children's plan two years on: a progress report*. London: DCSF. See http://publications.dcsf.gov.uk/default.aspx?PageFunction=productdetails&PageMode=publications&ProductId=DCSF-01099-2009

Department for Children, Schools and Families (2009c) *UNCRC: priorities for action*. London: DSCF. See http://publications.dcsf.gov.uk/default.aspx?PageFunction=productdetails&PageMode=publications&ProductId=DCSF-01099-2009

Department of Education and Skills (2002) *Listening to learn: an action plan for the involvement of children and young people*. See www.dcsf.gov.uk

Department of Health (1983) *The Mental Health Act.* London: DH.

Department of Health (1991) *The patient's charter.* London: HMSO.

Department of Health (1996) *The patient's charter: services for children and young people.* London: HMSO.

Department of Health (2000) *The NHS plan.* London: HMSO.

Department of Health (2001) *Seeking consent: working with children.* London: DH.

Department of Health (2002) *Listening, hearing and responding: Department of Health action plan – core principles for the involvement of children and young people.* London: DH.

Department of Health (2004) *The National Service Framework for children, young people and maternity services.* London: DH.

Department of Health (2007) *Annual report.* See www.doh.gov.uk

Department of Health and the Home Office (2003) *The Victoria Climbié Inquiry: report of an inquiry by Lord Laming.* London: HMSO.

F v West Berkshire HA [1990] 2 A.C. 1 ((HL)).

Flatman D (2002) Consulting children: are we listening? *Paediatric Nursing* **14**(7): 28–31.

Foley P, Roche J, Tucker T (eds) (2001) *Children in society: contemporary theory, policy and practice.* Basingstoke: Palgrave.

Gillick v West Norfolk and Wisbech AHA [1986] AC 112 ((HL)).

Glass v United Kingdom [2004] 1 FLR 1019.

Hall D, Elliman D (eds) (2003) *Health for all children,* 4th edn. Oxford: Oxford University Press.

Hill M, Davis J, Prout A, Tisdall K (2004) Moving the participation agenda forward. *Children and Society* **18**:77–96.

HM Government (2004) *Every child matters: change for children.* London: Department for Education and Skills.

Holt J (1975) *Escape from childhood, the needs and rights of children.* Hammondsworth: Penguin.

House of Commons (2001) *Children's Commissioner for Wales Bill.* London: HMSO. See http://www.parliament.the-stationery-office.co.uk/pa/cm200001/cmbills/003/2001003.htm

Hoyles M (1989) *The politics of childhood.* London: Journeyman.

J (A Minor) (Child in Care: Medical Treatment) [1993] Fam 15.

J (A Minor) (Prohibited Steps Order: Circumcision) [2000] 1 FLR 571.

James A, Jenks G, Prout A (1999) *Theorising childhood.* London: Policy Press.

James A, Prout A (eds) (1990) *Constructing and reconstructing childhood.* Basingstoke: Falmer Press.

Kempe CH (1962) The battered child syndrome. *Journal of the American Medical Association* **181**:17–24.

Kennedy I, Grubb A (2000) *Medical law: text and materials,* 3rd edn. London: LexisNexis.

Kennedy I, Grubb A (2002) *Principles of medical law.* Oxford: Oxford University Press.

Lansdown G (2001) *Promoting children's participation in democratic decision making.* Florence: UNICEF.

Lowden J (2002) Children's rights: a decade of dispute. *Journal of Advanced Nursing* **37**(1): 100–7.

Mayall B (ed.) (1994) *Children's childhoods observed and experienced.* London: Falmer Press.

Mayall B (1996) *Children, health and social order.* Milton Keynes: Open University Press.

Mayall B (1998) Towards a sociology of child health. *Sociology of Health and Illness* **20**: 269–88.

Muir J, Sidey A (2000) *Textbook of children's community nursing.* London: Baillière Tindall.

Neill AS (1962) *Summerhill.* Harmondsworth: Penguin.

Noyes J (2000) Are nurses respecting and upholding the human rights of children and young people in their care? *Paediatric Nursing* **12**(2): 23–7.

Nursing and Midwifery Council (2008a) *Code of professional conduct.* London: NMC.

Nursing and Midwifery Council (2008b) *The code: standards of conduct, performance and ethics for nurses and midwives.* London: NMC.

Office of Public Sector Information (1933) *The Children and Young Persons Act.* See http://www.opsi.gov.uk/RevisedStatutes/Acts/ukpga/1933/cukpga_19330012_en_1

Office of Public Sector Information (1969) *The Family Law Reform Act.* See http://www.opsi.gov.uk/RevisedStatutes/Acts/ukpga/1969/cukpga_19690046_en_1

Office of Public Sector Information (1976) *The Adoption Act.* See http://www.opsi.gov.uk/RevisedStatutes/Acts/ukpga/1976/cukpga_19760036_en_1

Office of Public Sector Information (1977) *The National Health Service Act.* See http://www.opsi.gov.uk/RevisedStatutes/Acts/ukpga/1977/cukpga_19770049_en_1

Office of Public Sector Information (1978) *The National Health Service Act (Scotland).* Edinburgh: Local Government Boundary Commission for Scotland. See http://www.statutelaw.gov.uk/content

Office of Public Sector Information (1987) *The Family Law Reform Act.* See http://www.statutelaw.gov.uk/leg

Office of Public Sector Information (1989) *The Children Act.* See http://www.opsi.gov.uk/acts/acts1989/ukpga_19890041_en_1

Office of Public Sector Information (1998) *The Human Rights Act.* http://www.opsi.gov.uk/acts/acts1998/ukpga_19980042_en_1

Office of Public Sector Information (2000) *The Care Standards Act.* See http://www.opsi.gov.uk/acts/acts2000/ukpga_20000014_en_1

Office of Public Sector Information (2002) *The Adoption and Children Act.* See http://www.opsi.gov.uk/acts/acts2002/ukpga_20020038_en_1

Office of Public Sector Information (2003) *The Sexual Offences Act.* See http://www.opsi.gov.uk/acts/acts2003/ukpga_20030042_en_1

Office of Public Sector Information (2004) *The Children Act.* See http://www.opsi.gov.uk/acts/acts2004/ukpga_20040031_en_1

O'Halloran K (1999) *The welfare of the child: the principle and the law.* Aldershot: Ashgate Arena.

Payne M (1995) Children's rights and needs. *Health Visitor* **68**(10): 412–14.

R (Axon) v Secretary of State For Health [2006] EWHC 37.

Re B (A Child) [2003] EWCA Civ 1148 ((CA)).

Re B (A Minor) (Wardship: Medical Treatment) [1981] 1 WLR 1421.

Re J [2000] 1 FLR 571 ((Fam)).

Re L (Medical Treatment: Gillick Competence) [1998] 2 FLR 810.

Re M (A Child) (Refusal of Medical Treatment) [1999] 2 FLR 1097 ((CA)).

Re R (A Minor) (Wardship Consent to Treatment) [1992] 1 FLR 190.

Re W (A Minor) (Medical Treatment Court's Jurisdiction) [1992] 3 WLR 758.

Rowse V (2007) Consent in severely disabled children: informed or an infringement of their rights? *Journal of Child Health Care* **11**(1): 70–8.

Royal College of Paediatrics and Child Health (1997) *Withholding or withdrawing life saving treatment in children: a framework for practice.* London: RCPCH.

Royal College of Paediatrics and Child Health (2000) Guidelines for the ethical conduct of medical research involving children. *Archives of Disease in Childhood* **82**: 177–82.

Scottish Government (2009) *Do the right thing.* A response by the Scottish Government to the 2008 concluding observations from the UN Committee on the Rights of the Child. Edinburgh: The Scottish Government.

Shakespeare T, Watson N (1998) *Theoretical perspectives of research with disabled children.* London: Jesscia Kingsley.

Shier H (2001) Pathways to participation: openings, opportunities and obligations. *Children and Society* **15**: 107–17.

Sidaway v Bethlem Royal Hospital [1985] AC 871.

Sinclair R (ed.) (1996) Special issue on research with children. *Children and Society* **10**(2): editorial.

Sinclair R (2004) Participation in practice: making it meaningful and sustainable. *Children and Society* **18**: 106–18.

Sinclair R, Franklin A (2000) *Young people's participation.* London: Department of Health.

Swansea University/University of Central Lancashire/Save the Children (2008) *Evaluating the Children's Commissioner for Wales.* Cardiff: Children's Commissioner.

Tait W (1883) *The works of Jeremy Bentham,* vol. 3. Edinburgh: Edinburgh University Press.

United Nations (1989) *Convention on the Rights of the Child adopted under General Assembly resolution 44/25.* Geneva: UN.

United Nations Committee on the Rights of the Child (2008) *Consideration of reports submitted by States Parties under Article 44 of the Convention. Concluding Observations of the Committee on the Rights of the Child: United Kingdom of Great Britain and Northern Ireland.* Geneva: UN.

US Census Bureau (2006) See http://www.census.gov/

Van de Mheen H, Stronks K, Looman C, Mackenbach J (1998) Role of childhood health in the explanation of socioeconomic inequalities in early adult health. *Journal of Epidemiology and Community Health* **52:** 15–19.

Verhellen E (ed.) (1996) *Monitoring children's rights.* The Hague: Martinus Nijhoff.

Wanless D (2003) *The review of health and social care in Wales.* Cardiff: Welsh Assembly Government.

Waterhouse R, Clough M, Le Fleming M (1999) *Lost in care: report of the tribunal inquiry into the abuse of children in care in the former county councils of Gwynedd and Clwyd since 1974.* London: The Stationery Office.

Welsh Assembly Government (2000) *Framework for partnership with children and young people.* Cardiff: WAG.

Welsh Assembly Government (2004) *Children and young people: rights to action.* Cardiff: WAG.

Welsh Assembly Government (2005a) *The national service framework for children, young people and maternity services.* Cardiff: WAG.

Welsh Assembly Government (2005b) *A study of advocacy services for children and young people in Wales.* Cardiff: WAG. See http://wales.gov.uk/caec/publications/childrenandyoungpeople/advocacystudy/advocacyen.pdf?lang=en

Welsh Assembly Government (2008a) *Rights in action.* Cardiff: WAG.

Welsh Assembly Government (2008b) *The new service framework for the future provision of advocacy services for children in Wales.* Cardiff: WAG. See http://new.wales.gov.uk/caec/report/cabinetstatements/2008/nsfdadvocacy/statemente.doc?lang=en

Welsh Assembly Government (2009) *Getting it right.* Cardiff: WAG.

Williams J, Jackson S, Maddocks A, *et al.* (2001) Case–control study of the health of those looked after by local authorities. *Archives of Disease in Childhood* **85**: 280–5.

Willow C (2002) The state of children's rights in 2002. *Childright* **187**: 120–9.

PART 2

Chapter 5

Safeguarding children and young people

Catherine Powell

Overview

This chapter is concerned with one of the most challenging and emotive aspects of child healthcare: that of child maltreatment. The chapter, which is underpinned by a children's rights perspective, introduces the professional roles and responsibilities of children and young people's nurses in safeguarding and promoting the welfare of children and young people and seeks to influence a positive and proactive approach. A number of anonymized case examples, drawn from the realities of practice, are provided to illustrate some of the challenges; please note that a chapter on safeguarding children is not an easy read, but it represents a vital competency for children and young people's nurses.

Introduction

It is argued from a critical standpoint that safeguarding children and young people is everyone's responsibility and that the universality of health provision in the UK and elsewhere should place children and young people's nurses at the forefront of prevention of maltreatment and early intervention to support families experiencing difficulties. The challenges faced in achieving this vision are exposed and solutions sought by drawing on the literature concerning child deaths from maltreatment including the highly publicized cases of Victoria Climbié and Peter Connelly.

Reflection points

★ How did you feel when you read the opening lines of this chapter?

★ How confident are you about your role in protecting children and young people?

★ What sources of advice and support on safeguarding children/young people are available to you in your current role?

Safeguarding children and young people is first and foremost everyone's responsibility; this includes children and young people themselves, their parents, their families and their communities. However, it is clearly also the remit of those whose professional lives bring them into contact with children, young people and

PART 2

their families. Ensuring that children and young people are safe is challenging work, but it can also be highly rewarding (Hall 2003). Professionals with responsibilities in safeguarding children and young people perform their roles within a range of different settings including health, early years, education, social care, police, probation and the voluntary sector. While working together in the best interests of children, young people and their families means that these professionals share both knowledge and responsibility, this chapter is written for 'children and young people's nurses' (chiefly, but arguably not exclusively, children and young people's nurses working in hospitals and community settings, child and adolescent mental health practitioners, midwives, health visitors and school nurses). The aim of the chapter is to provide the means to achieve the confidence and ability to successfully, and proactively, safeguard and promote the welfare of children and young people. Although knowledge and understanding of the subject matter is the key to success, it is also important to recognize the emotional burden of this work, and therefore the need to ensure robust clinical supervision and support.

Although deaths from child maltreatment (abuse and neglect) are relatively rare, much of the current direction of travel in terms of policy and practice improvement is linked to lessons learned from serious case reviews, including those related to high-profile enquiries. The chapter thus examines some of the key messages from such reviews within the context of child health practice. Finally, the chapter offers a consideration of how to achieve excellence in safeguarding children and young people practice, through enhanced understanding of the principles for practice, high-quality clinical supervision and new ways of working. It is hoped that readers will be helped to understand the very real potential for children and young people's nurses to make a positive difference to the lived experiences of children and young people and ensure that they achieve their potential into adulthood.

Principles for practice

- Safeguarding children and young people is everyone's responsibility.
- An understanding of the principles for practice is the key to success.
- Children and young people's nurses have an important safeguarding role within an interagency context.
- Practitioners need to ensure that they have access to high-quality clinical supervision.

Principles for safeguarding children practice

It is important to begin by defining some key terms, including 'child' and 'safeguarding', before discussing the primacy of the roles and responsibilities of parents. Children and young people's nurses, in particular, have done much to promote the notion of 'family-centred' care, and this has undoubtedly improved the healthcare experiences of children and young people over the past 20 years or so. However, I have previously suggested that 'child and family-centred care' may be a more appropriate concept (Powell 2007), especially because there is the ever-present danger that children and young people's nurses will be drawn to the pressing needs and difficulties of adults in the family, with the risk of a failure to consider a perspective on the daily lived experience of the child. Successful safeguarding children practice balances support for parents, and parenting, without losing the focus on the centrality of the child/young person, their needs and their *right* to be protected from harm. This is an approach that is enshrined within recent policy and legislation in the UK. Such policy and legislation reflects a more global initiative; the United Nations Convention on the Rights of the Child (United Nations 1989), which was ratified by the UK in 1991 (http://www2.ohchr.org/english/law/crc.htm). This is explored in more detail in Chapter 4.

Children and their right to protection

The four countries of the UK (England, Wales, Scotland and Northern Ireland) have adopted the legal definition of a child as being an individual who has not yet reached the age of 18 years. This is in line with the Convention and is the definition used within all of the UK's safeguarding guidance, policy and legislation (HM Government 2006; Welsh Assembly Government 2006; Children and Young People's Unit 2009; The Scottish Office, undated). The definition can present a challenge in relation to the client group typically served by paediatrics and child health, where young people over the age of 16 years may begin to choose to access, or to make a transition to, healthcare in a range of adult-centric settings. It is therefore essential that safeguarding children awareness reaches those working in 'adult' settings who will encounter 16 and 17 year olds in the course of their practice. A recent and notable exception to this age group accessing care in an adult environment is the move within Child and Adolescent Mental Health Services (CAMHS) to provide services up until the age of 18 years. This includes an explicit requirement to ensure that young people under this age who require inpatient care are not admitted to adult mental health facilities (Office of the Children's Commissioner 2007). It is timely to note that adult practitioners may also find themselves in a situation where they have to take action because of concerns that arise in relation to children and young people whose parents or carers are the primary service user. Ensuring that safeguarding children and young people is seen as everyone's responsibility, and being in a position to support and supervise practice, is arguably a vital component of the role of children's leads and children's champions across all healthcare organizations.

Reflection point

★ Think about the organization in which you practice. Is there 24/7 access to a practitioner with the qualifications and skills to support and advise on all aspects of the care of children and young people, including safeguarding?

It is also important to clarify the situation for unborn children. Although unborn children are not legally defined as children, their needs for safety and protection from harm must still be considered in cases where there is concern about expectant parents' ability to ensure the safety and well-being of their child. This would primarily be a responsibility of the midwife and others providing care in the antenatal period, but it is also pertinent to note that in some cases the 'parent to be' may be a child themselves, even if they are living independently from their own parents, in the armed forces or, indeed, married.

What is 'safeguarding children'?

It is notable that 'safeguarding children' is a term that has increasingly replaced the concept of 'protecting children' when referring to the prevention of, and response to, child abuse and neglect (for example I have held the role of Designated Nurse for Safeguarding Children since 2006; my predecessor was a Designated Nurse for Child Protection). However, as will be seen, safeguarding is a term that embraces additional activity surrounding the 'safety' of children and is therefore not a direct substitution for practice previously referred to as child protection. Safeguarding children[1] is perhaps best thought of as an umbrella term for a number of different, but related, actions that ensure the well-being of children and young people, all of which may be encompassed within the professional activities of children and young people's nurses.

A basic definition of safeguarding is provided in a joint inspectorates review of services for children, young people and their families; here, it is suggested that at its simplest safeguarding means 'keeping children safe from harm such as illness, abuse or injury' (Commission for Social Care Inspection *et al.* 2005, p.5). However, this definition says little about how this can be achieved. The current statutory guidance for England, *Working Together to Safeguard Children* (HM Government 2010), which was published in 2010, opens by emphasizing that safeguarding children and young people is primarily accomplished through good parenting:

Patterns of family life vary and there is no single, perfect way to bring up children.

Good parenting involves caring for children's basic needs, keeping them safe and protected, being attentive and showing them warmth and love, encouraging them to express their views and consistently taking these views into account, and providing the stimulation needed for their development and to help them achieve their potential, within a stable environment where they experience consistent guidance and boundaries.

(HM Government 2010, p. 29–30)

The guidance also recognizes that parenting can be challenging and that parents may require support and help. It notes that early engagement and partnership with professionals is of key importance and suggests that where parents seek help from the 'wide range of services available to families' this should be seen as a sign of responsibility, not of failure. The need for competent professional judgement, based on a sound assessment of the needs of the child or young person, and the parents' capacity to respond to these needs, is made clear at the outset. The guidance notes that the requirement for any compulsory intervention in family life should be seen as 'exceptional'. This is important because it supports the notion that universal

[1]Safeguarding adults is also currently an area of change and expansion.

services, such as those provided by health and education providers, have a key role to play in early intervention and support to families experiencing difficulties (Powell 2007). Other countries in the UK take a similar stance.

Reflection points

★ How do parents learn how to parent?

★ What might 'good parenting' look like?

★ At what point should agencies intervene when parenting is thought to be inadequate?

Safeguarding and promoting the welfare of children and young people is thus seen to encompass a number of separate, but interrelated, activities. According to the guidance this includes: protecting children from maltreatment; preventing impairment of their health and development; and ensuring that they are safe and well cared for (HM Government 2010). The overarching aim of safeguarding work is to make sure that children and young people are able to reach their potential and enter adulthood successfully, and that parents are supported as having key responsibility to ensure that this happens. The broader aspect of safeguarding children practice is perhaps best illustrated through a consideration of the objectives of the 'be safe' element of the *Every Child Matters* policy (more details are provided on this below), which include:

- *Being safe from maltreatment, neglect, violence and sexual exploitation;*
- *Being safe from accidental injury and death;*
- *Being safe from bullying and discrimination;*
- *Being safe from crime and anti-social behaviour in, and out of, school; and*
- *Having security, stability and being cared for.*

(HM Government 2004)

Child protection is clearly seen as an important part of safeguarding, but refers specifically to the actions undertaken to protect children who are at risk of, or suffering from, significant harm. Crucially, the *Working Together* guidance suggests that proactively safeguarding children and promoting their welfare will reduce the need for statutory interventions to protect children. Hence, it appears that in comparison with previous child protection guidance there is considerably more emphasis on *promoting welfare* and *ensuring safety* rather than simply recognizing and responding to child abuse and neglect. This has important implications for those children and young people's nurses who are engaged primarily in preventative services as well as for other, more specialist, health services that provide care for children, young people and their families in a variety of settings.

Reflection points

★ Which healthcare practitioners may a child/young person see on their healthcare journey?

★ What opportunities may this provide for supporting parents, offering early intervention where there are emerging concerns, or identifying signs of possible child maltreatment?

First, and foremost, however, is a need for practitioners to have an understanding of the nature of childhood and an appreciation that this is not necessarily reflective of a positive, creative, loving and caring experience that supports optimum health and development into adulthood. Although readers are encouraged to access the wider literature on the topic, a brief summary of the key issues is given below.

Childhood: a golden age?

The existence of childhood as a separate and distinct chronological stage to adulthood has raised some interesting debates in the literature; these embrace the notion of children's rights and the role of parents and the state in ensuring that they have a best possible upbringing (see, for example, Archard 2004). The debates on the nature of childhood have not always been favourable to the image of childhood as a golden age of innocence and purity. The following case example is drawn from practice.

Case study

Jodie, a bright and able girl who is 10 years old, often misses school and is beginning to fall behind with her learning; last term her recorded attendance demonstrated a drop from 87% to 62%. Many of these absences are recorded as being 'unauthorized'. Jodie's mother, June, is known to suffer from depression and anxiety, and in the past the police have notified agencies (health, social care and education) of some quite serious incidents of domestic abuse. Jodie's stepfather is thought to have a dependency on alcohol, and both parents smoke heavily. The school nurse visits the home to make an assessment of any health issues that may be preventing her from attending school. An education welfare officer is also in attendance. Jodie is noticed to be thin and unhappy, but anxious to please. It seems that June has been relying on her to be the main carer of her 17 month old half-sibling; this includes taking a key role in feeding, changing and bathing routines. Jodie explains that although she loves her baby brother she is missing her friends and worries about what her teachers will say when she returns to school. The toddler, who appears somewhat grubby and under-occupied, looks to Jodie for comfort in the presence of the two professionals.

Reflection points

★ What are the key healthcare needs for each of the members of this family and how can they be best met?

★ How might a child like Jodie be supported in returning to school?

The debates about the nature of contemporary childhood often highlight the *oppression* of children through a lack of human rights afforded to others; this has been linked to their vulnerability to child maltreatment. Examples of the oppression of children include their disenfranchisement, their lack of a say in issues that concern them and the continued use of corporal punishment (i.e. hitting, smacking, and beating) in many societies, including the UK (for a debate on these issues, see Powell 2004; Whiting *et al.* 2004). Other evidence of children as an oppressed group includes the expectations held by adults of subservience to their elders and their segregation from mainstream society. In 2006 The Children's Society commissioned a review of childhood in the UK (The Children's Society 2006). Citing family breakdowns, continuing child poverty, excessive pressure on children to succeed at school, poor provision of child and adolescent mental health services and the promotion of junk food diets that lead to obesity, the report concluded that 'excessive individualism' in society was ruining children's chances of a good childhood (Layard and Dunn 2009). A recent addition to the many sanctions the UK has against children and young people is the mosquito alarm, a device installed within some shopping malls to stop young people congregating in groups (as only infants, children and young people can hear the high-pitched and irritating sound). This initiative has led to a high-publicity campaign to ban their use by the Children's Commissioner for England. It is issues such as these that underpin the calls for children to have the same basic human rights as adults and feeds directly in to the children's rights lobby.

Arguably, however, while supportive of the notion of children's rights and especially those linked to equality and to choices made within healthcare arenas, there is a pragmatic stance to be taken in recognizing the need for children and young people to also have protective and welfare rights that recognize both their developmental vulnerability and their need for specialist service provision. This takes us back to the importance of the Convention.

Reflection points

★ Think about the language used by adults, including children and young people's nurses, in relation to children and young people. How often do we hear small human beings (i.e. infants) being described as 'it'; is this term applied to any other groups in our society?

★ What do you think about the negative connotation of the word 'childish'?

The United Nations Convention on the Rights of the Child

The United Nations (UN) Convention on the Rights of the Child (United Nations 1989) establishes the irrefutable rights of children and young people and outlines the actions and responsibilities of governments in ensuring that all services for children are offered in a child-centred, rights-based framework. The UN Convention has been ratified by every country in the world but two, these being Somalia and the

PART 2

USA. However, it is fair to say that at the time of writing there are indications that the US president (Barack Obama) is preparing to ratify the convention, albeit in the face of opposition from a large body of citizens who vigorously defend the principle of parents' rights to bring up children in the way in which they choose.

The UN Convention proposes both welfare rights (such as food, healthcare, housing and education) and protective rights (e.g. from child maltreatment) which are embodied in a series of clauses known as 'Articles'. There is a strong emphasis on ensuring that children and young people have a healthy and safe development into adulthood, together with the provision of extra support for parents and services to meet the needs of children in 'special circumstances'. This group includes children who are disabled, children in the care system and children who are refugees. In essence, the UN Convention aims to ensure the best outcomes for children and young people everywhere and provides a mandate for governments to achieve this. The right to freedom from child maltreatment is one of the protective rights and is enshrined in Article 19, which states:

> *State parties shall take all appropriate legislative, administrative, social and educational measures to protect the child from all forms of physical or mental violence, injury or abuse, neglect or negligent treatment, maltreatment or exploitation, including sexual abuse, while in the care of parent(s), legal guardian(s) or any other person who has care of the child.*
>
> *Such protective measures should, as appropriate, include effective procedures for the establishment of social programmes to provide necessary support for the child, and for those who have care of the child, as well as for other forms of prevention and for identification, reporting, referral, investigation, treatment and follow up of instances of child maltreatment described heretofore, and, as appropriate, for judicial involvement.*

> *(United Nations 1989, Article 19)*

Key points

- Safeguarding children guidance and legislation applies throughout childhood, i.e. until an individual has reached the age of 18 years. Although unborn babies are not included in the legal definition of 'a child', it may be necessary to consider safeguarding needs.
- The UN Convention on the Rights of the Child (United Nations 1989) explicitly promotes the rights of children to protection from harm, as well as outlining the welfare rights that support a healthy development into adulthood.
- Protecting children and young people from maltreatment is part of safeguarding, but safeguarding children is a broader concept.
- Safeguarding children and young people is primarily accomplished through good parenting.
- Contemporary children's policy is supportive of parenting and families and ensuring positive outcomes for children and young people; there is an emphasis on parental responsibility.

Principles from contemporary policy

The Convention is reflected in contemporary policy, legislation and guidance for the care of children, young people and their families. In the UK, the tragic death of Victoria Climbié in 2000 has been a key driver for a fundamental review of children's policy and the provision of services to children in recent years. In England, this is reflected in the *Every Child Matters* policy (HM Government 2004), the *National Service Framework for Children, Young People and Maternity Services* (Department of Health 2003; Department of Health and Department for Education and Skills 2004) and new legislation; the Children Act 2004 (Office of Public Sector Information 2004). The crux of the policy is that children and young people should be supported to grow up safe and well into adulthood. The *Every Child Matters* policy reflects a framework of objectives that is based on five key outcomes for children. These outcomes are reported to have been drawn from consultation with children and young people themselves and include the aspirations to:

- be healthy
- stay safe
- enjoy and achieve
- make a positive contribution and
- achieve economic well-being.

Importantly, each of the outcomes is co-dependent on the others; for example, a child who is not healthy can find it difficult to enjoy and achieve in his or her childhood; and a child who has not achieved is much less likely to achieve economic well-being, and so forth. Thus, children's nurses and other children and young people's nurses are seen to be increasingly crucial as key players within the children's workforce because of their important contribution in protecting and promoting health.

The government has continued to build on the progress of *Every Child Matters* (HM Government 2004) through a fundamental departmental reorganization and the publication of a *Children's Plan* for England (Department for Children, Schools and Families 2007). This has the aspirations to '… make this country [England] the best place in the world for children and young people to grow up in'.

The Children's Plan has five key principles which are broadly in line with the aims of *Every Child Matters*. These include overt recognition that parents are the ones to bring up children (not governments); that all children are seen to have potential; that more needs to be done to support parents and families; that children and young people should have the opportunities to enjoy their childhood and be prepared for adult life; that services need to be shaped by, and responsive to, children, young people and their families (i.e. not designed around professional boundaries); and that it is always better to prevent failure than deal with a crisis later on.

Reflection points

★ Think about the service that you practise in – how well do you and your team meet the needs of fathers?

★ Do you routinely engage with fathers and how do you ensure that information on their children's health needs is fed back to them, especially in situations where they are 'absent'?

The recently published child health strategy *Healthy Lives, Brighter Futures: the Strategy for Children and Young People's Health* (Department for Children, Schools and Families and Department of Health 2009) is part of a commitment from *The Children's Plan* and provides a real opportunity for the transformation of children's health services, including a growth in the numbers entering the child health professional workforce (most notably health visitors and midwives). However, it is vital that practitioners understand that the contemporary issues for child health and well-being may require some fundamental changes to patterns of working. These include an increasing requirement to work across professional boundaries and organizations (such as local authorities and the voluntary sector) and the need to ensure that health protection and improvement are part of every contact with children, young people and their families. The strategy also recognizes that there will be some groups of children who will require additional or 'targeted' services to ensure that they achieve good outcomes.

Reflection points

★ How can you support good outcomes for children and young people in your day-to-day practice?

★ How can you demonstrate an outcomes-based approach to the commissioners of your services?

The Children's Plan (Department for Children, Schools and Families 2007) also made a commitment to build on the 'stay safe' outcome and the ensuing *Staying Safe: Action Plan* (HM Government and Department for Children, Schools and Families 2008) is an important sister document to the *Child Health Strategy*. As such, it is essential that children and young people's nurses are familiar with the stated aims and direction. Heralded as the first ever action plan that seeks to improve the safety of children and young people, the action plan aims to reinforce the direction of travel of ensuring better outcomes for children by:

- raising awareness of the importance of safeguarding children and young people
- promoting better understanding of safeguarding issues and encouraging a change in behaviour towards children, young people, their safety and welfare
- ensuring that work in this area is coherent and effectively coordinated across government.

The action plan also outlines the different 'layers' of service provision to ensure children and young people are safeguarded. This is important because it ties in with the notion of universal, targeted and responsive services, as well as the broader definitions of safeguarding detailed above. The document suggests that universal safeguarding includes working to keep all children and young people safe and the creation of 'safe environments' to ensure that this happens. The next layer relates to services and policies that are targeted to groups at higher risk of harm and the final layer is linked to ensuring a prompt response to those children and young people who are suffering from harm. The work of children and young people's nurses touches on all the layers. For example, the work of health visiting teams to support parents in ensuring safe home environments for young children (universal

PART 2

safeguarding); the work of the Family Nurse Partnership programme practitioners with young and vulnerable first-time parents (targeted safeguarding); and the recognition and referral of child maltreatment by a children's emergency department practitioner (responsive safeguarding). The notion of responsive safeguarding can be illustrated by the following case study.

Case study

Ronald, aged 14 weeks, has been brought to the Emergency Department by his parents. His father explains that he has been 'off his feeds' and more sleepy than usual. Your first thought is that Ronald has a mild viral infection. However, when he is undressed to be weighed and examined you notice a small bruise on his upper arm. Mother thinks that he may have rolled onto a small toy.

Reflection points

★ At what age do children roll from front to back or back to front?

★ Why is an understanding of development important for assessment for possible child maltreatment?

★ What is the significance of bruising in a not independently mobile child (see National Collaborating Centre for Women's and Children's Health 2009)?

In keeping with their professional code (Nursing and Midwifery Council 2008) nurses and midwives are accountable for their actions and must do what they can to protect and promote health and well-being. As I have argued elsewhere, there are shared core attributes between nursing and safeguarding. These can be summarized as 'Assessing need and working in partnership with individual children and young people, their families and multi-disciplinary teams to promote physical and emotional well-being and ensure safety' (Powell 2007, pp. 15–16). These attributes, together with the universality of healthcare, mean that children and young people's nurses are well placed to make a major contribution to safeguarding.

The importance of the impact of child maltreatment on childhood morbidity and mortality cannot be overstated. While there may well be evidence that children have never been healthier (Department for Children, Schools and Families and Department of Health 2009), child maltreatment emerges as a 'new morbidity' that is widely unreported yet affects as many as one in 10 of children during the course of their childhood (Gilbert *et al.* 2009) and continues to present a major challenge to the health and well-being of children and young people.[8] This is particularly so for children and young people who are disabled, where the evidence suggests that this group is both at higher risk of maltreatment when compared with their non-disabled peers and less likely to be identified as victims (Murray and Osborne 2009).

Child maltreatment

Child maltreatment is a somewhat difficult concept to define (and measure), not least because of the temporal and cultural aspects that mean that what is, or is not, considered to be harmful to children can vary both over time and between individuals, according to knowledge, beliefs and values (Corby 2006). Some find it easier to consider child maltreatment as part of a spectrum of poor to 'good enough' parenting, whereas others would see a more clear-cut divide between behaviour that is indicative of abuse and behaviour which is not. Context and the longer term effects on the victim are also judged to be an important factor, especially where the nature of maltreatment is reflective of neglect or emotional abuse. Many in the field would have sympathy with what Parton *et al.* (1997) have described as *diagnostic inflation* in recognition that child maltreatment is now usually understood to embrace a more extensive range of behaviours and features than those initially identified (i.e. deliberate and severe physical maltreatment), with typical reference to four key (but not exclusive) categories of physical abuse, sexual abuse, emotional abuse and neglect.

Reflection points

★ Which of the following scenarios could indicate the possibility of child maltreatment?

☆ An expectant mother is smoking small quantities of cannabis.

☆ Timothy's father often tells him that he was not wanted; Timothy has Down's syndrome.

☆ A mother lashes out at her 4 year old who has wet the bed for the third time in three nights. She leaves a small bruise on his back.

☆ Sally, who is HIV positive, is refusing to allow her baby to be tested.

☆ Rosie and John who are 10 and 8 years old are often home before their mother in the evenings.

☆ Jim, aged 12 years, is missing school because he has to help to care for his disabled father.

☆ Tyler, aged 2, has sustained a fractured femur. There appears to be no history of how it happened.

☆ Joshua, aged 5 years, never seems to be appropriately dressed in cold weather.

☆ Usha, aged 14 years, is sleeping with her 19 year old boyfriend.

☆ The parents of Sam, who has cystic fibrosis, have rejected conventional medicine and are treating her with homeopathy.

☆ Abdul, aged 14 months, travels unrestrained in his parents' car. They report that they cannot afford a car seat.

☆ A father insists on tucking up his 7 year old stepdaughter, he says it is their 'special time'.

★ What else would you need to know? In all these cases further information needs to be gathered. The focus of decision-making, however, must always be on the impact on, and perspective of, the child (adapted from Powell 2007).

In England the policy and practice definitions of child maltreatment are set out in the *Working Together* guidance (HM Government 2010). The latest guidance, the fifth since 1988, has built upon previous definitions of the four 'categories' of child maltreatment mentioned above, i.e. physical abuse, emotional abuse, sexual abuse and neglect. Midwives should note that this current edition alludes to maternal substance misuse in pregnancy and neglect. Another new addition is 'overprotection' as a form of emotional abuse; and it is perhaps pertinent here to note that, despite popular opinion to the contrary, the greatest risk of maltreatment (including abduction and murder) is from those related to, or known to, the child. Reference is also made to neglect incorporating 'exclusion from home', reinforcing, perhaps, the enduring nature of parental responsibility until adulthood. The category for physical abuse is seen to include fabricated or induced illness as a form of abuse; this was previously described as Munchausen's syndrome by proxy.

Working Together (HM Government 2010, pp. 38–9) sets out the four categories of maltreatment as follows:

Physical abuse

Physical abuse may involve hitting, shaking, throwing, poisoning, burning or scalding, drowning, suffocating, or otherwise causing physical harm to a child. Physical harm may also be caused when a parent or carer fabricates the symptoms of, or deliberately induces, illness in a child.

Emotional abuse

Emotional abuse is the persistent emotional maltreatment of a child such as to cause severe and persistent adverse effects on the child's emotional development. It may involve conveying to children that they are worthless or unloved, inadequate, or valued only insofar as they meet the needs of another person. It may include not giving the child opportunities to express their views, deliberately silencing them or 'making fun' of what they say or how they communicate. It may feature age or developmentally inappropriate expectations being imposed on children. These may include interactions that are beyond the child's developmental capability, as well as overprotection and limitation of exploration and learning, or preventing the child participating in normal social interaction. It may involve seeing or hearing the ill-treatment of another. It may involve serious bullying (including cyberbullying), causing children frequently to feel frightened or in danger, or the exploitation or corruption of children. Some level of emotional abuse is involved in all types of maltreatment of a child, though it may occur alone.

Sexual abuse

Sexual abuse involves forcing or enticing a child or young person to take part in sexual activities, not necessarily involving a high level of violence, whether or not the child is aware of what is happening. The activities may involve physical contact, including assault by penetration (for example, rape or oral sex) or non-penetrative acts such as masturbation, kissing, rubbing and touching outside of clothing. They may also include non-contact activities, such as involving children in looking at, or in the production of, sexual images, watching sexual activities, encouraging children to behave in sexually inappropriate ways, or grooming a child in preparation for abuse (including via the internet). Sexual abuse is not solely perpetrated by adult males. Women can also commit acts of sexual abuse, as can other children.

Neglect

Neglect is the persistent failure to meet a child's basic physical and/or psychological needs, likely to result in the serious impairment of the child's health or development. Neglect may occur during pregnancy as a result of maternal substance abuse. Once a child is born, neglect may involve a parent or carer failing to:

- *provide adequate food, clothing and shelter (including exclusion from home or abandonment);*
- *protect a child from physical and emotional harm or danger;*
- *ensure adequate supervision (including the use of inadequate care-givers); or*
- *ensure access to appropriate medical care or treatment.*

It may also include neglect of, or unresponsiveness to, a child's basic emotional needs.

The significance of these definitions lies in their use within statutory safeguarding children procedures. Children and young people's nurses may be invited to make a contribution to a Child Protection Conference where a multiagency decision has to be made on whether or not a child (or children) should be subject to a Child Protection Plan, and if so what 'category' of abuse the child is at risk of, or has suffered from. It is thus important to have a working knowledge of the definitions provided for each category.

This first section of the chapter has considered the principles for safeguarding children practice. The principles for practice below summarize the learning thus far. The following section will add to the knowledge base for successful safeguarding children practice by exploring the learning from serious case reviews and includes reference to the cases of Victoria Climbié and Peter Connelly.

Principles for practice

- Children and young people's nurses can make a vital contribution to safeguarding children through universal, targeted and responsive services.
- Child maltreatment can be described as reflecting neglect, physical, sexual and emotional abuse, and includes fabricated or induced illness.

Learning from child maltreatment deaths

The death of a child or young person from maltreatment is a rare and tragic event that will always raise questions of preventability. The true incidence of child death from abuse or neglect remains unknown. The ways in which child deaths are classified, as well as difficulties of definition and reporting, make an assessment of accurate figures for children and young people who die from maltreatment very challenging. The National Society for the Prevention of Cruelty to Children (NSPCC) provides a helpful explanation of how child maltreatment death statistics are gathered, and have recently updated their information. They have considered the serious childcare incidents that are reported to Ofsted and currently suggest that up to four children die as a result of maltreatment each week in England and Wales; previously, they have been of the opinion that the number is one or two per week. The NSPCC also considers a possibility that ascertaining the figures may improve (and thus figures rise further) with the introduction of new child death review processes (see below). The NSPCC also notes that the risk of death from child maltreatment is greatest for younger children, especially those less than 1 year old, owing to their greater physical and developmental vulnerability. Parents, or those known to the child, are responsible for the majority of these deaths, and the younger the child the more likely it is that this will be the case. Despite a commonly held viewpoint, the NSPCC reports that the recorded numbers of children who die from abuse have remained broadly similar since the 1970s. The remainder of this section introduces the new child death review processes in England, the serious case review processes and the learning from biennial analyses of serious case reviews. It then considers some of the learning from the two most highly publicized and influential reviews of child deaths from maltreatment in modern times – Victoria Climbié and Peter Connelly.

Child death review processes

The *Working Together* (HM Government 2010) guidance now requires Local Safeguarding Children Boards to set up processes to review all childhood deaths, both expected and unexpected, that occur in each local authority area. The processes are outlined in Chapter 7 of the document and, in summary, include a 'rapid response' to unexpected deaths and the setting up of local Child Death Overview Panels to review all deaths. Children and young people's nurses need to be familiar with the aims and objectives of these processes, as it is highly likely that they will both be in a position to make a notification to a local Child Death Overview Panel coordinator and be approached to contribute case information to inform the Panel's work. Although these new processes are essentially a public health exercise and reflect the broader definitions of safeguarding outlined at the beginning of this chapter, there is also the opportunity to improve the ascertainment of child deaths from maltreatment. Work with 'early starters' and a review of the literature on the work of established panels (largely from the USA) has demonstrated how these processes have a potential to lead to improvements in child health and services to children, young people and their families, the prevention of future deaths and better bereavement care (Sidebotham *et al.* 2008).

Reflection point

★ Jenny and Isaac (2006, p. 265) note that 'The death of a child is a sentinel event in a community, and a defining marker of a society's policies of safety and health.' Discuss this statement with a professional colleague. What may change as a result of an untimely death of a child or young person?

Serious case review

When a child or young person dies and maltreatment is known or suspected, a local serious case review (SCR) may be commissioned by the Local Safeguarding Children

Board. This will consider lessons to be learned about the ways in which agencies and organizations work together to safeguard and promote the welfare of children, and to help to prevent similar tragedies in the future. The SCR process is detailed in Chapter 8 of *Working Together* (HM Government 2010); hence, these reviews are sometimes known as 'Part 8' reviews or inquiries.

Child health nursing professionals may be invited to make a contribution to SCRs and should be appropriately supported by their safeguarding children leads (usually the named and designated professionals) during the process. This includes being given full explanation of the need to 'secure records' and receiving feedback on their contribution and the recommendations that arise. SCR reports comprise individual management reviews from each agency (widely referred to as IMRs), an overview report (written by an independent author who is an expert in the field) and an executive summary, which is published (suitably anonymized) by Local Safeguarding Children Boards (typically on their website).

There is an expectation that a number of recommendations will be made and these are then translated into action plans, which will be closely monitored and scrutinized. An important recent finding is that practitioners do not feel as adequately involved as could be expected in the dissemination of learning from reviews (Brandon *et al.* 2009). Although the aims of the serious case review process are to prevent future tragedies and seek improvements in practice, there is an ever-present danger that the focus on SCR and 'what went wrong' can detract from learning lessons from the vast majority of safeguarding cases where daily improvements are being made to the lives, and the life chances, of some of our most vulnerable children, young people and their families, often in very challenging circumstances.

National overviews

The Department for Children, Schools and Families commissions biennial analyses of serious case reviews from across England, and these reports are highly influential in safeguarding policy and practice. Brandon *et al.* (2009) in the fourth biennial analysis, which examined 189 serious case reviews, demonstrate the complexities and challenges of working with families where there are multiple risk factors. This includes the reality that safeguarding children professionals will be working with many families who are either difficult to engage with or who act with disguised compliance. The demographics of the children who were the subject of the reviews point to the risks to very young children; two-thirds of the children were aged less than 5 years, and nearly half were under the age of 1 year, although there was also a subgroup of adolescents. Two-thirds of the cases involved child deaths, including, for the older age group, death by suicide. The majority of families lived in poor conditions, and had little family support. The issue of neglect was extremely common, and in the 17% of children who were subject to a child protection plan at the time of the incident, neglect was the most common reason for a plan to be in place. Three parental issues were frequently noted in these families and often coexisted: a history of domestic abuse, substance misuse and past or present adult mental health problems. Importantly, feeling overwhelmed was an emotion seen in both the parents and those whose role it was to protect the children. The case for high-quality support and supervision is self-evident.

The biennial analyses are of critical importance to children and young people's nurses because they can help to feed into a range of preventative actions that can better support children, young people and their families. They also help to inform areas of practice improvement and allocation of resources to address issues of inequality and access to services. Importantly, the reports reinforce the need to ensure that safeguarding children is seen as an important area for practice not only for child health but also for those working in services for vulnerable adults including adult mental health and substance misuse services. In addition to learning from the national biennial analyses of serious case reviews, children and young people's nurses should also have an understanding of the two high-profile child maltreatment deaths of recent times. An outline of these is given below.

Victoria Climbié

Victoria Adjo Climbié was born on the Ivory Coast on 2 November 1991. She was said to be a lovable and intelligent child who, in 1998, was taken by a great aunt to France, and then to England, to ensure that she had access to a good education and better opportunities for the future. What followed was an almost unbelievable sequence of escalating violence and maltreatment that led to her death on 25 February 2000, at 8 years of age. Her postmortem was undertaken by a Home Office pathologist, who described this as the 'worse case [of child abuse] he had ever dealt with … or heard of' (House of Commons Health Committee 2003, p. 1). A total of 128 separate injuries were found on her body. Victoria had been beaten with implements such as shoes, football boots, a coat hanger, a wooden cooking spoon and a bicycle chain. Furthermore, she was also said to have spent long periods of time tied up in a bin-bag, covered in urine and faeces and made to eat left-over food off a piece of plastic 'like a dog'. When Victoria was admitted to hospital in a moribund condition she was found to be bruised, deformed, hypothermic and malnourished. Kouao (the great aunt) and Manning (a boyfriend of the aunt) were both given life sentences for her murder.

The report of Lord Laming's Inquiry into the death of Victoria Climbié makes distressing reading, both in terms of the details of the appalling maltreatment she suffered and because it highlights the missed opportunities that a variety of agencies had to intervene. Laming described the extent of failures in the child protection system as 'lamentable' (p. 3). Victoria was seen at a general practice and admitted to two different hospitals; the first time because of concerns about various cuts and marks on her face and hands, and the second time following a scald to her face. The second admission was for nearly 2 weeks. In addition to the contact with statutory agencies (including health, social care and housing), she was seen from time to time by distant relatives and also members of the church. For a brief period of time Victoria was also cared for by a child-minder; however, she did not attend school. It is fair to report that the possibilities of child maltreatment were raised by individual health professionals during both hospital admissions. However, as the inquiry into her death noted:

> *The concerns that medical and nursing staff at the hospital told me [Laming]*
> *that they felt about Victoria never, in my view, crystallised into anything*
> *resembling a clear, well-thought-through picture of what they suspected had*

happened to her and that would have helped social services in determining how best to deal with her case.

(House of Commons Health Committee 2003, p. 274)

A number of children and young people's nurses were called to give evidence to the inquiry panel. Here they reported observing (although not documenting) indicators of physical abuse. These included lesions that they later considered to be indicative of intentional harm, such as burns, belt marks and bites. As worrying were their reports of witnessing Victoria's demeanour in the presence of Kouao and Manning. This was described as a 'master and servant' relationship. The Inquiry made a number of recommendations for health services, including the need for good record-keeping; the reconciliation of differences of opinion; proper planning for discharge; and arrangements for follow-up. A particularly challenging finding was the lack of opportunity for Victoria to communicate what was happening to her, and in reading the report it is clear that 'adult-centric' needs (e.g. for housing) took priority over the needs and wishes of this tragic child.

As indicated earlier, the case of Victoria Climbié has been instrumental in changing policy and practice in safeguarding children. The Victoria Climbié Foundation, which campaigned to support these changes, has opened a school in Victoria's memory in her home village of Abobo. Their website (http://www.victoria-climbie.org.uk) usefully provides links to the Inquiry Report and recommendations and subsequent key safeguarding policy documents.

Reflection points

★ How would you respond if you discovered unexplained injuries on a child?

★ To whom would you report?

★ How would you document your findings and your actions?

Peter Connelly

In May 2009, following the sentencing of his mother, mother's boyfriend and another male, for causing or allowing his death, Haringey Local Safeguarding Children Board published the Executive Summary of a serious case review of a child who had become known via the media as 'Baby P' or 'Baby Peter'. This contains details about the case, an exploration of how agencies worked together and a series of recommendations for improving practice. In addition to the serious case review, the Care Quality Commission (2009) has undertaken a review of the health services provided to Baby Peter and his family. Both documents are easily accessible and recommended reading.

Peter Connelly was born on 1 March 2006 and died on 3 August 2007, aged just 17 months. At the time of his death he was subject to a child protection plan following a series of injuries suggestive of physical abuse. He had also been failing to thrive and showing evidence of neglect. The postmortem revealed that Peter had bruising to his body, a torn frenulum and had swallowed a tooth (which was lodged in his colon). He had eight fractured ribs and a fractured spine. The provisional cause of death was given as a fracture/dislocation of the thoracolumbar spine (Haringey Local Safeguarding Children Board 2009). The Executive Summary contains some important messages for practice. Notably agencies were found to have low expectations and too low a level of concern for this family. A significant deficit was a failure to establish who was living in the household and what their relationships were. Concerns were expressed about the dangers of an unrelated man joining such a vulnerable single parent family. A number of assumptions were made by professionals that others were taking action in relation to the safeguarding needs. This led to missed opportunities to intervene. As the author suggests, 'It is simpler to lift the telephone than to live with the regret of not having done so' (p. 21).

The Care Quality Commission made five recommendations to health trusts. One recommendation was specific to one of the trusts involved in the case, but the others hold important messages for child health services. These relate to the need to ensure that health staff are clear about procedures and have been trained in safeguarding; that there are a sufficient number of appropriately qualified paediatric staff available when required; that there is a need to establish clear communication and working arrangements with relevant children's social care services and a requirement for boards to ensure that arrangements are in place for safeguarding supervision; attendance at child protection conferences and training; and that assurance on core standards can be provided (Care Quality Commission 2009).

As with Victoria Climbié, the case has led to a review of safeguarding children systems and processes. Lord Laming was invited to review progress made since he led and reported on the Public Inquiry into Victoria's death (Laming 2009). His report and recommendations have been accepted by the government. Lessons from the report will help to inform the final section of this chapter: achieving excellence in safeguarding children practice.

Key points

- One to four children die as a result of child maltreatment each week in England and Wales.
- The highest risk of fatal maltreatment is in infants and younger children. Most deaths are caused by parents, or those known to the child.
- New child death review processes reflect the broader definitions of safeguarding and provide an additional opportunity to improve the ascertainment of child deaths from maltreatment.
- Serious case reviews consider lessons to be learned about the ways in which agencies and organizations work together to safeguard and promote the welfare of children.
- Parental issues such as domestic abuse, substance misuse and mental health problems are important risks to children.
- The need to listen to children's views and wishes and have a child-centred approach to assessment is key.

Achieving excellence in safeguarding children practice

This chapter concludes with some messages to help children and young people's nurses to achieve excellence in safeguarding children practice. We begin with four key messages from Laming's (2009) review of safeguarding children. These are crucial messages and a very important aspect of the ability to deliver excellence:

- Put yourself in the place of the child and consider first and foremost how the situation must feel for them.
- Be aware of how easy it is to find yourself justifying and reassuring yourself that all is well, rather than taking a more objective consideration of what has occurred.
- Recognize that sympathy for the parents can lead to your expectations of their parenting being set too low.
- Remember that whatever role you have (i.e. working with the child or their parents/carers or as a member of the public) be clear that it is not acceptable to do nothing when a child may be in need of help.

These messages are at the heart of keeping children safe and should inform every contact with a child, young person and their family. Importantly, where concerns are emerging, there will be a need for those working with families to offer early help and support in a coordinated way. The *Every Child Matters* (HM Government 2004) policy promotes the notion of 'integrated working' to achieve better outcomes for children. This means that more than ever before it is important to ensure that services work with children and families in a 'joined up' way. The Common Assessment Framework can help to ensure targeted support to those families who need extra help.

The Common Assessment Framework

The Common Assessment Framework (or 'CAF') has been developed to ensure that the estimated 20–30% of children who have 'additional needs' receive timely support. The CAF is a shared assessment and planning framework that can be used across all children's services. It aims to help the early identification of additional needs and promote coordinated service provision to meet them. This process is managed by a 'lead professional' from one of the agencies who will work with the multiagency 'team around the child'. Children and young people's nurses are often ideally placed to undertake this role. Needs are assessed in relation to three domains of 'child', 'parents and carers' and 'family and environment'. 'Additional needs' may include risk factors for child maltreatment, and input at an early stage can reduce the risk of children being harmed – it may even save a child's life. However, where there are clear concerns about risk of, or actual, child maltreatment then practitioners need to be confident about both recognizing these and responding proactively.

Recognizing and responding to child maltreatment

In my experience children and young people's nurses and others working in health services are both well placed and well able to recognize children and young people who are at risk of, or suffering from, child maltreatment. There is a wealth of research and literature in the field that helps with the identification of child abuse and neglect, and many of you will be aware of the 'signs and symptoms'. The National Institute for Health and Clinical Excellence recently published clinical guidance on child maltreatment (National Collaborating Centre for Women's and Children's Health 2009). In addition to outlining the key health indicators of physical and sexual abuse, neglect and emotional abuse, the document also provides information on when to consider or suspect fabricated or induced illness and concludes with a useful section on harmful parent–child interactions.

However, there are acknowledged and important barriers to recognizing and responding to child maltreatment. These have been usefully summarized in a toolkit from the Royal College of General Practitioners and the NSPCC (2007). This highlights some of the barriers already mentioned in this chapter, such as the hidden nature of harm, the tendency for the child's needs to be overshadowed by those of the parents and the difficulties in taking an objective view. In addition, the toolkit also mentions the impact of the upsetting nature of child abuse, the feelings of a betrayal of the trust held in therapeutic relationships with the family and the practicalities and challenges of inter-agency working.

Good practice in safeguarding children reflects the importance of child-centred assessment, keeping clear and contemporaneous records in which you record your observations and what you have been told, by whom, and when and why this is of concern. There is no expectation that all practitioners should be experts on 'signs and symptoms' of child abuse and neglect, but it is crucially important to seek advice and support if you are worried about a child or young person. In many cases reviewing the concerns, together with child/young person and family information that may be known by other professionals, will help to build a picture that can more accurately determine whether or not a child/young person is at risk of harm. An understanding of the context of normal child care and development is particularly helpful and you have a head start in this respect!

Concerns about the safety and welfare of a child or young person should always be shared. In this respect it is important to avoid making a promise of confidentiality to a child or young person and to be clear with them on the need to share the concerns. A decision may be made to refer the child to children's social care for further assessment of need. Healthcare organizations will have internal procedures, which are in line with Local Safeguarding Children Board procedures and reflect *Working Together* guidance. It is important to understand how the statutory processes operate in your local area and to seek opportunities to attend inter-agency training and development events.

Children and young people's nurses may be asked to contribute their expertise to the assessment and planning for the child's future safety. Children's social care, which, with the police, is the lead agency in any child protection enquiries, may decide to convene an early 'strategy discussion', normally involving the referring agency and the police. Further enquiries may take place prior to a multiagency child protection conference, which may result in putting in place a 'child protection plan' to address concerns of risk of harm. Health professionals play a crucial role in contributing to child protection (or 's47') enquiries and child protection conferences. This will include the provision of a written report, which will normally be shared with parents in advance of the conference.

Reflection point

How may clinical supervision help to overcome some of the barriers listed above?

Reflection point

Do you know how to access your safeguarding leads for advice and support on the referral process?

Information sharing

If you are worried about a child, it is crucially important to be open and honest with parents, and, where age-appropriate, the child or young person, as to the nature of your concerns and the need to involve other agencies, unless to do so would place the child or others at greater risk. The vast majority of children who are subject to a child protection plan will remain in the family home and parents have the key role and responsibility for ensuring their future protection from harm. This means that they need to be fully involved in the process. There are now excellent guidelines available to help practitioners understand when and how to share information. The guidelines include the 'seven golden rules' for information sharing, which can readily be downloaded in a pocket-sized guide (see the list of Further Reading on p. 150). An important aspect is that, when possible, consent should be sought if you wish to share information with others. However, the notion of 'public interest' means that you can share information without consent if you make a balanced professional judgement that this is necessary to protect an individual, promote their well-being or prevent a crime. You will need to document your decision and the rationale for it.

This section has outlined the key aspects of achieving excellence in safeguarding children practice. Where possible children and young people's nurses should seek to intervene at an early stage to ensure additional help for children, young people and their families, and the CAF is an excellent tool to facilitate this. However, where there are concerns of a risk of, or actual, child maltreatment then it is important to make a referral to children's social care and to ensure that you are content with the actions that follow (escalating any continuing concerns to safeguarding leads (named or designated professionals)). The collaboration and contribution of children and young people's nurses to child protection plans and review conferences, together with the delivery of high standards of healthcare to the child, young person and their family, are an essential part of the protective net. This will deliver excellence. And as was noted at the outset of this chapter, this work can be highly rewarding.

Principles for practice

- Laming's (2009) four key messages are at the heart of keeping children safe and should inform every contact with a child, young person and their family.
- The Common Assessment Framework (CAF) can help to ensure targeted support to those families who need extra help.
- Children and young people's nurses are both well placed and well able to recognize children and young people who are at risk of, or suffering from, child maltreatment.
- It is important to understand how statutory child protection processes operate in your local area and to seek opportunities to attend inter-agency training and development events.
- Although it is good practice to seek consent to share information, 'public interest' means that you can share information without consent if you make a balanced professional judgement that this is necessary to protect an individual, promote their well-being or prevent a crime.
- Safeguarding children work can be highly rewarding.

Conclusion

This chapter has sought to introduce the challenging and emotive area of safeguarding children practice. Children and young people's nurses as well as other health and social care nursing practitioners can make a major contribution to the prevention and detection of children and young people at risk of, or suffering from, child maltreatment. While fatal maltreatment is rare, lessons from serious case reviews have played an important part in the development of policy and practice in the field. Provision of support with the challenges of parenting and openness and honesty with parents when there are concerns are vital. However, above all, it is crucial to ensure that assessment and delivery of care is centred on the well-being and interests of the child and their daily 'lived experiences'; this is the best way to ensure that they are healthy and safe and achieve optimum outcomes into adulthood.

Summary of principles for practice

- Children and young people's nurses have a responsibility to ensure that every child and young person is safeguarded in practice.
- Children and young people's nurses must be knowledgeable about maltreatment in all its forms.
- Children and young people's nurses have a duty to report any suspected case of maltreatment.
- Children and young people's nurses must always act in the interests of the child or young person.

Further reading

These websites give more background on some of the topics covered in this chapter:
- The Children Are Unbeatable! Alliance campaigns for the UK to satisfy human rights obligations by modernising the law on assault to give children the same protection as adults. http://www.childrenareunbeatable.org.uk
- For information about initiatives similar to Every Child Matters in Wales, Scotland and Northern Ireland, see http://www.ncb.org.uk/about_us/partnerships/4_nations_child_policy.aspx
- For details of the Family Nurse Partnership programme, see http://www.dcsf.gov.uk/everychildmatters/strategy/parents/healthledsupport/healthledsupport/
- The Lancet Series on Child Maltreatment (2008–9) offers an excellent range of papers summarizing current evidence (including statistics) and conceptual issues. http://www.thelancet.com/series/child-maltreatment
- Download the pocket-sized version of the guidelines on information sharing from: http://www.dcsf.gov.uk/everychildmatters/resources-and-practice/IG00340/
- The NSPCC campaigns to end child cruelty. The website gives statistics on child death and injuries and how these figures are gathered. http://www.nspcc.org.uk

References

Archard D (2004) *Children: Rights and Childhood.* London: Routledge.

Brandon M, Bailey S, Belderson P, *et al.* (2009) *Understanding serious case reviews and their impact: a biennial analysis of serious case reviews 2005-07.* London: Department for Children, Schools and Families.

Care Quality Commission (2009) *Review of the involvement and action taken by health bodies in relation to the case of Baby P.* London: CQC.

Children and Young People's Unit (2009) *Safeguarding children: a cross-departmental statement on the protection of children and young people.* Belfast: Office of the First Minister and Deputy First Minister. Northern Ireland.

Commission for Social Care Inspection, Her Majesty's Chief Inspector of Schools, Her Majesty's Chief Inspector of Court Administration, *et al.* (2005) *Safeguarding children: the Second Joint Chief Inspectors' Report on Arrangements to Safeguard Children.* London: Commission for Social Care Inspection.

Corby B (2006) *Child abuse: towards a knowledge base*, 3rd edn. Maidenhead: Open University Press.

Department for Children, Schools and Families (2007) *The Children's Plan: building brighter futures*. London: DCSF and Department of Health.

Department for Children, Schools and Families, Department of Health (2009) *Healthy lives, brighter futures: the strategy for children and young people's health*. London: DCSF and DH.

Department of Health (2003) *Getting the right start: national service framework for children– standard for hospital services*. London: DH.

Department of Health, Department for Education and Skills (2004) *National service framework for children, young people and maternity services: core standards*. London: DH.

Gilbert R, Kemp A, Thoburn J, *et al.* (2009) Recognising and responding to child maltreatment. *The Lancet* **373**(9658): 167–80. (doi:10.1016/S0140-6736(08)61707-9)

Hall D (2003) Protecting children, supporting professionals. *Archives of Disease in Childhood* **88**: 557–9.

Haringey Local Safeguarding Children Board (2009) *Serious case review: Baby Peter*. See www.haringeylscb.org/executive_summary_peter_final.pdf

HM Government (2004) *Every child matters: change for children*. London: Department for Education and Skills.

HM Government (2010) *Working together to safeguard children: a guide to inter-agency working to safeguard and promote the welfare of children*. London: Department for Children, Schools and Families.

HM Government, Department for Children, Schools and Families (2008) *Staying safe: action plan*. London: DCSF.

House of Commons Health Committee (2003) *The Victoria Climbié Inquiry Report (Laming Report)*. London: The Stationery Office.

Jenny C, Isaac R (2006) The relationship between child death and child maltreatment. *Archives of Disease in Childhood* **91**: 265–9.

Laming, Lord (2009) *The protection of children in England: a progress report*. London: The Stationery Office.

Layard R, Dunn J (2009) *A good childhood: searching for values in a competitive age*. London: The Children's Society.

Murray, M, Osborne C (2009) *Safeguarding disabled children: practice guidance*. London: Department for Education and Skills.

National Collaborating Centre for Women's and Children's Health (commissioned by the National Institute for Health and Clinical Excellence) (2009) *When to suspect child maltreatment*. London: RCOG Press.

Nursing and Midwifery Council (2008) *The code: standards of conduct, performance and ethics*. London: NMC.

Office of Public Sector Information (2004) *The Children Act*. London: OPSI. See http://www.opsi.gov.uk/acts/acts2004/ukpga_20040031_en_1

Office of the Children's Commissioner (2007) *Pushed into the shadows: young people's experience of adult mental health facilities*. London: The Children's Commissioner for England. See http://www.11million.org.uk/resource/m8vtedhs9cbqx3aid5stkdrk.pdf

Parton N, Thorpe D, Wattam C (1997) *Child protection, risk and the moral order*. Basingstoke: Macmillan.

Powell C (2004) Why nurses should support the 'Children are unbeatable!' Alliance. *Paediatric Nursing* **16**(8): 29.

Powell C (2007) *Safeguarding children and young people: a guide for nurses and midwives*. Maidenhead: Open University Press.

Royal College of General Practitioners, NSPCC (2007) *Safeguarding children and young people in general practice: a toolkit*. London: RCGP.

Sidebotham P, Fox J, Horwath J, *et al.* (2008) *Preventing childhood deaths: a study of 'early starter' child death overview panels in England*. London: Department for Children, Schools and Families.

The Children's Society (2006) *The good childhood: A National Inquiry*. London: The Children's Society.

The Lancet Series on Child Maltreatment (2008–9) See http://www.thelancet.com/series/child-maltreatment

The Scottish Office (undated) *Protecting children: a shared responsibility: guidance on inter-agency co-operation*. See http://www.scotland.gov.uk/library/documents-w3/pch-02.htm

United Nations (1989) *Convention on the Rights of the Child*. Adopted under General Assembly resolution 44/25. Geneva: UN.

Welsh Assembly Government (2006) *Working together under the Children Act 2004*. Cardiff: Welsh Assembly Government.

Whiting L, Whiting M, Whiting T (2004) Smacking: a family perspective. *Paediatric Nursing* **16**(8): 26–8.

Chapter 6

The use of restraint

Sally Williams

Overview

This chapter will discuss fundamental issues surrounding the use of restraint on children and young people and will touch on the complex moral, legal and ethical components associated with this. As will be shown, this is an issue that affects all those working with children and young people across a range of clinical settings and has sadly resulted in a number of deaths. Reference will also be made to the use of physical restraint across a range of settings, including remand centres, psychiatric units and acute hospitals, given that children's nurses may also practise in these areas. The lack of research into the use of restraint will also be highlighted and the consequences discussed. The chapter concludes that there is a need for national policy and guidelines for the use of physical restraint in children and young people (United Nations 1989), criminal law and not least nurses' own professional code of conduct (Nursing and Midwifery Council 2008). The case for this and training and education for all those involved in physical restraint is also put forward, as is the need for further research in this under-researched area of practice.

Defining restraint

The use and interpretation of what constitutes 'restraint' with patients/clients differs according to the type or remit of the clinical area. The term may be applied in mental healthcare settings to describe a several person 'pin down' strategy used to contain a violent patient, whereas in the care of the older person the literature describes the restraint of stroke patients when bed rails are applied to prevent the patient from falling out of bed. Therefore, it could be considered useful to analyse several definitions of 'restraint' and to consider these definitions as to their appropriateness for use within children and young people's nursing. Within children and young people's nursing healthcare professionals refer to the use of restraint specifically for the facilitation of clinical procedures, which would predominantly occur within an acute children's ward or generic care area such as the Emergency Department.

The *Oxford Concise English Dictionary* (1995) defines 'restrain' as to 'check or hold in; keep in check or under control or within bounds'.

This definition gives the reader the image of the maintenance of some sort of predetermined normality, yet also implies some use of force to suppress what might happen if the object were not restrained, i.e. a loss of control. The definition goes some way to recognizing that there may be a 'need' to restrain, suggesting a rationale for its use. This has some relevance in the use of restraint of a person, where there has to be a morally acceptable rationale and the purpose for use deemed 'necessary' in order to achieve some justifiable goal.

Within a care context, several definitions have been suggested, many of which have been developed from a psychiatric or penal basis. This could be a reflection on the lack of suitable research and literature into the subject of restraint by caring professions themselves. The lack of a unique body of literature regarding restraint within the field of nursing has led to the improvisation of alternative definitions being used. Wright (1999) suggests that:

> *… physical restraint implies the violation of other socially and professionally valued aspects of the helping relationship, such as the promotion of the client's dignity, autonomy and self determination, even if it is to preserve life and prevent suffering after other means of stopping the dangerous behaviour have failed.*

(Wright 1999, p. 462)

This definition identifies the difficult dichotomy of roles for caring staff which exist in many care settings. Many of the fundamental principles that nursing staff expressly herald as pivotal within the professional code of conduct (Nursing and Midwifery Council 2008) are in essence violated in many instances of care, where the rationale for such actions usually is supported by the premise that the member of staff is acting in accordance with prescribed medical care in ensuring that the best interests of the patient or client are served. This is further complicated in child health and children and young people's nursing where the majority of patients have

Case study

Thomas, a 3 year old boy, is admitted to hospital with suspected septicaemia. He is pale, lethargic and appears generally very unwell. The advanced nurse practitioner assesses Thomas and recognizes that intravenous access, bloods and cannulation are immediately necessary. Topical anaesthetic creams such as Ametop and Emla would normally be applied prior to cannulation or venepuncture of a child, to help minimize the pain experienced during the procedure. These creams take between 20 and 60 minutes to produce an effective topical anaesthetic response. Owing to a lack of time and the seriousness of the child's condition the paediatric nurse present during the admission procedure restrains Thomas by holding his arm firmly. This allows the nurse practitioner to safely and successfully perform the intravenous cannulation. Thomas would undoubtedly struggle during the experience as a result of the increased pain, and his inability to cognitively understand the necessity of the procedure and thus cooperate by keeping still. However, in this situation it is seen as 'in the best interests of the child' to immediately treat such a serious suspected infection; therefore, the use of restraint is deemed necessary and justified.

an altered view of what is in their best interests, according to their age and development. A child and young person's cognitive stage has a huge impact on their ability to understand the rationale for many medical and nursing procedures, many of which can cause pain and discomfort; for example, venepuncture and cannulation, which are often essential for the accurate diagnosis and treatment of an infection. As the case study on p. 153 demonstrates, in emergency situations children and young people's nursing staff may need to use restraint to ensure the safety of a child or young person during a necessary procedure.

In this respect Healy's (1997) definition of restraint may also be considered pertinent within a nursing context:

> *Restraint occurs whenever a client has his or her movement physically restricted by the use of intentional force by a member of staff. Restraint can be partial; restricting and preventing a particular movement; or total; as in the case of immobilisation.*

(Healy 1997, p. 8)

Many clinical interventions use only partial restraint for older children, whose cognitive development and understanding would enable some appreciation of the purpose of the intervention. The older child would generally be encouraged to collaborate with the nursing staff, allowing consent to be gained and therefore minimal restraint to be used.

However, as already identified in the above case study the degree of cooperation and compliance is drastically reduced in children under the age of 5 who may require total immobilization to allow clinical interventions. This is usually undertaken in conjunction with the parents or primary care giver, who would assist the nursing staff in actively restraining the child.

Within the literature reviewed the terms restraint and 'holding still' may be used to describe the necessary restraint of a child or young person. The Department of Health (1995) and the Royal College of Nursing (1999) provide some clarity on the differentiation between these two terms. Physical restraint is defined in terms of a minimum force necessary to overpower a child/young person with a guiding rationale of preventing the child/young person from harming themselves or others or from causing serious damage to property. In contrast, 'holding still' is identified as using necessary force to ensure the safety of a child/young person throughout a clinical procedure. This may not require the 'overpowering' of the child in totality, merely the restraint of only part of the child/young person's body. The Royal College of Nursing (1999) goes further to suggest that, essentially, the difference is related to the degree of force the nurse uses, as well as the intention of the nurse.

Therefore, for restraint to be justified in a children and young people's nursing context the nurse would have to use restraint for the purpose of holding a child still, with clearly identifiable intentions, which would be supported by the minimal use of force required for the intervention to be both successfully and safely performed. However, as recognized by Wright's (1999) definition, there are issues of violation of the 'helping relationship' which conflict with a nurse's ability to respect the child or young person's autonomy and self-determination. The act of restraint could therefore prove emotionally difficult for the nurse involved, even when the above criteria, the purpose and intention of the restraint, are clearly defined.

The term 'restraint' will be used throughout this chapter, and is intended to encompass the practices of what is also described in the literature as 'holding still', 'immobilizing' and 'clinical holding'.

Principles for practice

- The use, interpretation and definition of restraint within paediatric nursing vary. Other terms for restraint may include 'holding still', 'immobilizing' and 'clinical holding'.
- The physical restraint of children and young people may be justified in clinical practice, but on a case-by-case basis.
- The use of restraint by children and young people's nurses must involve clearly identified intentions supported by the use of minimal force.

The use of restraint across the clinical spectrum

The use of restraint in other areas of nursing is well documented. The fields of both adult psychiatry and care of the older person describe the difficulties associated with the use of restraint in a practical care context, acknowledging both the physical problems associated with restraint (Molassiotis 1995; Bell J 1997) and the potential psychological effects on the patient (Gallinagh *et al.* 2001). Patients were identified as feeling a sense of entrapment, and they described a loss of autonomy and felt controlled by the nursing staff who used restraint habitually on the ward. These detrimental effects on the psychosocial well-being of the patients are further compounded by physical problems identified by Molassiotis (1995), which include contractures of major joints of locomotion, oedema of lower extremities, pressure sores, changes to bone demineralization and electrolyte loss. Although these studies relate to adult patients, the consequences of restraint may be equally applicable to children and young people.

The issue of restraint clearly extends beyond the UK and has international implications. Cleary (2001) acknowledges the commonplace use of restraint in healthcare facilities in the USA, highlighting concerns over the lack of research supporting the efficacy of physical restraints in maintaining the safety of patients. Cleary (2001) suggests that the increasing development of legislation to protect patients' rights has been promoted as concern for the use of restraint among the elderly population is raised; in the context of this chapter, this is also relevant to children and young people. These changing trends are recognized and supported by other authors (Stilwell 1991; Tinetti *et al.* 1992; Mason *et al.* 1995). Cleary (2001) also identifies the role of individual members of the multidisciplinary team in considering the ethical and legal implications of using any prescribed restraint in practice.

There are clearly parallels to be drawn from the use of restraints in elderly care and in paediatrics. Although at differing ends of a chronological spectrum the loss of autonomy which exists within elderly patients with dementia often results in regression and inappropriate behaviour that cannot be reasoned with. This lack of understanding, abnormal actions and limited cognitive ability can cause an adult to display similar types of characteristics to a young child whose ability to comprehend context is limited to their own particular perception of the world. Both of these age groups become disempowered and lack the status and political leverage of the majority of the adult population. The public perception of the appropriateness of overpowering and controlling behaviour through restraint appears more socially acceptable than if nurses chose, for example, to restrain a normally functioning adult without any deficit in understanding. This would be regarded as a serious assault, as opposed to a necessary restraint.

Bell (Bell J 1997) concludes that restraint in care of the elderly has not been properly evaluated, nor have its full moral or legal implications been considered. The same criticism may be applied to children and young people's nursing practice and other settings where children and young people are cared for.

There is, however, a growing body of evidence that suggests that there are successful alternatives available in elderly care, which could be used in clinical practice, to reduce the need for restraint (Royal College of Nursing 1992; Molassiotis 1995; Bell J 1997). These can be differentiated into broadly two different categories: psychological approaches, such as reminiscence therapy, and environmental controls, e.g. electronic tagging and video monitoring. It has been suggested that these techniques could be easily incorporated into clinical areas through adequate staff training and education (Robbins 1986; Stilwell 1991; Royal College of Nursing 1992). The call for the use of alternatives to restraint is echoed in children and young people's nursing. This suggests that the nursing profession as a whole is beginning to question the routine use of restraint throughout practice and engaging in the process of identifying and questioning current standards, promoted by the quest for more evidence-based, patient-orientated practice.

Principles for practice

- There are clear parallels between the use of restraint in the elderly and that in children and young people.
- Detrimental effects on the physical and psychological well-being of the elderly caused by the use of physical restraint may be applied equally to its use on children/young people.
- The case for alternatives to physical restraint in the elderly is echoed in children and young people's nursing practice with regard to children and young people.

Methods of restraint and impact on children and young people

The use of restraint by adults to overpower children and young people in any context is an emotive subject which raises complex legal, ethical and practical issues. Clear guidance is required to help protect the rights of the child and those of the practitioner involved in restraining the child or young person. Current guidance within the UK is limited, with many institutions developing their own frameworks to help define best practice (Hart 2004). This has heralded a call for the UK government to undertake a comprehensive review of the practice of restraint by all institutions involved, to ensure compliance with the United Nations (UN) Convention on the Rights of the Child (Committee on the Rights of the Child 2002) set out below.

The UN Convention on the Rights of the Child (1989) states:

Article 12

1. Parties shall assure to the child who is capable of forming his or her own views the right to express those views freely in all matters affecting the child, the views of the child being given due weight in accordance with the age and maturity of the child.

Article 19

1. Parties shall take all appropriate legislative, administrative, social and educational measures to protect the child from all forms of physical or mental violence, injury or abuse, neglect or negligent treatment, maltreatment or exploitation, including sexual abuse, while in the care of parent(s), legal guardian(s) or any other person who has the care of the child.

2. Such protective measures should, as appropriate, include effective procedures for the establishment of social programmes to provide necessary support for the child and for those who have the care of the child, as well as for other forms of prevention and for identification, reporting, referral, investigation, treatment and follow-up of instances of child maltreatment described heretofore, and, as appropriate, for judicial involvement.

The developing interest in physical restraint has also been fuelled by already documented investigations into serious restraint-related injuries sustained by children at Aycliffe Children's Centre by the Department of Health (1993a). Such reviews have accelerated the call for a revision of techniques used by staff to restrain children (Department of Health 1993b), prohibiting control and restraint techniques which originated in the prison service (Epps 1999 *et al.*). In the government's response to coroners' recommendations following the inquests of Gareth Myatt and Adam Rickwood, restraint was identified as a contributing factor to both boys' deaths in secure units in England (Ministry of Justice 2008, p. 3). It states:

> *Gareth Myatt, aged 15, died in hospital on 19 April 2004, following a restraint incident at Rainsbrook secure training centre. Gareth's death revealed a number of shortcomings in relation to Physical Control in Care (PCC), the approved method of restraint in secure training centres, and wider safeguarding issues were highlighted at the inquest into his death. Several months afterwards, on 9 August 2004, Adam Rickwood, aged 14, committed suicide at Hassockfield secure training centre. The jury at the inquest into Adam's death found that a restraint incident some hours before Adam's death had not contributed to it and that staff at Hassockfield had behaved appropriately throughout the time he was at the centre – but it was clearly a distressing incident for Adam. A number of safeguarding issues arose from the inquest and the coroner made a number of recommendations.*

The physical restraint of children and young people for clinical procedures by nursing staff is common within healthcare settings (Bland 2002; Folkes 2005; Pearch 2005). The child's ability to comprehend the need for the procedure, and thus his or her compliance, is directly linked to the child's age and developmental stage, as set out in Table 6.1, which is based on Piaget's cognitive developmental stages.

Table 6.1 Cognitive development and main characteristics as described by Piaget (Bee and Boyd 2006)

Age of child in years	Piaget's stage of cognitive development	Main characteristics as described by Piaget
0–2	Sensorimotor	Simple reflexes, first habits, circular reactions, novelty and curiosity, internalization of schemes, object permanence
2–7	Preoperational	Magical thinking predominates, acquisition of motor skills, egocentrism, child cannot conserve or use logical thinking
7–12	Concrete operational	Child begins to think logically but only with practical aids, child is very concrete in his or her thinking, begins to conceive, no longer egocentric
12+	Formal operational	Development of abstract reasoning, children develop abstract thought, can easily conserve and think logically

Younger children, as exemplified in the above case study, are unable to understand the rationale for procedures such as venepuncture; their non-compliance is exhibited by behaviours associated with the primal responses to fear – fight and flight – making any procedure difficult to perform. It is common practice for parents, nurses, doctors and other multidisciplinary team members to engage in the forceful restraint of the uncooperative child to ensure the completion of a multitude of clinical procedures, e.g. taking the child's temperature, blood, X-rays. Nurses identify a need to hold the child to reduce the risk of additional injury from medical equipment being used to perform the task (Collins 1999). It can be argued that the moral rationale for holding the child still is 'for the greater good of the child', depending on the urgency underpinning the necessity of such clinical investigation (Robinson and Collier 1997; Collins 1999), with care being exercised to ensure that the child suffers no harm as a result.

However, it may be argued that in situations where the child does not require urgent therapeutic intervention the use of restraint becomes questionable. The taking of blood for non-urgent investigations, for example, means the use of excessive restraint can be seen as unjustified. In some circumstances the children and young people's nurse should consider and explore the use of alternative techniques, such as distraction, and the appropriate use of topical anaesthetics to manage the procedure, thus minimizing the use of restraint at all times.

Play specialists have the appropriate skills and knowledge to engage children of all ages with the use of appropriate techniques to understand even complex clinical interventions, minimizing the child's fear and engaging the child through the medium of play to increase cooperation. The simple use of blowing 'bubbles' around the clinical setting while children are undergoing venepuncture, combined with the adequate use of a topical anaesthetic gel or cream, can provide enough distraction to be able to perform the necessary investigation without the child really being aware of the procedure. This minimizes the use of restraint and allows the experience to be less traumatic for both the child and the parent.

Principles for practice

- The compliance of children and young people in clinical procedures is related to their stage of cognitive development.
- Although the use of restraint may be justified 'for the greater good of the child' care must be exercised to ensure that the child or young person does not suffer harm.
- When appropriate, the nurse must consider the use of suitable alternatives to restraint to minimize the need for inappropriate levels of restraint in all non-urgent procedures.

The use of restraint in psychiatric settings

There is a plethora of research into the restraint of children which exists within a psychiatric context (Bell L 1997; Allen 2002; Kenny 2004). However, the purpose behind some of the restraint used within this field is identified as a therapeutic treatment. Child psychotherapists use forceful restraint to help children express emotions through confrontation, as a treatment for conditions such as autism, schizophrenia and attachment disorders (Mercer 2002).

Other aspects of society, such as education, have also begun to grapple with some of the legal and moral dilemmas of restraining children (Hamilton 1997; Fletcher-Campbell *et al.* 2003; Gold 2004; Hart 2004). With the advent of the Education Act 1996 (Department for Education and Employment 1996), which prohibits the use of 'corporal punishment' within schools, teachers have sought clarity on the issue of using reasonable force in restraining pupils to prevent them committing crimes or causing disruption, injury or damage. There is much confusion and ambiguity surrounding how much 'force' can be considered 'reasonable' while restraining pupils. It is essential to define the concept of reasonable force, which has become the accepted theoretical moral ruler by which each case is measured and considered in light of an increasingly litigious society (Hantikainen and Kappeli 2000; Jeffery 2002; Charles-Edwards 2003). As the following case study shows, restraint may be ruled unlawful and has consequences for the individual patient/client, professionals involved and their organization.

Case study

The inquest into the death of 25 year old Godfrey Moyo, while on remand at HMP Belmarsh, concluded in July 2009 with the jury deciding that the medical cause of his death was (a) positional asphyxia with left ventricular failure following restraint and (b) epilepsy. The jury's verdict reflects the shocking evidence of what happened on 3 January 2005. In their damning narrative verdict the jury found that:

On 3 January 2005 at approximately 2.50am at Belmarsh prison Mr Godfrey Moyo suffered an epileptic fit in his cell. Prison officers were alerted and together with a nurse were dispatched to the cell. Upon regaining consciousness, Mr Moyo experienced post-ictal behavioural disturbance and attacked a cellmate. Prison officers entered the cell to bring Mr Moyo under control. A vigorous struggle ensued between Mr Moyo and five prison officers in which three officers sustained injuries. Prison officers brought Mr Moyo to the floor on the landing outside the cell. Full control was achieved immediately. Mr Moyo was then restrained in the face down prone position for approximately 30 minutes.

During this time Mr Moyo suffered at least two further fits, followed by periods of unconsciousness in which his breathing was restricted as a result of his position.

Mr Moyo began to suffer from the effects of positional asphyxia. The first nurse on the scene failed to adequately monitor Mr Moyo's condition during the restraint, which contributed to his death by neglect.

The prison officers also failed to recognize the signs of distress being shown by Mr Moyo during the restraint, as highlighted by their control and restraint training. At no time during the restraint by any persons present was an attempt made to move Mr Moyo off his front as per the control and restraint guidelines or place him in the recovery position during periods of unconsciousness.

Reflection point

Consider how the death of Mr Moyo could have been averted and the nurse's role in this situation as the client's advocate.

Other deaths caused by physical restraint have also been reported in the USA, as set out below:

Case study

Angellika Arndt suffocated while in a control hold at the Rice Lake Day Treatment Centre, Wisconsin, USA, in May 2006. The case went to trial and was reported in the local newspaper, *The Chronotype*, on 14 May 2009 (Coalition Against Institutionalized Child Abuse 2009).

Angellika was born in Milwaukee. She was subjected to severe physical and sexual abuse while living with her biological parents, stated the complaint. She was diagnosed with a variety of psychological disorders and developmental problems, including a short attention span. Her parents terminated their parental rights in 2004. She was placed with foster parents Donna and Daniel Pavlik in January 2005 and immediately became a part of their family. Angellika was placed in the Rice Lake Day Treatment Center for academic assistance on April 24, 2006.

From that day until May 25, 2006, Angellika was placed in the control hold at least a dozen times lasting from a minimum of 17 minutes up to a maximum of 98 minutes. She was placed in the control holds for such behavior as putting her hands down the front of her pants, putting her arms and head inside her shirt, not sitting properly, talking to others and gargling her drink.

Angellika was a client of the center, which provided intensive intervention and preventative mental health services for youths. The defendant, Ridout, with other staff members had placed Angellika in a control hold as a disciplinary measure at the clinic on May 25, 2006. She was forced to lie face down on the floor and was restrained by at least three staff members, including Ridout lying across the 67-pound girl's back and shoulders. She suffocated from the pressure and could not be revived. During the last control hold, Angellika lost consciousness, stopped breathing, sustained a tear to the cornea and had blunt trauma to the head. She went into cardiac arrest and sustained internal bleeding and brain death.

The clinic pleaded no contest to a subsequent charge of homicide under the patient abuse statute. It was fined $100,000. As part of the plea agreement, the Rice Lake center closed its doors. Ridout pleaded no contest to misdemeanour negligent patient abuse. He was placed on 1 year of probation with 60 days in jail.

Key points

- Physical restraint is used on children and young people in a psychiatric setting as part of therapy, in educational settings and the penal system.
- Deaths caused by physical restraint have been recorded in the UK and USA.

The need for guidelines on restraint to inform practice

Within children and young people's nursing little has been written and even less researched surrounding the issue of restraining children and young people for clinical procedure. Some authors suggest this could be due to the difficult nature of the topic, questioning whether restraining children/young people was tantamount to identifying poor practice within children and young people's nursing (Robinson and Collier 1997; Folkes 2005).

There is a clear acknowledgement of the lack of local and national policies regarding suitable techniques for use by nursing staff. This could be attributed to the lack of clarity currently available from relevant professional bodies, such as the Royal College of Nursing (2003), which itself highlighted the need for local organizations to undertake 'organisation wide risk assessments' regarding the use of restraint. It concluded that such assessments would need to include the identified risks within each area, to help ascertain staff training needs. It can be suggested that, as yet, no one has assumed responsibility for directing this aspect of professional practice within the UK, with both national and local institutions seeking guidance from each other.

There are only two examples in the children and young people's nursing literature that discuss the introduction of policies to guide practice within a specific clinical area: the introduction of a clinical holding policy within a teaching hospital in England (Lambrenos and McArthur 2003), and the use of clinical benchmarking in defining best practice concerning restraint in health authorities in north west England (Bland 2002). Both of these are good examples of local organizations taking the initiative in developing their own guidance to help define and guide best practice when restraining children for clinical procedures, as described in Table 6.2.

Table 6.2 Summary of key attributes associated with best practice in restraining children for clinical procedures

Lambrenos and McArthur (2003)	Bland (2002)
Flow chart to assist decision-making on clinical holding used in each procedure for each individual child	Development of an evidence-based clinical benchmark as a tool to be used to identify best practice in procedural restraint
Narrative document developed defining terms, responsibilities, training needs and need for audit	Promotes equal partnership with the child and family, ensures the rights of the child are maintained
A consent form and information document completed prior to the procedure	Assessment to minimize risk to the child and clear documentation of the processes involved to reduce potential for litigation
Professional training package developed specifically designed for the purpose of clinical procedural holding	Implementation of a formalized education and training package
Developmental needs of the child are highlighted as well as alternative approaches to consider	Physical and psychological developmental needs assessed and alternative techniques considered where possible

Reflection points

★ What guidelines or clinical protocols are used in your clinical area in relation to the physical restraint of children and young people?

★ Have the training needs of yourself and your professional colleagues have been met in relation to appropriate techniques for restraining children and young people and the use of alternatives such as distraction?

The development of a clinical protocol to help guide best practice is discussed by Bland (2002) in the use of 'clinical benchmarking' as a process used to develop an action plan to initiate best practice in restraining children for procedures. The process is similar to the research paradigm action research in its cyclical, re-evaluative approach to a clinical development. His work defines six core factors used to consider the most appropriate management of restraint within a clinical area (Bland 2002), as set out in Box 6.1.

Box 6.1	Six core factors in relation to physical restraint (Bland 2002)
1 Equal partnership with child and family	4 Training and education
2 Methods of restraint	5 Assessment and documentation
3 Alternatives to restraint	6 The rights of the child

A scoring system of statements identified along a continuum from A to E allows a practitioner to clearly isolate best practice (A on the scale), then in comparison highlight where the particular unit's practice lies.

For example, under training, best practice is defined as 'mandatory' on restraint management for all staff, whereas poor practice highlights that there would be no evidence of training or education surrounding the topic (Bland 2002). Staff training, education and implementation would need to be supported, both financially and practically, to ensure success of this type of local intervention. This type of local policy development can help ensure practice is evidence based.

Reflection points

★ Whose responsibility is it to ensure all healthcare professionals have training and education in restraint?

★ What may be the consequences of a lack of training and education?

The literature surrounding the development of local policies in the USA regarding restraint suggests that without clear national guidance a lack of parity can occur nationally. This can create problems for both staff and patients as experiences and expectations differ from area to area (Selekman and Snyder 1995).

There is at present very little practical guidance for children and young people's nurses in restraint techniques from a policy perspective either. In the UK, the Royal College of Nursing (RCN) has published two documents which help inform and guide nurses in practice. The first document, *Restraining, Holding Still and Containing Children and Young People* (Royal College of Nursing 2003), fails to give any direct advice in the practical management and correct procedures for restraining children or young people, choosing instead to clarify the need for locally based training programmes which will enable nursing staff to have greater knowledge and thus more confidence when restraining children/young people.

The second document, *Restraint Revisited: Rights, Risks and Responsibility* (Royal College of Nursing 2004), has a more moral and ethical remit, but its focus is not on restraining children or young people but rather on the older adult with challenging behaviour. This leaves nurses questioning the basis from which currently used techniques have been developed (Valler-Jones and Shinnick 2005).

Within the field of nurse education pre-registration nursing students are currently taught manual handling and receive violence and aggression training, but the issue of restraining children and young people is not directly addressed within the indicative content of most UK Fitness for Practice child nursing programmes.

Key points

- There is a lack of national policy or guidelines in relation to physical restraint in the USA and UK.
- Although the guidelines outlined so far may inform practice there is a need for national policies and guidelines applicable to all areas where physical restraint is used.

The restraint of children and young people across a range of settings

The literature has highlighted methods for the safe restraint of children and young people, and their appropriate use, in several areas of society which deal with children and young people, such as education, residential care, dentistry and radiography.

The Department for Education and Employment has sought to clarify the use of restraint as a means for controlling children within an education environment. The Education Act 1996 (Department for Education and Employment 1996) prohibits the use of 'corporal punishment' at any local education authority, independent, special or grant-maintained school. Circular 10/98, produced by the Department for Education and Employment (1998), seeks to address section 550A of the Education Act 1996 and discusses the issue of using 'reasonable force' to prevent pupils committing a crime, causing injury or damage, or causing disruption, stating that such powers have already existed under common law but have been misunderstood.

The concept of 'reasonable force' has been determined through a Court of Law and can be described as an objective test determined by the jury (Police National Legal Database 2004). A jury is asked to determine whether the amount of force used, under given circumstances, can be justified by the defendant, as detailed in Box 6.2. However, civil rights lawyers interpret 'reasonable' as meaning 'minimal' and, under the Human Rights Act 1998, have disputed the interpretation of 'reasonable'.

Box 6.2	Section 3(1) of the Criminal Law Act 1967, United Kingdom

A person may use such force as is reasonable in the circumstances in the prevention of a crime, or in effecting or assisting in the lawful arrest of offenders or suspected offenders or of persons unlawfully at large.

A jury must decide whether a defendant honestly believed that the circumstances were such as required him to use force to defend himself from an attack or threatened attack; the jury has then to decide whether the force used was reasonable in the circumstances.

Note that this is basically an 'objective test' determined by the jury. The jury does not have to consider whether the defendant thought his/her actions were reasonable in the circumstances. They just have to consider what *they* believe was reasonable.

The degree of force used to restrain a child or young person for clinical procedures is also of concern to professions allied to medicine. In radiographic examinations children and young people are required to undergo diagnostic tests which require immobilization, often against the will of the child (Hardy and Armitage 2002). There are concerns raised about the legal and moral implications for restraining children and young people within this field, acknowledging that the majority of radiographers lack any formal paediatric education and training, thus increasing the reliance on parents and other healthcare staff, namely nurses, to ensure adequate restraint of a child for radiographic imaging.

The same holds true for other professions. A quantitative questionnaire survey of 179 dental practitioners conducted by Newton *et al.* (2004) indicated that 39% felt that physical restraint was an acceptable practice for very young patients, with an even greater number acknowledging its appropriateness in handicapped children (62%). The results showed the decline in use of a previously more common practice – hand over mouth – which is broadly defined as a practitioner placing his or her hand over a patient's mouth while behavioural expectations are calmly explained to the child, and ensuring the airway remains patent. This decline is linked to increased education of practitioners, concerns over the legal status of the technique and increasing parental concerns. Interestingly, 51% of these dental practitioners felt that long-term psychological problems might occur, such as fear of further treatment, which has direct relevance to restraint in paediatric nursing and the potential long-term impact of such practices as described in the case study below.

Case study

An 8 year old girl attends a local paediatric admissions unit for removal of sutures following complex abdominal surgery performed in another district general hospital. The sutures were due to be removed 10 days postoperatively. However, the child attends the unit on day 15 postoperatively and her parents explain that she is very frightened about having the sutures removed owing to a previous 'bad experience' when she was caused considerable pain during suture removal after the last operation. The parents apologize, but explain that it has taken them 15 days to persuade their daughter to attend the hospital. They are now worried about the implications of trying to remove the sutures as the skin has already started to embed around the sutures, making any attempts at removal very difficult. Local anaesthetic and systemic pain relief appears ineffective. The anaesthetic medical team are reluctant to give a general anaesthetic to allow for suture removal, stating that it is medically too risky to give a second general anaesthetic to this particular child for such a minor procedure. They suggest holding the child down to enable suture removal. The child complains of extreme pain during the procedure and reacts in a physically and verbally aggressive manner to the restraint, resulting in five clinical staff being required to hold her still to enable safe suture removal. This action can be seen as compounding the fear and anxiety in a child who already suffers with procedural anxiety related to prior experience. The child will need further surgery and this experience will undoubtedly psychologically significantly affect the child and could lead to profound long-term effects.

Reflection points

★ What are your feelings and emotions after reading the above Case Study?

★ What other measures could staff have considered and employed to minimize the pain and distress experienced by the 8 year old girl having embedded sutures removed from her abdomen?

★ What may be the long-term consequences of this experience for the girl, her family and staff?

The use of restraint in psychotherapy

Within the psychotherapy field restraint can be used for a different purpose. Mercer (2002) reviews four main techniques used within child psychotherapy, whose long-term goal is to 'create family warmth and affection', but the action is described as 'Uncomfortable physical restraint and intrusive emotional confrontations that verge on violence' (Mercer 2002, p. 304).

The assumption behind these therapies is that they treat emotional problems by releasing accumulated negative emotions that would otherwise inhibit positive emotion and affection for others (Mercer 2002). The four techniques include Z-process therapy, Welch method attachment therapy, Colorado style attachment therapy and Feserici's therapeutic holding. In essence, the child is physically restrained by usually more than one adult and encouraged to express their emotions. They are then verbally and physically overpowered until the child becomes calm. These treatments were claimed to be successful for autism, schizophrenia, attachment and attention disorders (Mercer 2002). The potential for harming the child and the inappropriate use of the techniques as punishment are highlighted; there are, however, descriptions of extensive forceful restraint, coupled with emotional challenge, which exist far beyond the scope of the types of restraint used for clinical interventions within nursing, so are not clearly comparable. The author's description of 10 year old Candace Newmaker's death as a result of such psychotherapy restraint techniques does, again, bring the question of reasonable force to the forefront of restraint of children. Such cases, covered extensively by the media, have helped highlight the issue to a wider audience.

Case study

Candace Newmaker died on 18 April 2000 in Evergreen, CO, USA. She was the victim of child abuse as a young child and was 5 years old when she was removed from her parents. She was then adopted by Jeane Newmaker 2 years later; however, there were concerns about her behaviour and attitude at home. She was eventually enrolled in a 2 week intensive session of 'attachment therapy' involving a 70 minute 'rebirthing' session during which she was wrapped in a flannel sheet to simulate a womb and told to extract herself from the sheet, while four adults used their hands, feet and large pillows to push against her to prevent her from freeing herself. The experience of 'rebirthing' was supposed to help Candace 'attach' to her adoptive mother.

The session was videotaped and Candace repeatedly tells the adults involved that she is having difficulty breathing. She even states on the tapes that she thinks that she is dying.

Candace Newmaker died as a result of being asphyxiated during the restraint.

Mercer's (2002) conclusions regarding the appropriateness of such restraint techniques within child psychotherapy are supported by Sourander *et al.* (2002). This study examines the use of restraints, holding, seclusion and time-out within child and adolescent psychiatric inpatient units in Finland from the perspective of the consultant psychiatrist responsible for the child/young person's care. About 40% of the sample (*n* = 504) had experienced some form of restraint procedure during an inpatient stay, with 'aggressive acts' being the rationale for instigating the restraint of the child or young person. This study again raises concern surrounding the lack of 'research based understanding' of the impact of restraining children and young people.

Key points

- There are legal implications for the use of 'physical restraint' in practice.
- Research and real life case studies identify worrying practices such as the use of 'hand over mouth' and questionable psychotherapeutic techniques.

Probably the most comprehensive review of the topic to date is by Hart and Howell (2004), which consists of a report commissioned by the National Children's Bureau. The report states:

> *The use of direct physical contact in order to overpower a child raises complex legal, ethical and practical issues. There are times when such intervention is necessary in order to protect the child or others from harm but clear guidance is essential in order to safeguard both the child concerned and the practitioner exercising the restraint. It is debatable whether such clarity currently exists in the UK.*
>
> *(Hart and Howell 2004, p. 4)*

Hart and Howell (2004) call for more research into the implications of restraint on children and the safety and effectiveness of techniques, most of which are derived from adult control and restrain policies originating from prisons and which can be considered an inappropriate basis that fails to acknowledge the different physical and psychological status of children and young people. The authors also highlight the need for research into the actual incidence of restraint within a variety of contexts, including healthcare, and the effectiveness of their use.

The concerns about the lack of research are compounded by Epps *et al.* (1999), who suggest that most childcare organizations are left to develop techniques and procedures with little external support or guidance. They blame the deficit in research for the lack of systematic practice development. The lack of clear policy and practical guidelines appears to be an issue across many childcare facilities and is not therefore regarded as uniquely a deficit in children and young people's nursing. These findings compound Hart and Howell's (2004) conclusion that at present there is a lack of guidance surrounding the issue of restraining children across many institutions.

Key points

- The use of physical restraint in children has been questioned by the National Children's Bureau, UK.
- A lack of research into the use of physical restraint has been identified.

Restraining children in nursing practice: a review of recent research

Selekman and Snyder (1995) describe local policies which already exist in the USA regarding restraint in clinical practice. Their quantitative research study examines the reasons for the use of restraint, and possible alternatives, and compares the use of restraint across general paediatric, psychiatric and rehabilitation centres. This chapter has already demonstrated that the use and types of restraint varies so much within these different settings. The psychiatric unit staff in this study perceived an increased need for restraints for managing agitation, preventing self-injury and protecting staff and others from physical abuse, compared with general children and young people's nurses whose primary reason for the use of restraint is described as 'to prevent interference' with tubes, intravenous lines and dressings. This study concludes by suggesting that there should be increased parity between local policies on the safe restraint of children, to address the problems of local variations which cause confusion for practitioners as well as patients. The findings have particular relevance for children and young people's nurses in the UK, where at present local NHS trust-specific policies are beginning to emerge without clear national guidelines. This will undoubtedly lead to guidance which lacks rigour and cannot cross geographical boundaries, and emphasizes the need for national if not international guidelines on restraint.

In the UK, Collier and Pattison (1997) examined the attitudes of 52 nurses and 67 doctors towards 12 stipulated myths surrounding children's experiences of pain. The majority of respondents (68.9% doctors, 61.1% nurses) agreed that the process of being restrained for a clinical procedure distressed children more than the pain involved in the procedure itself. This is supported by several other authors (Robinson and Collier 1997; Stephens *et al.* 1999). The discussions conclude that there is a perceived and real lack of credible research into the field of restraint (Collier and Pattison 1997), highlighting that adequate preparation of the children may help address the issue in a practical context. The authors conclude that restraint does appear to be a neglected issue within children and young people's nursing. Likewise, Robinson and Collier (1997) researched the opinions and experiences of 153 children and young people's nurses working within hospitals in Nottingham and Grantham, UK. They investigated the use of restraint within a general paediatric context. The results supported the idea that in most cases children became distressed as a result of being restrained rather than the pain involved in the procedures (69.3% of the sample).

One way of reducing the need for restraint is to consider the use of pharmacological agents to sedate the child prior to the procedure. Young (2000) studied the effectiveness of two pharmacological sedatives, ketamine and midazolam, in minimizing the need for restraint of 644 children during interventions such as suturing, stapling, Steri-Strips and gluing of minor wounds in the Emergency Department. The results show that ketamine was more effective, with children requiring less restraint and reporting an overall better behavioural experience throughout the whole procedure (Young 2000). There is, however, an acknowledgement that some children and young people will be unsuitable for sedation and will continue to be restrained for procedures.

When practitioners are unable to use sedation or other alternative techniques and restraint is deemed necessary to ensure the safety of the child or young person during a procedure, it is vitally important that nurses have clear guidance available to help ensure best practice. A clinical tool is necessary to help guide practitioners in the safe and appropriate choice of techniques and to ensure consent is properly gained from the parents and documented prior to the procedure. The effect of the experience on the parents must be recognized and their needs also taken into consideration at all stages of the procedure.

Principles for practice

- There would seem to be a need for national and even international guidance in relation to the use of physical restraint.
- Research shows that the use of physical restraint on the child can cause more distress than the actual clinical procedure.
- To minimize distress clinical staff could consider the use of sedation in children.

The impact of restraint: understanding parents' experiences

Prolonged exposure to events such as traumatic restraints of children can alter the nurse's perception (Benner and Wrubel 1989). Student nurses and parents are often well placed to describe the potential impact of traumatic restraint experiences as they have yet to be overexposed to such emotionally difficult situations and often perceive the experience differently from a more experienced nurse.

As noted by Benner and Wrubel (1989, p. 60):

> *Stress management approaches that deal only with the altering emotional states by dampening, controlling or distracting may be helpful in the short term to interrupt a stressful response set, but in the long run, such strategies foster an alienated stance towards emotion.*

Perhaps this explains why a student's response can appear so emotionally raw to more experienced staff who, over time, can become more emotionally detached. Maybe this is why more experienced practitioners have been slow to question their actions during such episodes of restraint, after prolonged exposure has dampened their response to such situations as part of a developing coping strategy. Again such apathy towards the issue of restraining children and young people could be part of the reason why policy and guidance has been so slow to evolve surrounding the topic.

In previous research 98% of nurses questioned felt that the parent's presence was beneficial to the child during a procedure (Robinson and Collier 1997), yet extreme emotional responses by the parents would probably only upset the child further. This is a difficult professional decision when deliberating at the time of the event: whether a parent should stay with the child and be involved in the restraint or merely be present while the nurse holds the child.

Such an ad hoc approach to the preparation of the parents and child could be minimized if staff were encouraged to formally assess and document the patient's individual needs prior to the restraint for any necessary procedures (Lambrenos and McArthur 2003). This would automatically require discussion between parents, the child/young person and the nursing staff on how best to approach the patient.

The need for documentation and assessment has been highlighted by several authors (Bland 2002; Jeffery 2002; Lambrenos and McArthur 2003; Royal College of Nursing 2003). When children and young people are deemed unable to reliably give consent for the use of the restraint, the parents should at least have an opportunity to discuss and agree on the types of restraint to be used and the degree of force appropriate. This would serve only to improve the communication between parents and the nursing staff concerned. If the nurse involved is obliged to discuss and gain prior consent for the restraint from the parents, this at least should serve as a period of time for psychological preparation of the parents, forewarning them what to expect.

Ideally, the staffing levels on the children and young people's ward need to reflect sufficient personnel to help support parents through these difficult experiences rather than rely on them to physically help with the restraint of their own child. There is an acknowledged need for parents to remain with their children wherever possible during clinical procedures to ensure their child has emotional support. Parents become essentially compromised, both emotionally and physically, when giving hands-on help to restrain their child. Without proper risk assessment and documentation of this role for parents there also appear considerable risks for the trusts and ward managers concerned.

There is a clearly identified need for children and young people's nurses to gain the consent of the parents and, if possible, the child to ensure the ethos of collaborative family-centred care. Many of the procedures and restraints that are undertaken could be considered as intimately invasive, and respecting the need for consent for such events is essential in defining best practice for children and young people's nursing, as highlighted in Table 6.2. There could also be benefits from staff training in the risk and potential of any litigation through improvements in child safety (Bland 2002; Royal College of Nursing 2003). This might also address the astounding lack of awareness of the legal responsibility of the children and young people's nurse when restraining a child (Robinson and Collier 1997).

Principles for practice

- All staff involved in clinical procedures must carefully assess whether the use of physical restraint is necessary and consider all other approaches.
- Parents must be involved in any discussion and be supported by staff.
- If physical restraint is used, consent must be sought from parents.

Legal, ethical and moral issues

Issues surrounding the perceived use of power to overcome a child who chooses not to comply with treatment such as the child in the case study where sutures were removed with sedation/anaesthesia on p. 165 are raised by Charles-Edwards (2003), who illustrates how both a child and the parent can be overawed in the power-coercive environment of a hospital. She suggests that individual practitioners should examine the ethical principles followed by a workplace in determining when restraint can be justified.

Nurses have been described as feeling 'uncomfortable' in their role when actively restraining children (Lambrenos and McArthur 2003). This feeling is echoed by student nurses (Valler-Jones and Shinnick 2005), and supported by the experiences of practitioners in other fields of nursing (Bonner *et al.* 2002). Again this could be attributed to the violation of other socially and professionally valued aspects of the 'helping relationship', as suggested by Wright (1999), and the basis of the code of conduct (Nursing and Midwifery Council 2008), beneficence and non-maleficence. This is often coupled with concerns over the dichotomy of their relationship with children they provide care for, which is developed through a gradual formation of mutual trust, only to have that fragile bond shattered through the need to restrain a child for a painful clinical procedure (Bricher 1999).

There are obvious consequences to the restraining of older children without their prior consent. The dangers of harming not only the child but also the staff involved are real and even accentuated owing to the size of the child. There are also ethical implications for restraining children for the purpose of undertaking procedures, without the child's consent, which is described as a last resort practice in a child of this age (Jeffery 2002; Royal College of Nursing 2003).

Gaining a child's consent for the restraint and the procedure has been identified as the ideal (Collins 1999; Department of Health 2003; Lambrenos and McArthur 2003; Royal College of Nursing 2003). This can possibly be achieved with older children who could be defined as 'Gillick competent' in the UK and therefore able to understand and rationalize the need for treatment. However, it can be argued that the majority of children who require restraining for a clinical procedure are cognitively unable to comprehend adequately the need for treatment. This is supported by Robinson and Collier (1997), whose study identified the age of less than 6.7 years as those most likely to require restraint.

Summary of Gillick competence, UK

In UK law, a person's 18th birthday draws the line between childhood and adulthood, so that in healthcare matters an 18 year old enjoys as much autonomy as any other adult. To a more limited extent 16 and 17 year olds can also take medical decisions independently of their parents. The right of younger children to provide independent consent is proportionate to their competence, but a child's age alone is clearly an unreliable predictor of his or her competence to make decisions. See also p. 103.

A judgment in the High Court in 1983 (Wheeler 2006) laid down criteria for establishing whether a child, irrespective of age, had the capacity to provide valid consent to treatment in specified circumstances. Two years later these criteria were approved in the House of Lords and became widely acknowledged as the 'Gillick test' after the name of a mother who had challenged health service guidance that would have allowed her daughters aged under 16 to receive confidential contraceptive advice without her knowledge. For many years the criteria that have been referred to as the test for Gillick competence have provided clinicians with an objective test of competence. This identifies children aged under 16 who have the legal capacity to consent to medical examination and treatment, providing they can demonstrate sufficient maturity and intelligence to understand and appraise the nature and implications of the proposed treatment, including the risks and alternative courses of action (Wheeler 2006).

The issue of consent could be partially addressed if nurses were obliged to formally assess and document their rationale for restraining a child, with collaboration from the parents (Bland 2002; Jeffery 2002; Royal College of Nursing 2003). This could be structured to show a deliberated assessment of the child's age and understanding, the rationale for use of specified and agreed techniques as well as details of alternatives which could be considered appropriate and shown as being tried before resorting to restraint, which should only be considered as a last resort (Lambrenos and McArthur 2003; Royal College of Nursing 2003). Examples of these have been developed by Lambrenos and McArthur (2003) and Folkes (2005), both of which take the form of a clinical flowchart to aid the decision-making process, coupled with supporting documentation for recording, explaining and gaining consent for the process. However, Lambrenos and McArthur (2003) acknowledge that the increasing legal knowledge gained through implementation of teaching sessions accompanying the implementation of the new policy has 'heightened' some practitioners' concerns regarding their vulnerability to litigation.

The legality of restraining children and young people has to be viewed in light of any pertinent legislation which seeks to promote children's rights within society. The UN Convention on the Rights of the Child (United Nations 1989), although not a 'law', has been ratified by the UK, which is committed to its implementation. The latest report by this committee specifies a request for a review of all uses of restraint of children (Hart and Howell 2004). This has implications for the health service, which has been identified as one such area which needs to review current procedures and guidance, and has special relevance for all areas involved in the regular care and subsequent restraint of children and young people.

The Human Rights Act (1998) and criminal law also seek to protect the rights of children and young people from abuse and excessive unjustifiable physical force to restrict them, their liberty and their autonomy. Again clear guidance on permissible forms of restraint are urgently needed by practitioners to help them clarify their role in restraining children and young people for clinical procedures, ensuring that minimal force is utilized. The Royal College of Nursing (2003) suggests practitioners seek guidance on the legal implications of any locally produced restraint policies. There is some evidence of use of the Education Act 1996 (Department for Education and Employment 1996) and mental health and mental handicap recommendations being used for guidance in formulation of teaching sessions on restraint (Valler-Jones and Shinnick 2005) owing to the lack of specific guidance for children and young people's nursing at present.

In the UK, the nurses' professional code of conduct (Nursing and Midwifery Council 2008) also provides guidance on a nurse's role within his or her professional capacity. It identifies a practitioner as personally accountable for ensuring that the nurse promotes and protects the interests and dignity of patients and clients. The code also reminds the professional to deliver safe and competent care, and to respect patients' and clients' autonomy. While guidance on restraining children appropriately for clinical procedures remains inadequate, nurses might be considered at risk of breaching their own code of conduct (Nursing and Midwifery Council 2008).

The code of conduct (Nursing and Midwifery Council 2008) also reinforces the nurse's role in obtaining clear documented consent for treatment from the patient or a person with parental responsibility. Good record-keeping is identified as helping to protect patients and clients by providing an accurate account of treatment and care planning and delivery (Nursing and Midwifery Council 2009). With the current lack of documentation regarding the assessment, management and evaluation of restraint techniques used, nurses cannot prove that they comply with their professional and legal duty of care. The Nursing and Midwifery Council (2009) states that accurate documentation provides evidence that a nurse has honoured his or her duty of care, and that he or she has taken all reasonable steps to care for a patient and not compromise the patient's safety in any way. The Nursing and Midwifery Council (2009) reminds nurses to use their professional judgement to decide what is relevant and what to record. With the difficulties that arise from ensuring consent from children, young people and their parents, and the physical contact nature of restraining children and young people against their will, it would seem logical that this should be considered a vital area to clearly document within children and young people's nursing.

Principles for practice

- The use of physical restraint raises important questions in relation to the UN Convention on the Rights of the Child (United Nations 1989).
- The legal implications of any local guidelines or policies on physical restraint need to be considered.
- Children's nurses need to be aware of their professional responsibilities with regard to taking part in physical restraint on children and young people.

Nurses can experience feelings of guilt that are difficult to explain without further in-depth research focusing on why nurses feel guilty when restraining children. This could be partly attributed to what Bricher (1999) refers to as the perceived loss of trust within the nurse–patient relationship which has been carefully formed while caring for a child or young person. The nurse then has to abuse that trust by causing the child pain or distress during a necessary procedure.

The feeling of guilt could also be linked to the interpersonal conflict with our professional and personal self-images, or as Wright (1999) terms as a result of the 'violation' of other socially and professionally valued aspects of the helping relationship. To cause intentional harm to a child in any other context could be construed as physical abuse; this behaviour also conflicts with any inherent nurturing instinct the nurse may have which encourages him or her to protect the child.

This moral sense of wrongdoing is reflected in the literature by both paediatric authors (Lambrenos and McArthur 2003) and authors writing about other fields of nursing (Bonner *et al.* 2002). It was also one of the issues raised through informal discussions with child branch nursing students by Valler-Jones and Shinnick (2005).

Nurses involved in the restraint of children for clinical procedures can feel they need to have a moral 'rationale' for their actions. They describe the moral dilemma of restraining the child to enable clinical procedures as a need to 'be cruel to be kind'. This kind of rationale is supported by the findings of Robinson and Collier (1997), who found that the majority of nurses used restraint as a means to protect the child from accidental injury and out of necessity for the procedure to be undertaken safely. However, this rationale can still be seen as causing moral and professional dilemmas for the individual nurse.

Robinson and Collier's (1997) study also highlights the ambiguity of the nurse's understanding regarding legal and professional responsibilities. Only 12% of their sample (n = 153) identified the nurse as legally responsible when restraining a child for a clinical procedure, and 52% of the study sample stated that they 'didn't know' who was responsible. Such confusion in the legal and ethical aspects of restraint can be clearly attributed to a lack of formal training and national/local guidance surrounding the issue.

Education and training of professionals involved in restraint

The need for further training was highlighted in the literature by several authors (Bland 2002; Lambrenos and McArthur 2003; Willock *et al.* 2004), whose findings all suggest a lack of knowledge into perceived alternatives to restraint by qualified nursing staff currently working with children. This is highlighted as contributing to the high reliance on the use of restraint within children and young people's nursing at present in the UK. Most of the authors highlight a need for staff training which needs to be evidence based and developed from national guidelines (Collier and Pattison 1997; Robinson and Collier 1997; Collins 1999; Jeffery 2002; Valler-Jones and Shinnick 2005). Even the policy put forward by the Royal College of Nursing (2003), *Restraining, Holding Still and Containing Children and Young People*, highlights the need for adequate staff training and refers practitioners to their designated workplace risk managers and named executive directors to implement the provision of locally based training programmes, of which, to date, none are specifically designed (Lambrenos and McArthur 2003; Folkes 2005; Pearch 2005; Valler-Jones and Shinnick 2005).

The National Service Framework for Children (Department of Health 2003) suggests that practitioners use the guidance from the Royal College of Nursing (2003) when restraining a child, which again causes confusion for practitioners when the guidance fails to be the prescriptive clinically detailed advice they urgently need in practice. Valler-Jones and Shinnick (2005) conclude that with the current lack of guidance it is pertinent to question what guidelines practitioners are currently working to. And who has designated the current techniques used as safe and acceptable? Does current policy and practice breach the UN Convention (Hart and Howell 2004)?

What training exists at present has been classed as 'lacking in quality' (Robinson and Collier 1997), and lacking clear application to the specific situation of clinical restraint for procedures (Lambrenos and McArthur 2003). With 90.8% of their study group identifying a clear need for guidance, Robinson and Collier (1997) are supported in raising this as an important issue for the profession. The issue of 'credibility of trainers' again raises concern (Lambrenos and McArthur 2003; Valler-Jones and Shinnick 2005) with some evidence in the literature of individual areas developing their own training programmes (e.g. Valler-Jones and Shinnick 2005) to meet the specific needs for pre-registration child branch nurses. Again, although this is admirable, the lack of clear guidance nationally will lead to differing standards and educational preparation which may disadvantage other students. The training needs of current practitioners must also be recognized, as they serve as clinical mentors to the students during clinical practice.

The evidence suggests that clear guidance and training will not only benefit the staff, but ultimately improve the hospitalization experience for the child and family (Collier and Pattison 1997; Robinson and Collier 1997; Collins 1999). This experience could be further improved if the educational training programmes sought to raise nurses' awareness of possible alternatives, such as distraction techniques and guided imagery (Willock *et al.* 2004), which many nurses feel unable to use because of limited training in their use and application (Bland 2002; Lambrenos and McArthur 2003). Another reason for limited use of alternatives is a lack of resources; low staffing levels might encourage nurses to restrain rather than spend time with the child using explanations and play therapies to adequately prepare a child for an intervention (Collins 1999). Collins (1999) argues that parents might be taught to use distraction prior to admission, under certain circumstances, which would be assessed as ideal practice under Bland's (2002) clinical benchmark criteria, supporting the nursing ethos of collaborative 'family-centred care'.

Use of alternatives to physical restraint

The use of restraint of younger patients for necessary clinical procedures has been described as problematic. When patient-restraining techniques are used without proper pharmacological support this potentially makes the procedures more difficult to perform. The use of alternative techniques, for example distraction by a nurse or play therapist, can prove valuable but also have to be viewed as only part of any solution to avoid or minimize use of physical restraint (Table 6.3).

Table 6.3 Alternative techniques and their application in practice.

Technique	Example
Play/distraction techniques	Use of bubbles, noisy toys, TV, conversation, cuddly toys, mimicry, role play
Guided imagery	Use of pictures, images, sounds, smells
Relaxation techniques	Use of deep breathing, progressive muscular relaxation, relaxation imagery and meditation
Pharmacological management	Use of sedatives/hypnotics

Reflection points

★ Are any of the alternative techniques to restraint listed above used in your clinical area?

★ If not, why not?

★ What may be some of the barriers to using these techniques in clinical practice?

As previously discussed in this chapter children and young people's nurses need adequate training, preparation and support within clinical areas to enable confidence in utilizing the above techniques. Other multidisciplinary members could also be trained to use these techniques within clinical areas such as medical staff, play staff and other therapists. With correct training and support parents could also be taught how to use these alternative techniques both at home and within the clinical environment.

Key points

• Training and education in the use of physical restraint and the use of alternatives is urgently required in practice.
• Training and education will improve the hospitalization experience for children and their parents.

Conclusion

This chapter has discussed some of the fundamental issues surrounding the use of restraint of children for clinical procedures. The complex moral, legal and ethical components which are weaved throughout the topic have been critically analysed and their implications explored. A clear lack of research into the issues pertinent to the use of restraint in paediatric nursing has been highlighted and the consequences discussed.

There is a need for clear national policy as well as national guidelines from which educational and training programmes for nurses in pre- and post-registration could be developed. The current situation of locally developed guidance could prove problematic in the future, when a lack of national parity could create confusion for practitioners, parents and patients, as has occurred in the USA (Selekman and Snyder 1995).

Educational and training programmes on the safe restraint of children and young people in all settings could potentially benefit students and professionals as well as families. The current situation of poorly informed practitioners which lack adequate preparation within this field of practice cannot persist. Training and education in the use of alternative techniques could be expanded to include other multidisciplinary members and parents.

Above all, parents need to be supported in their role as emotional aids to their children, and not coerced into participation involving emotionally and physically alien roles as collaborators to their child's distress during restraint for a procedure. A need for assessment and documentation of the types and situations within which restraint could be used can also be deemed essential from both a practitioner's and the patient's/family's perspective. This would also help to clarify the necessary informed consent prior to the actual experience occurring.

Lastly, it is questionable whether the current use of restraint in children and young people's nursing as described and explored within this chapter complies with current guidance from the UN Convention on the Rights of the Child (United Nations 1989), the Human Rights Act (1998) and criminal law. With calls for the government to undertake a comprehensive review of the practice of restraint by all institutions involved (Committee on the Rights of the Child 2002), children and young people's nursing must identify the urgency of this issue. Practitioners are best placed to instigate change within this area, by highlighting current practice and their concerns to those responsible for risk assessment within their areas (Royal College of Nursing 2003).

It is clear that restraint is used on children and young people across a range of settings and that children and young people's nurses as well as other health and social care practitioners need to be aware of all the issues surrounding this.

Summary of principles for practice

- Children and young people's nurses must avoid using restraint wherever possible.
- Children and young people's nurses must advocate other means that do not involve restraint and view actual restraint as the last resort.
- Children and young people's nurses must ensure that any method of restraint does not cause the child or young person actual harm.
- Children and young people's nurses must consider the legal issues involved and receive training and education in restraint.

References

Allen B (2002) *Ethical approaches to physical interventions: responding to challenging behaviour in people with intellectual disabilities.* Kidderminster: British Institute of Learning Disabilities, p. 239.

Bee H, Boyd D (2006) *The developing child*, 11th edn. London: Pearson Education.

Bell J (1997) The use of restraint in the care of elderly patients. *British Journal of Nursing* **6**: 504–8.

Bell L (1997) The physical restraint of young people. *Child and Family Social Work* **2**: 37–47.

Benner P, Wrubel J (1989) *The primacy of caring: stress and coping in health and illness.* Reading, MA: Addison-Wesley.

Bland M (2002) Procedural restraint in children's nursing: using clinical benchmarks. *Professional Nurse* **17**(12): 712–15.

Bonner G, Lowe T, Rawcliffe D, Wellman N (2002) Trauma for all: a pilot study of the subjective experience of physical restraint for mental health inpatients and staff in the UK. *Journal of Psychiatric and Mental Health Nursing* **9**: 465–73.

Bricher G (1999) Paediatric nurses, children and the development of trust. *Journal of Clinical Nursing* **8**: 451–8.

Charles-Edwards I (2003) Power and control over children and young people. *Paediatric Nursing* **15**(6): 37–42.

Cleary KK (2001) The use of restraint in health care: background, regulations, ethical implications and legal considerations. *Acute Care Perspectives* **10**(4): 11–14.

Coalition Against Institutionalised Child Abuse (2009) See http://www.caica.org/angelika_arndt_lawsuit_filed_over_child's_death_5-14-09.htm

Collier J, Pattison H (1997) Attitudes to children's pain: exploding the 'pain myth'. *Paediatric Nursing* **9**(10): 15–18.

Collins P (1999) Restraining children for painful procedures. *Paediatric Nursing* **11**(3): 14–16.

Committee on the Rights of the Child (2002) *Consideration of reports submitted by States Parties under Article 44 of the Convention. Concluding observations of the Committee on the Rights of the Child: United Kingdom of Great Britain and Northern Ireland.* Geneva: United Nations.

Department for Education and Employment (1996) *Education Act, Section 548.* See http://www.legislation.hmso.gov.uk/acts/acts1996/96056-cn.htm

Department for Education and Employment (1998) *Section 550A of the Education Act 1996: the use of Force to Control or Restrain Pupils.* Circular 10/98. London: DfEE.

Department of Health (1993a) *A place apart: an investigation into the handling and outcomes of serious injuries to children and other matters at Aycliffe Centre for Children Country Durham.* London: Social Services Inspectorate, DH.

Department of Health (1993b) *Guidance on permissible forms of control in children's residential care.* London: DH.

Department of Health (1995) *Support force for children's residential care. Good care matters: ways of enhancing good practice in residential child care.* London: DH.

Department of Health (2003) *Getting the right start: national service framework for children 'standards for hospital services'.* London: DH.

Epps K, Moore C, Hollin C (1999) Prevention and management of violence in a secure youth centre. *Nursing and Residential Care* **1**(5): 261–7.

Fletcher-Campbell F, Springall E, Brown E (2003) *Evaluation of circular 10/98 on the use of force to control or restrain pupils.* National Foundation for Educational Research. London: Department of Education and Skills.

Folkes K (2005) Is restraint a form of abuse? *Paediatric Nursing* **17**(6): 41–4.

Gallinagh R, Nevin R, McAleese L, Campbell L (2001) Perceptions of older people who have experienced physical restraint. *British Journal of Nursing* **10**(13): 852–9.

Gold K (2004) Dark shadows. *TES Extra: Special Needs* **June**: 6–7.

Hamilton C (1997) Physical restraint of children: a new sanction for schools. *Childright* **138**: 14–16.

Hantikainen V, Kappeli S (2000) Using restraint with nursing home residents: a qualitative study of nursing staff perceptions and decision making. *Journal of Advanced Nursing* **32**(5): 1196–205.

Hardy M, Armitage G (2002) The child's right to consent to x-ray and imaging investigations: issues of restraint and immobilisation from a multi-disciplinary perspective. *Journal of Child Health Care* **6**(2): 107–19.

Hart D (2004) Forcing the issue. *Community Care* **1519**: 38–40.

Hart D, Howell S (2004) Report on the use of physical intervention across children's services. London: National Children's Bureau. See http://www.ncb.org.uk/resources/res

Healy A (1997) The prevention and management of violence. In Hayden C (ed.) *Physical restraint in children's residential care.* Report no. 37. Portsmouth: Social Services Research and Information Unit, University of Portsmouth.

Human Rights Act (1998) London: The Stationery Office.

Jeffery K (2002) Therapeutic restraint of children: it must always be justified. *Paediatric Nursing* **14**(9): 20–2.

Kenny C (2004) Can mental health nursing ever give up the option of restraint? *Community Care* 1553: 14–15.

Lambrenos K, McArthur E (2003) Introducing a clinical holding policy. *Paediatric Nursing* **15**(4): 30–3.

Mason R, O'Conner M, Kemble S (1995) Untying the elderly: response to quality of life issues. *Geriatric Nursing* **16**: 68–72.

Mercer J (2002) Child psychotherapy involving physical restraint: techniques used in the four approaches. *Child and Adolescent Social Work Journal* **19**(4): 303–14.

Ministry of Justice (2008) *The government's response to coroners' recommendations following the inquests of Gareth Myatt and Adam Rickwood.* See http://www.justice.gov.uk/publications/docs/response-coroners-inquest-web.pdf

Molassiotis A (1995) Use of physical restraints 2: alternatives. *British Journal of Nursing* **4**(4):201–2, 219–20.

Newton JT, Patel H, Shah S, Sturmey P (2004) Attitudes towards the use of hand over mouth (HOM) and physical restraint amongst paediatric specialist practitioners in the UK. *International Journal of Paediatric Dentistry* **14**: 111–17.

Nursing and Midwifery Council (2008) *Code of professional conduct*. London: NMC.

Nursing and Midwifery Council (2009) *Guidelines for records and record keeping*. London: NMC.

Oxford Concise English Dictionary, 9th edn (1995). Oxford: Oxford University Press.

Pearch J (2005) Restraining children for clinical procedures. *Paediatric Nursing* **17**(9): 36–8.

Police National Legal Database (2004) See http://fis-search/pnldb/docs/d386.htm

Robbins LJ (1986) Restraining the elderly patient. *Clinical Geriatric Medicine* **2**(3): 5919.

Robinson S, Collier J (1997) Holding children still for procedures. *Paediatric Nursing* **9**(4): 12–14.

Royal College of Nursing (1992) *Focus on restraint*, 2nd edn. London: Scutari Press.

Royal College of Nursing (1999) *Restraining, holding still and containing children: guidance for good practice*. London: RCN.

Royal College of Nursing (2003) *Restraining, holding still and containing children and young people. Guidance for nursing staff*. See www.rcn.org.uk

Royal College of Nursing (2004) *Restraint revisited: rights, risks and responsibility. Guidance for nursing staff*. See www.rcn.org.uk

Selekman J, Snyder B (1995) Nursing perceptions of using physical restraints on hospitalized children. *Pediatric Nursing* **21**(5): 460–4.

Sourander A, Ellila H, Valimaki M, Piha J (2002) Use of holding, restraints, seclusion and time out in child and adolescent psychiatric in-patient treatment. *European Child & Adolescent Psychiatry* **11**: 162–7.

Stephens B, Barkey M, Hall H (1999) Techniques to comfort children during stressful procedures. *Accident and Emergency Nursing* **7**(4): 226–36.

Stilwell E (1991) Nurses education related to the use of restraint. *Journal of Gerontology Nursing* **17**(2): 236.

Tinetti ME, Wen-Liang Lui, Ginter SF (1992) Mechanical restraint use and fall related injuries among residence of skilled nursing facilities. *Annals of Internal Medicine* **116**(5): 369–76.

United Nations (1989) *Convention on the Rights of the Child*. Adopted under General Assembly resolution 44/25. Geneva: UN.

Valler-Jones T, Shinnick A (2005) Holding children still for invasive procedures: preparing student nurses. *Paediatric Nursing* **17**(5): 20–2.

Wheeler R (2006) Gillick or Fraser? A plea for consistency over competence in children. *British Medical Journal* **332**: 807.

Willock J, Richardson J, Brazier A, *et al.* (2004) Peripheral venepuncture in infants and children. *Nursing Standard* **18**(27): 43–50.

Wright S (1999) Physical restraint in the management of violence and aggression in in-patient settings: a review of issues. *Journal of Mental Health* **8**(5): 459–72.

Young S (2000) Comparing the use of ketamine and midazolam in emergency settings. *Paediatric Nursing* **12**(2)18–21.

Chapter 7

Principles of pain management and entitlement to pain relief

Alison Twycross

Overview

Within this chapter the reasons for managing pain effectively and why it is important will be identified. An individual nurse's accountability to practice in an evidence-based manner will also be discussed, as will the need for evidence-based practice. An historical overview of how well pain has been managed in the past will be provided, followed by a review of studies demonstrating how well pain is currently managed. Drawing on current best practice guidelines, the steps that need to be taken to manage pain effectively will be identified. Finally, the obstacles to optimal pain management practices will be identified and strategies proposed to ensure that these barriers are overcome.

Why managing pain in children is important

Reflection point

What are the consequences of unrelieved pain?

Painful experiences are part of life for every child (Fearon *et al.* 1996; Van Cleve *et al.* 1996; Perquin *et al.* 2000; McGrath and Hillier 2003). Pain has an important purpose, serving as a warning or protective mechanism; people who are unable to feel pain often suffer extensive tissue damage (Melzack and Wall 1996). However, unrelieved pain has a number of undesirable physical and psychological consequences (see below). When these adverse effects are considered the need to manage children's pain effectively is clear.

Physical effects of unrelieved pain

- Rapid, shallow, splinted breathing, which can lead to hypoxaemia and alkalosis
- Inadequate expansion of lungs and poor cough, which can lead to secretion retention and atelectasis
- Increased heart rate, blood pressure and myocardial oxygen requirements, which can lead to cardiac morbidity and ischaemia
- Increased stress hormones (e.g. cortiosol, adrenaline, catecholamines), which in turn increase the metabolic rate, impede healing and decrease immune function
- Slowing or stasis of gut and urinary systems, which leads to nausea, vomiting, ileus and urinary retention
- Muscle tension, spasm and fatigue, which leads to reluctance to move spontaneously and refusal to ambulate, further delaying recovery

Psychological effects of unrelieved pain

Behavioural disturbances: fear, anxiety, distress, sleep disturbance, reduced coping, developmental regression

At this point it is worth noting the effects of unrelieved pain on a child in a hospital setting, as set out in the case study below.

Case study

Tallulah is 18 months old and has had recurrent admissions to hospital following surgery when she was a neonate. She currently has a wound infection and returns to the ward every 3–4 days to be reviewed by the surgeons and to have her dressing changed. Tallulah's pain has not always been managed effectively and she particularly hates dressing changes. On many occasions she starts crying as the car pulls into the hospital grounds and is often hysterical by the time she and her parents arrive on the ward.

Reflection point

How could Tallulah's pain (physical and psychological) be managed?

Poor pain management in early life can affect children when older. This has been demonstrated in several studies. Taddio *et al.* (1997) looked at data from a clinical trial studying the use of EMLA during routine vaccinations at 4 or 6 months to ascertain whether the effect of having a circumcision affected boys' pain response. Boys who had been circumcised without anaesthesia as neonates were observed to react significantly more intensely to vaccinations than uncircumcised boys ($P > 0.001$). This supports the findings from a previous study (Taddio *et al.* 1995). In a prospective cohort study, babies ($n = 21$) born to mothers with diabetes were compared with babies ($n = 21$) born to mothers with an uneventful pregnancy. Infants of diabetic mothers had repeated heel sticks in the first 24–36 hours of life (Taddio *et al.* 2002). Babies of diabetic mothers demonstrated significantly greater pain behaviours at venepuncture for newborn blood screening ($P = 0.04$).

A study by Grunau *et al.* (1998) examined the pain-related attitudes in two groups of children, aged 8–10 years (extremely low birthweight children ($n = 47$); full birthweight children ($n = 37$)). The extremely low birthweight group of children had been exposed to painful procedures as neonates; the other group had not. Children were shown the Pediatric Pain Inventory, which comprises 24 line drawings, each depicting a potentially painful event. The two groups of children did not differ in their overall perceptions of pain intensity. However, the very low birthweight children rated medical pain intensity significantly higher ($P < 0.004$) than psychosocial pain, suggesting that their early experiences affected their later perceptions of pain.

The relationship between the dose of morphine administered during a child's hospitalization for an acute burn and the course of post-traumatic stress disorder

(PTSD) symptoms over the 6 month period following discharge was investigated by Saxe *et al.* (2001). Children (*n* = 24) admitted to the hospital for an acute burn were assessed twice with the Child PTSD Reaction Index: while in the hospital and 6 months after discharge. All patients received morphine while in the hospital. The mean dose of morphine (mg/kg/day) was calculated for each child. There was a significant association between the dose of morphine received while in the hospital and a 6 month reduction in PTSD symptoms. Children receiving higher doses of morphine had a greater reduction in PTSD symptoms ($P < 0.05$).

When the consequences of unrelieved pain are taken into account, it is clear that managing children's postoperative pain effectively should be considered an ethical imperative. Failing to provide children with satisfactory pain relief can be considered a violation of their human rights. Indeed, the United Nations (UN) (1989), in its Convention on the Rights of the Child, states that 'children should in all circumstances be among the first to receive protection and relief, and should be protected from all forms of neglect, cruelty and exploitation'. It is, of course, entirely possible to manage a child's postoperative pain effectively, as shown in the Case study below.

Case study

Dexter is 7 years old and has been admitted to hospital for planned surgery. On admission the nurse takes a pain history from Dexter and his parents, identifying previous experiences of pain, the words used for pain and which pain-relieving interventions have been effective in the past. The nurse then explains that, following surgery, Dexter may have some pain. She introduces Dexter and his parents to the faces pain scale and explains how it is used to assess pain. The nurse tells Dexter and his parents that there are several drugs that can be used to manage his pain postoperatively. After the surgery Dexter has his pain assessed every hour for the first 6 hours after surgery. The nurses encourage Dexter and his parents to let them know if his pain 'gets bad'. Regular analgesic drugs are given to ensure that Dexter's pain is kept below a score of 3 out of 10. After the first 6 hours Dexter's pain appears well controlled and so it is assessed every 4 hours. The nurses continue to administer regular analgesic drugs. On discharge Dexter's parents are given verbal and written advice about how to manage his pain at home.

Principle for practice

Not managing pain in children effectively has adverse physical and psychological effects.

This principle can be applied to the management of pain, particularly as good practice guidelines are available. Further, the UNICEF (1999, p. 8) Child-Friendly Hospital Initiative highlights the importance of pain management, stating that 'A team will be established in the hospital whose remit is to establish standards and guidance in the control of pain and discomfort (psychological as well as physical) in children'.

Despite this there is evidence that children still experience moderate to severe unrelieved pain postoperatively (Health Care Commission 2004, 2007; Vincent and Denyes 2004; Johnston *et al.* 2005; Taylor *et al.* 2008).

Evidence-based practice and professional accountability

Principle for practice

Nurses should ensure that the care they provide is guided by the evidence available.

Current healthcare policy across the UK recognizes the need for evidence-based practice (Department of Health 1999, 2000, 2004; Scottish Executive 2000, 2001). Indeed, the (English) National Service Framework for Children, Young People and Maternity Services (Department of Health 2004) states that children and young people should receive high-quality evidence-based hospital care. Registered nurses are accountable for their actions. In the UK nurses' professional conduct must conform to the Nursing and Midwifery Council's (NMC) Code (Nursing and Midwifery Council 2008). The Code makes it clear that nurses should use evidence in practice and keep their knowledge and skills up to date (see below).

Using the best evidence available

- You must deliver care based on the best available evidence or best practice
- You must ensure any advice you give is evidence based if you are suggesting healthcare protocols or services

- You must ensure that the use of complementary or alternative therapies is safe and in the best interests of those in your care

(Nursing and Midwifery Council 2008)

Keep your skills and knowledge up to date

- You must have the knowledge and skills for safe and effective practice when working without direct supervision
- You must recognize and work within the limits of your competence

- You must keep your knowledge and skills up to date throughout your working life
- You must take part in appropriate learning and practice activities that maintain and develop your competence and performance

(Nursing and Midwifery Council 2008)

Historical overview of pain management in children

Historically pain in children was not managed effectively. Indeed, in 1968 Swafford and Allan (in)famously stated that 'Pediatric patients seldom need medication for the relief of pain after general surgery. They tolerate discomfort well' (p. 133).

The belief that children did not experience as much pain as adults is demonstrated by the results of several studies which found that children were experiencing unrelieved pain postoperatively and not receiving sufficient analgesics. In one study,

75% of children were in pain on the day of surgery, and 40% in severe pain with only slightly fewer patients reporting moderate to severe pain on the first postoperative day (Mather and Mackie 1983). Further, Eland (1985) reports that 66% of children (*n* = 2000), aged 4–10 years, undergoing surgery received no analgesic drugs.

Comparisons between the amount and type of analgesic drugs given to children and adults, in several studies, indicated that children received significantly less pain-relieving drugs (mg/kg) than adults did. Eland and Anderson (1977) compared the postoperative pain management of 18 adults with 25 children. Twelve of the children received a total of 24 doses of analgesics (13 non-opioids and 11 opioids), while the remaining 13 children were not given any analgesics. In contrast the adults received 372 doses of opioid and 299 non-opioid analgesics. Schechter *et al.* (1986) reviewed the charts of 90 children and 90 adults with identical diagnoses, and found that, in general, adults received twice as many doses of opioids as the children per hospital day. The longer the hospital stay the greater became the difference between adults and children. Beyer *et al.* (1983) compared the administration of analgesics to 50 children and 50 adults who had undergone cardiac surgery. Six children were prescribed no postoperative analgesics; adults received 70% of the analgesics administered; children received 30%. Clearly children's pain has not been managed well in the past. Indeed, the Royal College of Surgeons and College of Anaesthetists report (1990) on *Pain After Surgery* concluded that weaker oral analgesics were relied upon more frequently in children and fewer and relatively smaller doses of opioids were given compared with those of adults. In the next section the current situation regarding how well pain is managed in children will be discussed.

One reason that pain was not always managed effectively in the past was due to several misconceptions relating to pain in children. These are listed in Table 7.1 along with the evidence that proves their mythological status.

Table 7.1 Misconceptions about pain in children

Misconception	Evidence
Infants do not feel as much pain as adults	Pain pathways (although immature) are present at birth and pain impulses are able to travel to and from the pain centres in the brain (Wolf 1999; Coskun and Anand 2000; Fitzgerald 2000) Neonates exhibit behavioural, physiological and hormonal responses to pain (Franck 1986; Hogan and Choonara 1996; Carter 1997; Abu-Saad *et al.* 1998; Stevens 1999)
Infants cannot feel pain because of an immature nervous system	Complete myelination is not necessary for pain to be felt (Volpe 1981) Painful stimuli are transmitted by both myelinated and unmyelinated fibres (Volpe 1981; Craig and Grunau 1993) Incomplete myelination implies only a slower conduction speed in the nerves, which is offset by the shorter distances the impulse has to travel (Volpe 1981; Anand and Hickey 1987) Noxious stimuli have been shown to produce a cortical pain response in preterm babies (Bartocci *et al.* 2006; Slater *et al.* 2006)
Young children cannot indicate where pain is located	Children as young as 4 years old can demonstrate on a body chart where they hurt without knowing the names of body parts (Van Cleve and Savedra 1993) Children are able to report the intensity of pain by the age of 3–4 years (Harbeck and Peterson 1992)
Active children are not in pain A child engaged in playing activities cannot be in pain	Increased activity is often a sign of pain (Eland 1985) Children are particularly gifted in the use of distraction and use play as a diversion and as a coping mechanism (Eland 1985; McCaffery and Beebe 1989)
Sleeping children cannot be in pain	Sleep may be the result of exhaustion because of persistent pain (Hawley 1984)

Misconception	Evidence
Pain pathways in young infants are not developed sufficiently for them to experience pain	Neural pathways are in place *in utero* and maturation continues into adulthood; consequently, pain responses exist even in the very premature neonate (Fitzgerald and Howard 2003) Immature synapses within the spinal cord may cause activation of nerve impulses below the normal threshold increasing the pain response (Fitzgerald and Howard 2003) Immature gating mechanisms in the neonate result in an inability to distinguish between some types of stimuli, which may result in an exaggerated pain response (Fitzgerald and Howard 2003)
Lack of myelination prevents young infants from feeling pain	Myelin does not influence the generation of a nerve impulse (Fitzgerald and Howard 2003) The presence of myelin increases the speed of the impulse (Fitzgerald and Howard 2003) The process of myelination begins at about 22 weeks gestation (Fitzgerald and Howard 2003)
A young child's lack of previous experiences limits their ability to experience pain	Emotional processing and cognitive abilities develop over time, which may influence pain coping mechanisms (Fitzgerald and Howard 2003) Infants and young children have not yet developed these coping strategies and therefore they express pain differently (Fitzgerald and Howard 2003)
All children are sensitive to analgesic drugs	Infants and children require the same categories of analgesic drugs as adults; however, age-appropriate dosing must be considered (Charlton 2005)
Children are at greater risk (than adults) of addiction from opioids	The fear of opioid addiction in children has been greatly exaggerated with the incidence <1% (Charlton 2005)
Opioids are not safe to use for infants and children	Opioids are no more dangerous to infants and children than they are to adults (Charlton 2005) The risk of respiratory depression is no greater for infants and children provided the dose is appropriate (Charlton 2005)

Key point

- Historically, pain in children has not always been managed effectively. This was due, in part, to several misconceptions about pain in children which appear to influence practice despite evidence that demonstrates their methodological status.

Current situation

Pain is a bio-psycho-social experience. One individual cannot predict what another person will feel during a painful episode. When considering children's painful experiences it is, therefore, essential to explore children's views. Indeed the UN Convention of the Rights of the Child (1989) states that 'Children's views must be taken into account in all matters affecting them, subject to children's age and maturity'.

This is supported by current policy (e.g. Department of Health 2004). However, children's perceptions of how well their postoperative pain is managed have been examined in only three studies. In Alex and Ritchie's (1992) study children (*n* = 24), aged 7–11 years, were asked about their postoperative pain. Children rated their pain three times a day for the first three postoperative days using a vertical visual analogue scale and were then interviewed about their pain. Children felt that nurses needed to take a more active role in pain management. They suggested, for example, that nurses need to communicate with children about their pain.

Doorbar and McClarey (1999) collected data from children ($n = 61$) who gave in-depth interviews. The children ($n = 45$) drew pictures or completed sentence and/or picture sheets and they also ($n = 67$) took part in a *pain conference*. The children indicated that they felt that pain was poorly managed in hospital and that healthcare professionals needed to listen to what children were saying about their pain. Children, again, felt that nurses needed to communicate with them about their pain and felt that better explanations about what to expect were needed. Some children found it difficult to convince others that they were in pain.

Children ($n = 52$), aged 8–12 years, were asked about their postoperative pain experiences and to suggest what nurses could do to improve postoperative pain management in a study by Polkki et al. (2003). Children indicated that they wished the nurses had given them more or stronger analgesic drugs, as soon as they asked for them, and that they would like nurses to ask them about their pain on an hourly basis. Children would also like nurses to provide them with *meaningful things to do* to distract them from their pain. Despite the limited number of studies in this area it is evident that from the child's perspective there is a need to evaluate practices. Given the evidence cited earlier indicating that children continue to experience unrelieved moderate to severe pain postoperatively, it appears that current guidelines are not being implemented effectively into practice.

Key point

- Studies show that children feel nurses could be more proactive in managing pain. Suggestions have included that nurses should communicate with children about their pain and administer analgesic drugs as soon as they requested them.

Parents' views about how well their child's pain is managed postoperatively have been explored in three studies. In the study by Simons et al. (2001) 20 parent–nurse dyads were interviewed about their perceptions of children's postoperative pain management in the UK. Nurses felt that there was adequate involvement of parents and an acceptable standard of pain management for children whereas parents felt their involvement in their child's pain management was superficial and limited. In Simons and Roberson's (2002) study parents ($n = 20$) were interviewed about their perceptions of their child's postoperative pain management in the UK. Parents felt that nurses' communication about their child's pain was poor. Parents stated that they needed more information about pain management but felt that nurses were often dismissive of their concerns. This is regrettable for, as the following Case study taken from practice shows, parents play a crucial role in communicating their child's pain to nurses.

A questionnaire was completed by parents ($n = 192$) regarding their perceptions of their child's pain management while in hospital in Finland in Polkki et al.'s (2002) study. Ninety-eight per cent of parents felt they had adequate opportunities to participate in their child's care, with 86% of parents agreeing that they had a clearly defined role in relation to their child's pain-relieving interventions. Factors reported to hinder parents' involvement in their child's pain management included nurses' lack of time (32% of parents) and negative feelings of the nurses towards parental involvement (19%). However, parents would like more information about their

Case study

Joe is an 8 month old who has had a cleft lip and palate repair 4 days ago. The nurses had told his mother that the paracetamol he had been given should be sufficient to manage his pain. However, his mother felt that Joe wasn't himself and thought he was in pain, particularly as Joe cried every time he tried to smile or was offered a drink. At his mother's insistence the nurses eventually administered some Oramorph; after this Joe started drinking and was able to smile.

Reflection points

★ How should Joe's care and pain have been managed?

★ What would have been best practice?

child's pain management. Parents also suggested that nurses could pay heed to children's individuality or need for rest (especially after surgery), give appropriate pain medication, appreciate the child's and parent's opinions and involve them in decision-making. The results of these studies suggest that parents also feel there is a need for pain management practices to improve.

Principle for practice

• Parents would like more information about their child's pain management and how they could be involved in ensuring their child's pain is managed appropriately.

Few studies have focused on exactly how nurses manage children's pain. In Jacob and Puntillo's (1999) study, nurses ($n = 260$) in the USA completed a questionnaire about their pain management practices. Nurses reported that they were not consistently assessing pain in children, and pain management practices were not based on systematic assessment. The most frequently reported tool for assessing pain was the numerical rating scale. Nurses reported that they were not consistently administering analgesics for painful procedures. Nurses rarely used distraction and relaxation techniques. In another study, nurses ($n = 162$) completed a questionnaire about their use of non-drug methods of pain relief in five Finnish hospitals (Polkki *et al.* 2001). Distraction and preparatory information were reported as being used frequently and imagery was only used occasionally. Almost all nurses indicated that they used positioning. Massage and the application of heat/cold were used less frequently.

Observational data were collected about the verbal interaction of nurses ($n = 13$) with children ($n = 16$) in Byrne *et al.*'s (2001) study. Standardized open-ended interviews were also carried out with the nurses, children and parents. Data were analysed using discourse analysis and indicated that children were required to

Key point

Nurses' practices often do not appear to conform to current best practice guidelines.

> **Reflection point**
>
> Why do you think nursing practice does not always conform to best practice guidelines?

conform to ward routines and schedules of recovery. Rather than asking the child how much pain they were in, nurses appeared to manage pain using a set of behavioural milestones. In another observational study, registered nurses ($n = 13$) on a children's surgical ward in the English Midlands were each observed for a period of 5 hours per shift for two to four shifts (Twycross 2007a). The results of the study indicated that, although nurses administered analgesic drugs when a child complained of pain, in most other areas practices did not conform to current recommendations and were in need of improvement. Nurses did not, for example, routinely assess a child's pain, nor use non-drug methods of pain relief on a regular basis. The results of these studies indicate that nursing practices do not always conform to current best practice guidelines.

What is best practice when managing pain in children?

Clinical guidelines have been published in several countries to promote best practice. In England, the National Service Framework for Children, Young People and Maternity Services (NSF) (Department of Health 2004) includes six pain standards (Box 7.1), making it clear that pain management is an essential component of quality care for children in hospital. A list of key best practice guidelines and details of how to access them are provided below. These guidelines provide us with the knowledge about how pain should be managed.

Box 7.1	**Pain standards from the English National Service Framework (Department of Health 2004)**

- Standard 4.28
  - Pain is unpleasant, delays recovery, and adds to the trauma of illness, injury and clinical procedures
  - Historically, pain has been underestimated and undertreated
  - There is evidence that pain remains inadequately dealt with for children in hospital
- Standard 4.29
  - Where procedures are planned children should be prepared through play and education, pain relief should be planned for use during the procedure
  - The use of psychological therapies, including distraction, coping skills and cognitive–

behavioural approaches should be used for procedural pain and for pain from illness or trauma
- Standard 4.30
  - To treat children's pain effectively, a thorough pain assessment is necessary, and a number of guides are available to do this
  - These guides offer different options for communication, and can be completed in different ways by the child, family or professionals
  - Particular attention should be given to children who cannot express their pain because of their level of speech or understanding, communication difficulties, and those with altered consciousness or serious illness

- Standard 4.31
  — The treatment of children's pain using medicines requires appropriate choice of drug, dose, frequency and route
  — Research has found that some hospital staff may be reluctant to prescribe at all, and they tend to use a dose that is too small to address the child's pain adequately
  — Protocols, education and training can support staff in their management of children's pain, which should be reviewed regularly through audit
  — The involvement of pharmacists in the development of pain management guidelines is encouraged
- Standard 4.32
  — Children with long-term pain need a similar approach, spanning prevention, assessment and treatment
  — Special consideration should be given to children recovering from trauma and burns, and children with cancers, joint conditions, sickle cell disease, and those needing palliative care
- Standard 4.33
  — Hospital policies for managing children's pain should apply to all children in every hospital department, including newborns in neonatal units
  — Special focus should be given to children in accident and emergency departments, postoperative pain, pain related to procedures, and long-term pain in cancer

Principle for practice

There are a number of clinical guidelines available which identify best practice in relation to managing pain in children.

Selected current best practice guidelines: managing pain in children

Australia and New Zealand

- Australian and New Zealand College of Anaesthetists and Faculty of Pain Medicine (2010) *Acute pain management: scientific evidence*, 3rd edn. Melbourne: Australian and New Zealand College of Anaesthetists. See http://www.anzca.edu.au/resources/books-and-publications/Acute%20pain%20management%20-%20scientific%20evidence%20-%20third%20edition.pdf

North America

- American Academy of Pediatrics and American Pain Society (2001) The assessment and management of acute pain in infants, children and adolescents. *Pediatrics* **108**: 793–97. See http://www.ampainsoc.org/advocacy/pediatric2.htm
- American Academy of Pediatrics, Committee on Fetus and Newborn and Section on Surgery; Canadian Pediatric Society and Fetus and Newborn Committee (2006) Prevention and management of pain in the neonate: an update. *Pediatrics* **118**: 2231–41. See http://pediatrics.aappublications.org/cgi/reprint/118/5/2231

UK

- Association of Paediatric Anaesthetists of Great Britain and Ireland; Howard R, Carter B, Curry J, *et al.* (2008) Good practice in postoperative and procedural pain management. *Pediatric Anesthesia* **18**: 1–81. See http://www.blackwell-synergy.com/toc/pan/18/s1
- Royal College of Nursing (2009) *The recognition and assessment of acute pain in children*. London: RCN Publishing. See http://www.rcn.org.uk/__data/assets/pdf_file/0004/269185/003542.pdf

How should pain in children be managed?

Pain management means applying the stages of the nursing process to the treatment of pain. The four stages of pain management are:

1   assessment of pain (using a developmentally, validated pain assessment tool)
2   planning which pain-relieving interventions to use (analgesic drugs and non-drug methods)
3   implementing pain-relieving interventions
4   evaluating the effectiveness of the interventions used (by reassessing pain).

The cyclical nature of these stages is demonstrated in Fig. 7.1.

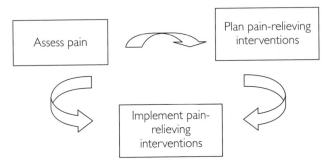

Figure 7.1 The pain management cycle.

Clinical guidelines relating to the management of pain in children and young people

A review of clinical guidelines relating to the management of pain in children and young people indicates that effective management of pain requires nurses to:

- Take a pain experience history from a child or young person and parent on admission
- Assess children and young people's pain using a valid and reliable, age-appropriate pain assessment tool
- Take into account children and young people's behavioural cues and physiological indicators of pain when assessing pain
- Administer appropriate analgesic drugs

- Use non-drug methods of pain relief
- Involve parents in their child's pain management
- Document pain scores and interventions
- Reassess pain having given time for pain-relieving interventions to take effect and, if necessary, alter the plan of care
- Communicate with children, young people and their parents about all aspects of pain management

(Developed from: American Academy of Pediatrics and American Pain Society 2001; Australian and New Zealand College of Anaesthetists 2010; Howard et al. 2008; Royal College of Nursing 2009)

How should pain in children be managed? Page 191

PART 2

Pain assessment tools

Table 7.2 details the various tools that can be used to assess children's pain.

Pain assessment tools for cognitively impaired children

While there are several pain assessment tools for this population, the most well validated measure is the Non-Communicating Children's Pain Checklist – Revised (Breau *et al.* 2002, see: http://www.aboutkidshealth.ca/Shared/PDFs/AKH_Breau_everyday.pdf). The paediatric pain profile has also been developed for use with this group of children (Hunt *et al.* 2004; Hunt *et al.* 2007) (see http://www.ppprofile.org.uk/).

Table 7.2 Pain Assessment Tools for Use with Children (adapted from Stinson 2009)

Tools for use with school-aged children and adolescents	
Verbal Rating Scales (VRS)	Consist of a list of simple word descriptors or phases to denote varying degrees or intensities of pain. Each word or phrase has an associated number. Children are asked to select a single word or phrase that best represents their level of pain intensity and the score is the number associated with the chosen word. One example of a VRS is using word descriptors of *not at all* = 0, *a little bit* = 1, *quite a lot* = 2 and *most pain possible* = 3 (Goodenough et al. 1997).
Faces Pain Scales	Faces pain scales present the child with drawings or photographs of facial expressions representing increasing levels of pain intensity. The child is asked to select the picture of a face that best represents their pain intensity and their score is the number (rank order) of the expression chosen. Faces scales have been well validated for use in children aged 5–12 years (Champion et al. 1998; Stinson et al. 2006). There are two types of faces scales – line drawings (e.g. Wong-Baker) and photographs (e.g. OUCHER). Faces pain scales with a happy and smiling *no pain* face or faces with tears for *most pain possible* have been found to affect the pain scores recorded. For example, the smiling lower anchor of the Wong-Baker FACES Pain Scale has been found to produce higher pain ratings than those with neutral faced anchors (Chambers and Craig, 1998).
Numerical Pain Scales (NRS)	A numerical rating scale (NRS) consists of a range of numbers (e.g. 0–10 or 0–100) that can be represented in verbal or graphical format. Children are told that the lowest number represents *no pain* and the highest number represents *the most pain possible*. The child is instructed to circle, record or state the number that best represents their level of pain intensity. Verbal NRSs tend to be the most frequently used pain intensity measure with children over eight years old in clinical practice. They have the advantage that they can be verbally administered without a print copy and are easy to score. They do require numeracy skills and, therefore, should be used in older school-aged children and adolescents. While there is evidence of their reliability and validity in adults, verbal NRS have undergone very little testing in children. An example of a well validated scale incorporating a graphic NRS is the OUCHER (Beyer 1984). The OUCHER comprises two separate scales; photographic faces scale and a 0–10 vertical NRS. Older school-aged children and adolescents are meant to use the NRS.

Tools for use with preverbal children	
Children's Hospital of Eastern Ontario Pain Scale (CHEOPS) (McGrath et al. 1985)	Intended for use in children 1-7 years of age but has been used in children 4 months to 17 years to assess procedural and postoperative pain. Indicators are scored on a four-point scale (0, 1, 2, 3) The indicators are: crying, facial expression, verbalizations, torso activity, whether and how child touches wound, leg position Range of total scores is 4–13, but there is no indication of what mild, moderate or severe pain score ranges would be CHEOPS has well-established evidence of reliability, validity and ability to detect change (von Baeyer and Spagrud, 2007) Length of tool and confusing scoring system makes it complicated to use in everyday clinical practice *(low to medium clinical utility)* Cannot be used in intubated or paralysed patients
FLACC (Malviya et al. 2005)	Intended for use in children 2 months to 8 years of age but has been used in children 0–18 years Procedural and postoperative pain Five categories scored on a 0–2 scale, which results in a total score between 0 and 10 Categories: facial expression, leg movement, activity, cry and consolability Well-established evidence of reliability and validity; however inconsistent ability to detect change (von Baeyer and Spagrud, 2007) Simple to use, score and interpret *(high clinical utility)* Cannot be used in intubated or paralysed patients Important to note that consolability requires (a) an attempt to console, and (b) a subjective rating of response to that intervention, which complicates the scoring Limited use in disabled children with altered limb/leg movement
Neonatal tools	
Premature Infant Pain Profile (PIPP) (Stevens et al. 1996)	Preterm and term infants (e.g. 28–40 weeks gestation) Initially developed for procedural pain, requires further evaluation with very low birth weight neonates and with non-acute and post-surgical pain populations Includes contextual indicators (e.g. gestational age and behavioural state) Indicators: gestational age, behavioural state, heart rate and oxygen saturation, brow bulge, eye squeeze, and nasolabial furrow Each indicator is evaluated on a four-point scale (0, 1, 2, 3) for a possible total score of 18–21 based on the gestational age of the infant; Total score of 6 or less generally indicates minimal or no pain, while scores greater than 12 indicate moderate to severe pain Most rigorously evaluated tool; evidence of reliability, validity and ability to detect change Pain assessments take 1 minute *(high clinical utility)*
CRIES (Crying, Requires O$_2$ for saturation above 95, Increased vital signs, Expression, and Sleeplessness) (Krechel and Bilder 1995)	Full-term neonates (32–60 weeks gestational age) Postoperative pain measure Each indicator is rated on a three point scale (0, 1, 2) that results in a total score ranging from 0–10 Indicators: cry, oxygen saturation, heart rate/blood pressure, expression and sleeplessness Evidence of reliability and validity (Duhn and Medves 2004) and some evidence of ability to detect change Easy to remember and use *(high clinical utility)* Uses oxygenation as a measure, which can be affected by many other factors BP measurements may upset neonates
Neonatal Infant Pain Scale (NIPS) (Lawrence et al. 1993)	Preterm and term infants Procedural pain measure Operational definitions for indicators are provided Each indicator is scored on a two-point (0, 1) or three-point (0, 1, 2) scale at one-minute intervals, before, during, and following a procedure Indicators: facial expression, cry, breathing patterns, arms, legs, state of arousal Evidence of reliability and validity (Duhn and Medves 2004) Hard to remember *(limited clinical utility)* Cannot be used in intubated or paralysed patients

Further reading on pain assessment tools

Further information about the pain assessment tools available for use with children can be found in:

- Royal College of Nursing (2009) *The recognition and assessment of acute pain in children*. London: RCN Publishing.
- Stinson J (2009) Pain assessment in children. In: Twycross A, Dowden SJ, Bruce L (eds) *Pain management in children: a clinical guide*, pp. 85–108. Oxford: Wiley-Blackwell.

- Stinson J, Yamada J, Kavanagh T, *et al.* (2006) Systematic review of the psychometric properties and feasibility of self-report pain measures for use in clinical trials in children and adolescents. *Pain* **125**(1–2): 143–57.
- von Baeyer CL, Spagrud LJ (2007) Systematic review of observational (behavioural) measures for children and adolescents aged 3 to 18 years. *Pain* **127**: 140–50.

Specific pain-relieving interventions

For details about specific pain-relieving interventions, see
- Twycross A, Dowden SJ, Bruce L (eds) (2009) *Pain management in children: a clinical guide*. Oxford: Wiley-Blackwell.

Barriers to best practice

Several factors have been suggested as reasons why children and young people's pain is still not managed effectively. These include knowledge deficits; incorrect or outdated beliefs about pain and pain management; the decision-making strategies used; ward culture; and organizational culture (Fig. 7.2). These will be discussed in turn.

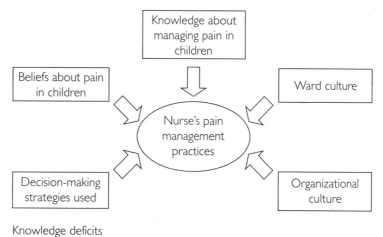

Figure 7.2 Factors having an impact on nurses' management of pain.

Knowledge deficits

Limited theoretical knowledge about managing pain in children and young people has been suggested as one reason nurses do not manage pain effectively. Seven studies have examined children's nurses' theoretical knowledge about pain in children. A study carried out with paediatric oncology nurses ($n = 106$) in the USA found a lack of understanding of basic pharmacological principles in relation to analgesic drugs (Schmidt *et al.* 1994). Salantera *et al.* (1999) developed a questionnaire which was completed by paediatric nurses ($n = 265$) in Finland; gaps were found in nurses' knowledge about managing pain in children in relation to analgesic drugs and non-drug methods of pain relief. Final-year student nurses ($n = 73$) also completed the questionnaire and demonstrated knowledge deficits in relation to analgesic drugs and pain assessment (Salantera and Lauri 2000). Twycross (2004) used a modified version of Salantera's questionnaire (as part of a larger study) and found that nurses ($n = 12$) had gaps in their knowledge and that these were especially noticeable in relation to analgesic drugs, non-drug methods and the physiology of pain as well as the psychology and sociology of pain.

The Pediatric Nurses' Knowledge and Attitudes Regarding Pain Survey was completed by nurses ($n = 274$) in Manworren's (2000) study. The mean score for the questionnaire was 66% (range 31–98%), with knowledge deficits particularly apparent in relation to pain assessment, the pharmacology of analgesic drugs, the use of analgesic drugs and non-drug methods. Further, nurses ($n = 67$) completed an adapted version of the Nurses' Knowledge and Attitudes Regarding Pain Survey in Vincent's (2005) study. Nurses had knowledge deficits in relation to non-drug methods of pain relief, analgesic drugs and the incidence of respiratory depression.

Rieman and Gordon (2007) surveyed children's nurses ($n = 295$) using a revised version of the Pediatric Nurses' Knowledge and Attitudes Regarding Pain Survey. The mean survey score was 74%. The 10 questions answered incorrectly by most participants related to pharmacology and the incidence of respiratory depression. Limited knowledge about many aspects of analgesic drugs was also found by Ellis *et al.* (2007). The results of these studies suggest that gaps remain in nurses' knowledge about pain in children, and in particular in relation to pain assessment, analgesic drugs and non-drug methods. These gaps in knowledge provide a partial explanation for suboptimal pain management practices.

However, looking at nurses' theoretical knowledge alone does not provide information about the impact of knowledge deficits on practice; this has been explored in two studies. Vincent and Denyes (2004) examined the relationship between knowledge and attitudes about children's pain relief and nurses' analgesic administration practices. They observed the care of children ($n = 132$), aged 3½ to 17 years, by nurses ($n = 67$) and found that nurses with a better theoretical knowledge about pain were not more likely to administer analgesia. In the second study by Twycross (2007b), nurses ($n = 13$) on one children's surgical ward were shadowed for a 5 hour period for two to four shifts. Data about postoperative pain management practices were collected using a pain management checklist and field notes. Nurses ($n = 12$) also completed the revised pain management knowledge test. Questionnaire scores were compared with the observational data. No positive relationship between individual children's nurse's level of knowledge and how well they actually managed pain was found. Even when the nurses had a good level of theoretical knowledge, this was not reflected in their pain management practices.

The findings of Vincent and Denyes (2004) and Twycross (2007b) support those of Watt-Watson *et al.* (2001), who collected data from 80 (adult) nurse–patient pairs. No relationship was found between nurses' knowledge and patients' ratings of pain and the amount of analgesia administered, even though the nurses had moderately good knowledge levels about pain management. Nurses do not appear to apply their theoretical knowledge in practice.

Key point

- Nurses will always need to be educated about managing pain in children. However, gaps in nurses' theoretical knowledge levels do not appear to provide the sole explanation for deficits in pain management practices.

Beliefs about pain in children

Nurses' beliefs about pain and, particularly, the priority nurses attribute to pain management have also been suggested as reasons for suboptimal pain management practices. Nurses' beliefs about pain management have been examined in several studies. Nurses ($n = 22$) completing a training needs questionnaire about several aspects of nursing attributed a significantly lower priority to pain management than to other aspects of their role, such as communication and teamwork, and management and supervision ($P < 0.001$) (Twycross 1999). Hamers *et al.* (1994) describe the results of two studies which examined the factors affecting nurses' assessment of pain and implementation of pain-relieving interventions in the Netherlands. Data were collected using semistructured interviews with nurses ($n = 20$), by observing participants and by examining nursing records. Nurses seemed to assume (incorrectly) that some pain was to be expected during a hospital stay, and used their past experiences (both bad and good) to determine what to do when managing pain. If nurses believe pain is to be expected during a hospital stay it is perhaps not surprising that relieving it is given a low priority.

The lack of priority attributed to pain management by children's nurses is supported by the findings of two observational studies. In Woodgate and Kristjanson's (1996) study, nurses ($n = 24$) were shown to concentrate on technical aspects of care and saw comforting the child as the parent's role. As discussed previously, Byrne *et al.* (2001) in their observational study found that nurses appeared to negate (ignore) children's pain. Children were required to conform to ward routines and schedules of recovery. Rather than asking the child or young person how much pain they were in, nurses appeared to manage pain using a set of behavioural milestones. Nurses' beliefs about managing pain in children and young people and how these affect practice clearly need exploring further.

One study has explored the link between the perceived importance of pain management and the priority nurses actually attribute to managing pain in practice (Twycross 2008). Participant observational data were collected about children's nurses' ($n = 13$) postoperative pain management practices on a children's surgical ward in the English Midlands. Nurses ($n = 12$) also completed a questionnaire to provide a measure of the importance they attributed to pain management tasks. The importance nurses attributed to the pain management task did not reflect the likelihood of the task being undertaken in practice. Indeed, the perceived importance of a pain management task bore little relationship to observed practices. There is evidence from the studies reviewed in this section that outdated and incorrect beliefs about pain management, and not making pain a priority, contribute to suboptimal practices but they do not provide a complete explanation.

Key point

- Outdated and incorrect beliefs about pain management, and not making pain a priority, may be contributing factors, but do not provide a complete explanation for suboptimal pain management practices.

Reflection points

★ Is pain relief a priority in your present clinical placement/ward?

★ Are up-to-date guidelines and practice a feature of your present clinical placement/ward?

★ What other factors do you feel may be responsible for suboptimal pain management practices in your present clinical placement/ward?

Decision-making strategies

Only three studies have explored children's nurses decision-making strategies when managing pain in children. Twycross and Powls (2006) examined children's nurses' decision-making when managing postoperative pain in children using the think-aloud technique. Nurses ($n = 12$) appeared to use an analytical model of decision-making. All the nurses used backward reasoning strategies[1] and collected similar types and amounts of information before making a decision about appropriate nursing care. This is indicative of non-expert decision-making. No differences were noted between nurses with 5 or more years of experience in paediatric surgery and less experienced nurses. Nor were there any differences apparent between graduate and non-graduate nurses. The complexity of managing pain could have affected nurses' decision-making, although as similar results were found among nurses working in a paediatric medical ward this is unlikely to be the case (Twycross and Powls 2006).

[1]In forward reasoning an individual works forward from a hypothesis to find a solution to a problem, whereas in backward reasoning an individual works backwards from a hypothesis to evaluate different options or find a solution (Lamond *et al*. 1996).

The influence of expertise on nurses' pain assessments and decisions regarding analgesia administration in children was explored by Hamers *et al.* (1997). First-year nursing students (*n* = 271), fourth-year nursing students (*n* = 222) and registered nurses (*n* = 202) were presented with video vignettes. Participants were asked to rate on a 100 mm visual analogue scale: the pain experienced by the child in the case; how sure they were that their pain assessment was correct; and whether they would administer analgesia to the child in the case. The results indicated that, while registered nurses were most confident and more inclined to administer analgesics than less experienced nurses, expertise (i.e. years of experience) did not influence the assessment of pain intensity.

Clinical scenarios were used to explore influences on nurses' (*n* = 334) decision-making about which analgesic drugs and non-drug methods to implement when managing children's pain (Griffin *et al.* 2008). The personal attributes of nurses (*n* = 334) such as education level, race/ethnicity, age, years of clinical experience, or having had continuing education about pain did not appear to have an impact on decision-making. Indeed, nurses in the study indicated that they would administer the maximum prescribed dose of analgesic drugs. This contradicts the results of other studies (Hamers *et al.* 1998; Vincent and Denyes 2004). This is perhaps attributable to a social desirability response affecting participants' responses; alternatively the introduction of pain standards by the Joint Commission on Accreditation of Healthcare Organizations (2000) may have had an impact on pain management practices in the USA. The studies discussed in this section provide some insight into how nurses make decisions and the factors that affect this process. Further research is needed in this context. However, suboptimal decision-making strategies might explain, at least in part, why children continue to experience unrelieved pain.

Key point

- Suboptimal decision-making strategies might explain, at least in part, why children continue to experience unrelieved pain. Further research is needed about the factors affecting children's nurses' decision-making.

Ward culture

Ward culture may also be an important factor in relation to pain management practices. This relates particularly to nurses, and other healthcare professionals, who have a tendency to learn through role modelling and professional socialization.

Role modelling

Evidence that nurses copy the behaviours of more senior staff has been found in several studies. Novice nurses (*n* = 15) in Taylor's (1997) study commented that 'they just followed the [more experienced] nurse's lead'. Student nurses (*n* = 99) interviewed by Fitzpatrick *et al.* (1996) discussed modelling their practices on those of more experienced nurses. In Twycross' (2004) study two participants indicated that they had learnt about pain management by observing/working with more senior staff, and another participant reported that she had had no formal education 'except what I picked up as I've gone along'.

If nurses learn by copying the behaviours of role models, the quality of their practice will depend on the practices of the role model. If role models have, for example, poor pain assessment skills or use limited non-drug methods of pain relief and merely administer analgesic drugs when a child complains of pain, the novice nurse is likely to develop a similar approach. Thus, even if a nurse has a good level of theoretical knowledge, this is unlikely to be applied in practice. Junior staff modelling their pain management practices on those of more senior staff who have suboptimal practices offers another explanation as to why pain management practices remain poor.

Professional socialization

Wanting to be part of a social group is part of being human (Furnham 1997; Fincham and Rhodes 1999). When starting a placement or job in a new ward or hospital, nurses undergo a period of socialization, during which they learn the rules (formal and informal) that guide the behaviour of staff. This has been explored in several studies. Gray and Smith (1999) found that there were rewards for student nurses ($n = 17$) for conforming to the norms of the ward, such as the increased likelihood of a good placement and feeling part of the team. In Philpin's (1999) study nurses ($n = 18$), half of whom had undergone traditional training and half of whom had received Project 2000 education, were interviewed. The results indicated that if new nurses did not conform to the area's norms they were excluded, shouted at in front of everyone and bullied. Neonatal nurses ($n = 4$) demonstrated a tendency to conform to ward practices rather than what they knew to be research-based best practice (Greenwood *et al.* 2000). In a study examining the effects of occupational socialization on nurses' ($n = 23$) moving and handling practice, Kneafsey (2000) found that nurses did not use their theoretical knowledge in practice but rather conformed to ward practices.

A nurse's need to *fit in* may mean that they adopt the ward's (poor) pain management practices, despite having (some) theoretical knowledge about how children's pain should be managed and believing that pain management is important. If nurses acting differently from the ward culture are *picked on* this is likely to discourage them from using their own discretion, or from questioning practice. Professional socialization may allow non-evidence-based practices to be perpetuated.

> **Key point**
> - Nurses role modelling the practices of more senior nurses and/or adopting (poor) ward pain management practices may explain, at least in part, why pain management practices do not conform to current best practice guidelines.

Organizational aspects

Organizational culture has been identified as the key to changing pain management practices (Bucknall *et al.* 2001; Treadwell *et al.* 2002; Botti *et al.* 2004; Jordan-Marsh *et al.* 2004; Bruce and Franck 2005) but can be difficult to achieve (Megens *et al.* 2008). Several studies have examined the impact of implementing organizational pain management strategies on practice.

In Treadwell *et al.*'s (2002) study staff were educated about the use of pain assessment tools and a standardized pain assessment protocol was implemented. Data were collected from children and parents (time 1, $n = 36$; time 2, $n = 49$) before and 12 months after the implementation of the protocol; staff also completed a questionnaire (time 1, $n = 68$; time 2, $n = 82$). Children, parents and staff all reported increased pain assessment ($P = 0.05$) and improved staff responsiveness to pain ($P < 0.001$) following the intervention. A chart audit demonstrated compliance with the assessment protocol.

An action research study was carried out to improve the management of acute pain in children through the systematic assessment of pain and the administration of appropriate analgesia in one US hospital (Jordan-Marsh *et al.* 2004). Pain management procedures for postoperative and procedural pain were implemented; a pain assessment tool was implemented; and analgesic drug regimes were standardized. Patient care rounds focusing on pain management also took place. Chart audits were carried out and demonstrated an increase in documented pain assessments; reassessment of pain; and the amount of analgesia administered.

An organization-wide comprehensive pain management programme was implemented in one Canadian hospital (Ellis *et al.* 2007). A statistically significant increase was found in the use of pain assessment tools ($P = 0.005$) and documentation of pain assessment in nursing notes ($P < 0.001$) 6 months after the start of the programme. Improvements in pain management practices have also been found in other studies (Megens *et al.* 2008; Oakes *et al.* 2008). These studies, together, provide evidence that making pain management an organizational priority can improve pain management practices. However, many of these studies are small scale and change is not always evaluated over a prolonged period.

Further evidence of the impact of organizational culture on pain management practices can be found in Lauzon Clabo's (2008) ethnographic study on two (adult) wards in one hospital in the USA. Participants described a clear pattern of pain assessment on each ward; these patterns were different from each other. The social context appeared to heavily influence nurses' pain assessment practices. The impact of organizational culture on pain management practices clearly needs exploring further.

Key point

- Organizational culture appears to have an impact on pain management practices. Further research is needed in this area.

Overcoming the barriers

Clearly, there is no easy answer to improving the management of pain in children. However, if the factors identified are addressed simultaneously practices may improve. Strategies for improving practices will now be discussed.

PART 2

Educational issues

There will always be a need to educate nurses about pain management. However, there is increasing evidence that children's nurses are not using their theoretical knowledge in practice (Vincent and Denyes 2004; Twycross 2007b). Several studies have found evidence that gaps in nurses' theoretical knowledge may mean that they do not understand the rationale for pain-relieving interventions (Schmidt *et al.* 1994; Salantera *et al.* 1999; Manworren 2000; Salantera and Lauri 2000; Twycross 2004; Vincent 2005; Rieman and Gordon 2007), which may explain why nurses do not use their knowledge in practice. If this is the case pre- and post-registration course content needs evaluating to ensure that nurses have a thorough knowledge of pain (e.g. pain as bio-psycho-social phenomenon, anatomy and physiology of pain, pain assessment, pharmacological and non-drug pain-relieving interventions and understand the rationale for pain-relieving interventions).

Reflection points

★ During your pre-registration programme how much of the curriculum was devoted to pain relief in children and was this enough?

★ During your postgraduate or post-registration programme how much of the curriculum was devoted to pain relief in children and was this enough?

★ Do you feel you need to update your knowledge and skills and how would you set about doing this?

One reason for the limited use of theoretical knowledge in practice could be that, because of their knowledge deficits, nurses do not understand the rationale for using specific interventions. Indeed, a review of pain content in pre-registration diploma courses in England found that most child branch curricula included less than 10 hours of education on pain, providing students with little more than a whistle-stop tour of pain management (Twycross 2000). It is perhaps not surprising that knowledge deficits remain. Further research is needed to ascertain the optimum time and content required on pain management in pre-registration nursing curricula.

Several educational strategies have been suggested that promote the use of theoretical knowledge in practice. Ochieng (1999) describes the use of reflective practice as a method of changing pain management practices. Three months after the start of the project, practices did appear to have changed but there was no evaluation of whether this was sustained long term. Other suggestions for improving the use of knowledge in practice, which have not yet been tested, include:

• the clinical discussion of individual patients and their care (Graffam 1990)
• incorporating clinical scenarios and simulations into teaching (Lee and Ryan-Wenger 1997; Cioffi 1998, 2001; Jones and Sheridan 1999)
• teaching rounds (Segal and Mason 1998)
• journal clubs (Kessenich *et al.* 1997; Khalid and Gee 1999).

Some methods of learning (e.g. *confluent education*) emphasize the importance of integrating left-brain knowledge with right-brain creativity. These teaching methods may help ensure the integration of theory and practice. The use of scenario-based or problem-based learning seems to support the integration of theoretical knowledge into practice; however, this needs further research. Future research should focus on identifying the educational strategies which facilitate the incorporation of theoretical knowledge into practice.

Supporting decision-making

A review of the decision-making literature provides no definitive answers about ways to improve nurses' decision-making strategies or how to ensure that current best practice guidelines are used when making clinical decisions. One possible method would be the use of a decision-making algorithm. The effectiveness of an algorithm in conjunction with the administration of regular multimodal analgesia was tested by Falanga *et al.* (2006). When the algorithm was used children received more analgesia and had lower pain intensity scores. Developing and using algorithms from best practice guidelines would remove much of the stress associated with decision-making and would guide nurses through the process in a step-by-step way. This might help ensure that best practice guidelines are adhered to and thus improve pain management practices.

Making pain an organizational priority

Several strategies have been put forward as ways of ensuring pain is an organizational priority. These are outlined in Fig. 7.3. Making pain an organizational priority will also help address the issues relating to ward culture.

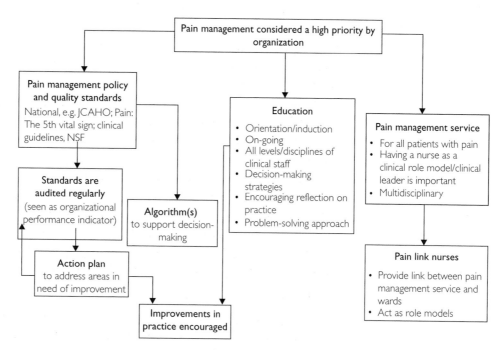

Figure 7.3 Improving pain management practices: organizational aspects (Redrawn from Twycross and Dowden 2009, with permission).

Setting and auditing pain standards

The first step in making effective pain management an organizational priority is to audit current practice against selected best practice guidelines. These pain management standards should be audited on a regular basis (at least every 6 months). Following completion of the audit an action plan should be drawn up. Once sufficient time has been given for changes to be implemented, practice should be re-audited. Figure 7.4 outlines the process of auditing pain management practices.

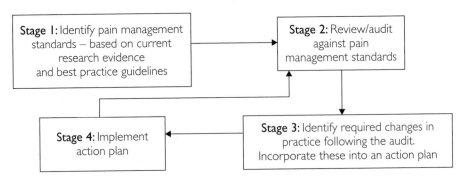

Figure 7.4 Auditing pain management practices (Redrawn from Twycross and Dowden 2009, with permission).

Pain management services

Another organizational strategy for improving pain management is the development of a pain service. Guidance on the provision of paediatric anaesthetic services by the Royal College of Anaesthetists in the UK emphasizes the need for a properly staffed and funded acute pain service covering the needs of children (Royal College of Anaesthetists 2001). The Royal College of Anaesthetists recommends that a member of the acute pain service should visit all children's surgical wards every day and see all children having major surgery. This is also supported by the UNICEF Child-friendly Hospital Initiative, which states that a team should be established whose remit is to establish standards and guidance in the control of pain and discomfort in children (UNICEF 1999). Usually newly established pain services initially manage only acute pain, but as the service develops many expand to include procedural pain, chronic pain and palliative pain management.

A pain nurse visiting the wards each day can provide support to the nurses caring for children and young people in pain. This could reduce the stress associated with decision-making and caring for children and young people in pain and may also increase nurses' confidence regarding pain management. Indeed, a study in Wales found that the introduction of an acute pain service led to considerable improvement in the level of adults' postoperative pain (assessed by visual analogue scores) (Gould *et al.* 1992). This concurs with the findings of other studies (Stratton 1999; Bardiau *et al.* 2003; McDonnell *et al.* 2005).

PART 2

Pain link nurses

Human sources of information have been shown to be important in changing practices and in the dissemination of research evidence into practice (Thompson *et al.* 2001; McCaughan 2002). Indeed, facilitators have been described as having a key role in relation to getting evidence into practice (Harvey *et al.* 2002; Rycroft-Malone *et al.* 2002). The use of link nurses has been suggested as a way of increasing the application of research in practice both generally (Thompson *et al.* 2001) and in relation to pain management (Ferrell *et al.* 1993; McCleary *et al.* 2004), but such roles need to be resourced adequately.

> ## Key point
>
>
> - Changing pain management practices requires a multifaceted approach. Several issues need addressing, including: the methods used to educate nurses about pain management; beliefs about pain management; nurses' decision-making strategies when managing pain in children; and organizational culture. Further research is needed to evaluate the effectiveness of interventions proposed to address these areas.

> ## Reflection points
>
> ★ Does your clinical placement/ward have access to a dedicated paediatric pain nurse or pain link nurse?
> ★ Do you think children and young people would benefit from such a service?
> ★ Would you consider a career as one in the future?

Conclusion

Pain management practices have improved over the past 25 years. However, there is still room for improvement, with many children and young people still experiencing moderate to severe unrelieved pain postoperatively. Several factors contribute to continuing poor pain management practices including: knowledge deficits; incorrect or outdated beliefs about pain and pain management; the decision-making strategies used; ward culture; and organizational culture. Improving pain management thus requires a multifactorial approach with all of these areas being addressed. Possible ways forward have been suggested in this chapter, but further research needs to be done to determine the effectiveness of the proposed interventions.

This chapter has shown that children and young people's nurses play a crucial role in managing pain in children and young people.

Summary of principles for practice

- Children and young people's nurses must make the management of pain in children and young people a priority.
- Children and young people's nurses must communicate with children and young people about their pain and administer analgesia as soon as it is requested.
- Children and young people's nurses must ensure that parents are given information about their child's pain and management.
- Children and young people's nurses have a duty to comply with best practice guidance in pain management.
- Children and young people's nurses must be competent in the assessment and management of pain.
- Children and young people's nurses must work with other healthcare professionals to ensure optimum pain management for the child or young person.

References

Abu-Saad HH, Bours GJ, Stevens B, Hamers JP (1998) Assessment of pain in the neonate. *Seminars in Perinatology* **22**(5): 402–16.

Alex M, Ritchie J (1992) School-aged children's interpretation of their experience with acute surgical pain. *Journal of Pediatric Surgery* **7**(3): 171–88.

American Academy of Pediatrics and American Pain Society (2001) The assessment and management of acute pain in infants, children and adolescents. *Pediatrics* **108**(3): 793–7.

American Academy of Pediatrics, Committee on Fetus and Newborn and Section on Surgery; Canadian Pediatric Society and Fetus and Newborn Committee (2006) Prevention and management of pain in the neonate: an update. *Pediatrics* **118**: 2231–41. See http://pediatrics.aappublications.org/cgi/reprint/118/5/2231

Anand KJS, Hickey PR (1987) Pain and its effects in the human neonate and fetus. *New England Journal of Medicine* **317**: 1321–9.

Association of Paediatric Anaesthetists of Great Britain and Ireland; Howard R, Carter B, Curry J, *et al.* (2008) Good practice in post-operative and procedural pain management. *Pediatric Anesthesia* **18**: 1–81. See http://www.blackwell-synergy.com/toc/pan/18/s1

Australian and New Zealand College of Anaesthetists and Faculty of Pain Medicine (2010) *Acute pain management: scientific evidence*, 3rd edn. Melbourne: ANZCA.

Bardiau FM, Taviaux NF, Albert A, *et al.* (2003) An intervention study to enhance postoperative pain management. *Anesthesia and Analgesia* **96**(1): 179–85.

Bartocci M, Bergqvist LL, Lagercrantz H, Anand KJS (2006) Pain activates cortical areas in the preterm newborn brain. *Pain* **122**: 109–17.

Beyer JE (1984) *The Oucher: a user's manual and technical report*. Hospital play equipment, Evanston, Illinois.

Beyer JE, DeGood DE, Ashley LC, Russell GA (1983) Patterns of postoperative analgesic use with adults and children following cardiac surgery. *Pain* **17**: 71–81.

Botti M, Bucknall T, Manias E (2004) The problem of postoperative pain: issues for future research. *International Journal of Nursing Practice* **10**(6): 257–63.

Breau LM, McGrath PJ, Camfield C, Finley GA (2002) Psychometric properties of the non-communicating children's pain checklist (revised). *Pain* **99**: 349–57.

Bruce E, Franck LS (2005) Using the worldwide web to improve children's pain care. *International Nursing Review* **52**(3): 204–9.

Bucknall T, Manias E, Botti M (2001) Acute pain management: implications of scientific evidence for nursing practice in the postoperative context. *International Journal of Nursing Practice* **7**(4): 266–73.

Byrne A, Morton J, Salmon P (2001) Defending against patients' pain: a qualitative analysis of nurses' responses to children's postoperative pain. *Journal of Psychosomatic Research* **50**: 69–76.

Carter B (1997) Pantomimes of pain, distress, repose and lability: the world of the preterm baby. *Journal of Child Healthcare* **1**(1): 17–23.

Chambers CT, Craig KD (1998) An intrusive impact of anchors in children's faces pain scales, *Pain* **78**(1): 27–37.

Champion GD, Goodenough B, von Baeyer CL, Thomas W (1998) Measurement of pain by self-report. In: Finley GA, McGrath PJ (eds) Measurement of pain in infants and children: progress in pain research and management. Vol. 10, pp. 123–60. Seattle: IASP Press.

Charlton JE (ed.) (2005) *Core curriculum for professional education in pain*, 3rd edn. IASP Task Force on Professional Education. Seattle: IASP Publications.

Cioffi J (1998) Decision making by emergency nurses in triage assessments. *Accident and Emergency Nursing* **6**: 184–91.

Cioffi J (2001) Clinical simulations: development and validation. *Nurse Education Today* **21**: 477–86.

Coskun V, Anand KJS (2000) Development of supraspinal pain processing. In: Anand KJS, Stevens BJ, McGrath PJ (eds) *Pain in neonates*, 2nd edn, pp. 23–54. Amsterdam: Elsevier.

Craig KD, Grunau RVE (1993) Neonatal pain perception and behavioural measurement. In: Anand KJS, Stevens BJ, McGrath PJ (eds) *Pain in neonates*, 2nd edn, pp. 67–105. Amsterdam: Elsevier.

Department of Health (1999) *Making a difference*. London: The Stationery Office.

Department of Health (2000) *The NHS plan*. London: The Stationery Office.

Department of Health (2004) *The National Service Framework for Children, Young People and Maternity Services*. London: The Stationery Office.

Doorbar P, McClarey M (1999) *Ouch! Sort it out: children's experiences of pain*. London: RCN Publishing.

Duhn LJ, Medves JM (2004) A systematic integrative review of infant pain assessment tools. *Advances in Neonatal Care* **4**(3): 126–40.

Eland J (1985) *Myths about pain in children*. Leeds: The Candlelighters Childhood Cancer Foundation.

Eland JM, Anderson JE (1977) The experience of pain in children. In: Jacox AK (ed.) *Pain: a sourcebook for nurses and other health care professionals*, pp. 453–73. Boston: Little, Brown and Company.

Ellis JA, McCleary LM, Blouin R, *et al.* (2007) Implementing best practice pain management in a pediatric hospital. *Journal for Specialists in Pediatric Nursing* **12**(4), 264–77.

Falanga IJ, Lafrenaye S, Mayer SK, Tetrault J-P (2006) Management of acute pain in children: safety and efficacy of a nurse-controlled algorithm for pain relief. *Acute Pain* **8**(2): 45–54.

Fearon I, McGrath PJ, Achat H (1996) 'Booboos': the study of everyday pain among young children. *Pain* **68**: 55–62.

Ferrell BR, Grant M, Ritchey KJ, *et al.* (1993) The pain resource nurses training program: a unique approach to pain management. *Journal of Pain and Symptom Management* **8**(8): 549–56.

Fincham R, Rhodes P (1999) *Principles of organizational behaviour*. Oxford: Oxford University Press.

Fitzgerald M (2000) Development of the peripheral and spinal pain system. In: Anand KJS, Stevens BJ, McGrath PJ (eds) *Pain in neonates*, 2nd edn, pp. 9–22. Amsterdam: Elsevier.

Fitzgerald M, Howard RFM (2003) The neurobiologic basis of pediatric pain. In: Schechter NL, Berde CB, Yester M (eds) *Pain in infants, children and adolescents,* 2nd edn, pp. 19–42. Philadelphia: Lippincott, Williams & Wilkins.

Fitzpatrick JM, While AE, Roberts JD (1996) Key influences on the professional socialisation and practice of students undertaking different pre-registration nurse education programmes in the United Kingdom. *International Journal of Nursing Studies* **33**(5): 506–18.

Franck L (1986) A new method to quantitatively describe pain behavior in infants. *Nursing Research* **35**(1): 28–31.

Furnham A (1997) *The psychology of behaviour at work*. Hove: Psychology Press.

Goodenough B, Thomas W, Champion G, *et al.* (1997) Pain in 4 to 6 year old children receiving intramuscular injections: a comparison of the faces pain scale with Oucher self-report and behavioural measures. *Clinical Journal of Pain* **13**(1): 60–73.

Gould TH, Crosby DI, Harmer M, *et al.* (1992) Policy for controlling pain after surgery: effect of sequential changes in management. *British Medical Journal* **305**(14): 1187–93.

Graffam S (1990) Pain content in the curriculum: a survey. *Nurse Educator* **15**(1): 20–3.

Gray M, Smith LN (1999) The professional socialization of diploma of higher education in nursing students (Project 2000): a longitudinal study. *Journal of Advanced Nursing* **29**(3): 639–47.

Greenwood J, Sullivan J, Spence K, McDonald M (2000) Nursing scripts and the organizational influences on critical thinking: report of a study of neonatal nurses' clinical reasoning. *Journal of Advanced Nursing* **31**(5): 1106–14.

Griffin RA, Polit DE, Byrne MW (2008) Nurse characteristics and inferences about children's pain. *Pediatric Nursing* **34**(4): 297–307.

Grunau RVE, Whitfield MF, Petrie J (1998) Children's judgements about pain at aged 8–10 years: do extremely low birthweight children differ from their full birthweight peers. *Journal of Child Psychology and Psychiatry* **39**(4): 587–94.

Hamers J, Abu-Saad H, Halfens RJG, Schumacher JNM (1994) Factors influencing nurses' pain assessment and interventions in children. *Journal of Advanced Nursing* **20**: 853–60.

Hamers JPH, van den Hout MA, Halfens RJD, *et al.* (1997) Differences in pain assessment and decisions regarding the administration of analgesics between novices, intermediates and experts in pediatric nursing. *International Journal of Nursing Studies* **34**(5): 325–34.

Hamers JPH, Abu-Saad HH, van den Hout MA, Halfens RJG (1998) Are children given insufficient pain-relieving medication postoperatively? *Journal of Advanced Nursing* **27**: 37–44.

Harbeck C, Peterson L (1992) Elephants dancing in my head: a developmental approach to children's concepts of specific pains. *Child Development* **63**: 138–49.

Harvey G, Loftus-Hills A, Rycroft-Malone J, *et al.* (2002) Getting evidence into practice: the role and function of facilitation. *Journal of Advanced Nursing* **37**(6): 577–88.

Hawley D (1984) Postoperative pain in children: misconceptions, descriptions and interventions. *Pediatric Nursing* **10**(1): 20–3.

Health Care Commission (2004) *Patient survey report 2004 – young patients.* London: Health Care Commission.

Health Care Commission (2007) *Improving services for children in hospital.* London: Health Care Commission.

Hicks CL, von Baeyer CL, Spafford PA, *et al.* (2001) The Faces Pain Scale – Revised: toward a common metric in pediatric pain measurement. *Pain* **93**: 173–183.

Hogan M, Choonara I (1996) Measuring pain in neonates: an objective score. *Paediatric Nursing* **8**(10): 24–7.

Howard R, Carter B, Curry J, *et al.* (2008) Good practice in post-operative and procedural pain management. *Pediatric Anesthesia* **18**: 1–81.

Hunt A, Wisbeach A, Seers K, *et al.* (2004) Clinical validation of the pediatric pain profile. *Developmental Medicine and Child Neurology* **46**(1): 9–18.

Hunt A, Wisbeach A, Seers K, *et al.* (2007) Development of the paediatric pain profile: role of video analysis and saliva cortisol in validating a tool to assess pain in children with severe neurological disability. *Jounal of Pain and Symptom Management* **33**(3): 276–89.

Jacob E, Puntillo KA (1999) A survey of nursing practice in the assessment and management of pain in children. *Pediatric Nursing* **25**(3): 278–86.

Johnston CC, Gagnon AJ, Pepler CJ, Bourgault P (2005) Pain in the emergency department with one-week follow-up of pain resolution. *Pain Research and Management* **10**(2): 67–70.

Joint Commission on Accreditation of Healthcare Organizations (2000) *Pain assessment and management standards.* Oakbrook Terrace, IL: JCAHO.

Jones DC, Sheridan ME (1999) A case study approach: developing critical thinking skills in novice pediatric nurses. *The Journal of Continuing Education in Nursing* **30**(2): 75–8.

Jordan-Marsh M, Hubbard J, Watson R, *et al.* (2004) The social ecology of changing pain management: do I have to cry? *Journal of Pediatric Nursing* **19**(3):193–203.

Kessenich C, Guyatt G, DiCenso A (1997) Teaching nursing students evidence-based nursing. *Nurse Educator* **22**(6): 25–9.

Khalid SK, Gee HA (1999) A new approach to teaching and learning in journal clubs. *Medical Teacher* **21**: 289–93.

Kneafsey R (2000) The effect of occupational socialization in nurses' patient handling practices. *Journal of Clinical Nursing* **9**(4): 585–93.

Krechel SW, Bildner J (1995) CRIES: a new neonatal postoperative pain measurement score. Initial testing of validity and reliability. *Pediatric Anesthesia* **5**: 53–61.

Lamond D, Crow RA, Chase J (1996) Judgements and processes in care decisions in acute medical and surgical wards. *Journal of Evaluation in Clinical Practice* **2**(3): 211–16.

Lauzon Clabo LM (2008) An ethnography of pain assessment and the role of social context on two postoperative units. *Journal of Advanced Nursing* **61**: 531–9.

Lawrence J, Alcock D, McGrath P, *et al.* (1993) The development of a tool to assess neonatal pain. *Neonatal Network* **12**: 59–66.

Lee JEM, Ryan-Wenger N (1997) The 'think aloud' seminar for teaching clinical reasoning: a case study of a child with pharyngitis. *Journal of Pediatric Health Care* **11**: 101–10.

Malviya S, Voepel-Lewis T, Burke C, *et al.* (2005) The revised FLACC observational pain tool: improved reliability and validity for pain assessment in children with cognitive impairment. *Pediatric Anesthesia* **16**: 258–65.

Manworren RCB (2000) Pediatric nurses' knowledge and attitudes survey regarding pain. *Pediatric Nursing* **26**(6): 610–14.

Mather L, Mackie J (1983) The incidence of post-operative pain in children. *Pain* **15**: 271–82.

McCaffery M, Beebe AB (1989) *Pain: clinical manual for nursing practice.* St Louis: CV Mosby.

McCaughan D (2002) What decisions do nurses make? In: Thompson C, Dowding D (eds) *Clinical decision making and judgement in nursing,* pp. 95–108. Edinburgh: Churchill Livingstone.

McCleary L, Ellis JA, Rowley B (2004) Evaluation of the pain resource nurse role: a resource for improving pediatric pain management. *Pain Management Nursing* **5**(1): 29–36.

McDonnell A, Nicholl J, Read S (2005) Exploring the impact of Acute Pain Teams (APTs) on patient outcomes using routine data: can it be done? *Journal of Research in Nursing* **10**(4): 383–402.

McGrath PA, Hillier LM (2003) Modifying the psychological factors that intensify children's pain and prolong disability. In: Schechter NL, Berde CB, Yaster M (eds) *Pain in infants, children and adolescents,* 2nd edn, pp. 85–104. Baltimore: Lippincott, Williams & Wilkins.

McGrath PJ, Johnson G, Goodman JT, *et al.* (1985) CHEOPS: a behavioural scale for rating postoperative pain in children. In: Fields HL, Dubner R, Cervero F (eds) *Proceedings of the fourth world congress on pain. Advances in Pain Research and Therapy,* Vol. 9. pp. 395–401. New York: Raven Press.

Megens JHAM, van der Werff D, Knape JTA (2008) Quality improvement: implementation of a pain management policy in a university pediatric hospital. *Pediatric Anesthesia* **18**: 620–7.

Melzack R, Wall P (1996) *The challenge of pain,* updated 2nd edn. London: Penguin.

Nursing and Midwifery Council (2008) *The Code: standards of conduct, performance and ethics for nurses and midwives.* London: NMC.

Oakes LL, Anghelescu DL, Windsor KB, Barnhill PD (2008) An institutional quality improvement initiative for pain management for pediatric cancer inpatients. *Journal of Pain and Symptom Management* **35**(6): 656–69.

Ochieng BMN (1999) Use of reflective practice in introducing change on the management of pain in a paediatric setting. *Journal of Nursing Management* **7**: 113–18.

Perquin CW, Hazebroek-Kampschreur AAJM, Hunfield JAM, *et al.* (2000) Pain in children and adolescents: a common experience. *Pain* **87**: 51–8.

Philpin SM (1999) The impact of 'Project 2000' educational reforms on the occupational socialization of nurses: an exploratory study. *Journal of Advanced Nursing* **29**(6): 1326–31.

Polkki T, Vehvilamen-Julkunen K, Pietila A-M (2001) Nonpharmacological methods in relieving children's postoperative pain: a survey on hospital nurses in Finland. *Journal of Advanced Nursing* **34**(4): 483–92.

Polkki T, Pietila AM, Vehvilamen-Julkunen K, *et al.* (2002) Parental views on participation in their child's pain relief measures and recommendations to health care providers. *Journal of Pediatric Nursing* **17**(4): 270–8.

Polkki T, Pietila A-M, Vehvilamen-Julkunen K (2003) Hospitalized children's descriptions of their experiences with postsurgical pain relieving methods. *International Journal of Nursing Studies* **40**: 33–44.

Rieman MT, Gordon M (2007) Pain management competency evidenced by a survey of pediatric nurses' knowledge and attitudes. *Pediatric Nursing* **33**(4): 307–12.

Royal College of Anaesthetists (2001) *Guidance on the provision of paediatric anaesthetic services.* London: Royal College of Anaesthetists.

Royal College of Nursing (2009) *The recognition and assessment of acute pain in children.* London: RCN Publishing.

Royal College of Surgeons and College of Anaesthetists (1990) *Pain after surgery.* London: RCS.

Rycroft-Malone J, Kitson A, Harvey G, *et al.* (2002) Ingredients for change: revisiting a conceptual framework. *Quality and Safety in Health Care* **11**(2): 174–80.

Salantera S, Lauri S (2000) Nursing students' knowledge of and views about children in pain. *Nurse Education Today* **20**: 537–47.

Salantera S, Lauri S, Salmi TT, Helenius H (1999) Nurses' knowledge about pharmacological and non-pharmacological pain management in children. *Journal of Pain and Symptom Management* **18**(4): 289–99.

Saxe G, Stoddard F, Courtney D, *et al.* (2001) Relationship between acute morphine and the course of PTSD in children with burns. *Journal of the American Academy of Child & Adolescent Psychiatry* **40**(8): 915–21.

Schechter NL, Allen DA, Hanson K (1986) Status of paediatric pain control: a comparison of hospital analgesic usage in children and adults. *Pediatrics* **77**(1): 11–15.

Schmidt K, Eland J, Weller K (1994) Pediatric cancer pain management: a survey of nurses' knowledge. *Journal of Pediatric Oncology* **11**(1): 4–12.

Scottish Executive (2000) *Our national health. A plan for action. A plan for change.* Edinburgh: The Stationery Office.

Scottish Executive (2001) *Caring for Scotland: the strategy for midwifery and nursing in Scotland.* Edinburgh: The Stationery Office.

Segal S, Mason DJ (1998) The art and science of teaching rounds. *The Journal for Nurses in Staff Development* **14**(3): 127–36.

Simons J, Roberson E (2002) Poor communication and knowledge deficits: obstacles to effective management of children's postoperative pain. *Journal of Advanced Nursing* **40**(1): 78–86.

Simons J, Franck L, Roberson E (2001) Parent involvement in children's pain care: views of parents and nurses. *Journal of Advanced Nursing* **36**(4): 591–9.

Slater R, Cantarella A, Gallella S, *et al.* (2006) Cortical pain response in human infants. *The Journal of Neuroscience* **26**(14): 3662–6.

Stevens B (1999) Pain in infants. In: McCaffery M, Pasero C (eds) *Pain: clinical manual*, 2nd edn, pp. 626–73. St Louis: Mosby.

Stevens B, Johnston C, Petryshen P, Taddio A (1996) Premature infant pain profile: development and initial validation. *Clinical Journal of Pain* **12**: 13–22.

Stinson J (2009) Pain assessment in children. In: Twycross A, Dowden SJ, Bruce L (eds) *Pain management in children: a clinical guide*, pp. 85–108. Oxford: Wiley-Blackwell.

Stinson J, Yamada J, Kavanagh T, *et al.* (2006) Systematic review of the psychometric properties and feasibility of self-report pain measures for use in clinical trials in children and adolescents. *Pain* **125**(1–2): 143–57.

Stratton L (1999) Evaluating the effectiveness of a hospital's pain management project. *Journal of Nursing Care Quality* **13**(4): 8–18.

Swafford LI, Allan D (1968) Pain relief in the pediatric patient. *Medical Clinics of North America* **52**(1): 131–6.

Taddio A, Goldbach M, Ipp M, *et al.* (1995) Effect of neonatal circumcision on pain responses during vaccination in boys. *The Lancet* **345**: 291–2.

Taddio A, Katz J, Ilersich AL, Koren G (1997) Effect of neonatal circumcision on pain response during subsequent routine vaccination. *The Lancet* **349**: 599–603.

Taddio A, Shah V, Gilbert-MacLeod C, Katz J (2002) Conditioning and hyperalgesia in newborns exposed to repeated heel lances. *Journal of the American Medical Association* **288**(7): 857–61.

Taylor C (1997) Problem solving in clinical nursing practice. *Journal of Advanced Nursing* **26**(2): 329–36.

Taylor EM, Boyer K, Campbell FA (2008) Pain in hospitalized children: a prospective cross-sectional survey of pain prevalence, intensity, assessment and management in a Canadian pediatric teaching hospital. *Pain Research and Management* **13**(1), 25–32.

Thompson C, McCaughan D, Cullum N, *et al.* (2001) The accessibility of research-based knowledge for nurses in the United Kingdom acute care settings. *Journal of Advanced Nursing* **36**(1): 11–22.

Treadwell MJ, Franck LS, Vichinsky E (2002) Using quality improvement strategies to enhance pediatric pain assessment. *International Journal for Quality in Health Care* **14**(1): 39–47.

Twycross A (1999) Pain management: a nursing priority? *Journal of Child Health Care* **3**(3): 19–25.

Twycross A (2000) Education about pain: a neglected area? *Nurse Education Today* **20**: 244–53.

Twycross A (2004) Children's nurses' pain management practices: theoretical knowledge, perceived importance and decision-making. Unpublished PhD Thesis, University of Central Lancashire, Preston.

Twycross A (2007a) Children's nurses' postoperative pain management practices: an observational study. *International Journal of Nursing Studies* **44**(6): 869–81.

Twycross A (2007b) What is the impact of theoretical knowledge on children's nurses' postoperative pain management practices? An exploratory study. *Nurse Education Today* **27**(7): 697–707.

Twycross A (2008) Children's nurses' pain management practices: theoretical knowledge and perceived importance. *Journal of Clinical Nursing* **17**(23): 3205–16.

Twycross A, Dowden S (2009) Where to from here? In: Twycross A, Dowden SJ, Bruce L (eds) *Pain management in children: a clinical manual*, pp. 219–34. Oxford: Wiley-Blackwell.

Twycross A, Powls L (2006) How do children's nurses make clinical decisions? Two preliminary studies. *Journal of Clinical Nursing* **15**: 1324–35.

UNICEF (1999) Global millennium targets: UNICEF Child-Friendly Hospital Initiative. *Paediatric Nursing* **11**(10): 7–8.

United Nations (1989) *Convention on the rights of the child*. New York: United Nations.

Van Cleve LJ, Savedra MC (1993) Pain location: validity and reliability of body outline markings by 4 to 7 year old children who are hospitalized. *Pediatric Nursing* **19**(3): 217–20.

Van Cleve L, Johnson L, Pothier P (1996) Pain responses of hospitalised infants and children to venipuncture and intravenous cannulation. *Journal of Pediatric Nursing* **11**(3): 161–8.

Vincent CVH (2005) Nurses' knowledge, attitudes, and practices regarding children's pain. *MCN* **30**(3): 177–83.

Vincent CVH, Denyes MJ (2004) Relieving children's pain: nurses' abilities and analgesic administration practices. *Journal of Pediatric Nursing* **19**(1): 40–50.

Volpe J (1981) *Neurology of the newborn*. Philadelphia: W.B. Saunders.

von Baeyer CL, Spagrud LJ (2007) Systematic review of observational (behavioural) measures for children and adolescents aged 3 to 18 years. *Pain* **127**: 140–50.

Watt-Watson J, Stevens B, Garfinkel P, *et al.* (2001) Relationship between nurses' pain knowledge ad pain management outcomes for their postoperative cardiac patients. *Journal of Advanced Nursing* **36**(4): 535–45.

Wolf AR (1999) Pain, nociception and the developing infant. *Paediatric Anaesthesia* **9**: 7–17.

Woodgate R, Kristjanson L (1996) A young child's pain: how parents and nurses 'take care'. *International Journal of Nursing Studies* **33**(3): 271–84.

PART 3
Care settings

Chapter 8

School nursing

Carwen Earles and Susan Jones

Overview

The school health nurse has a vital role to play in the seamless provision of a comprehensive health service to children and young people and makes an invaluable contribution in the field of public health and health promotion. This chapter will begin with an overview of the history of school nursing from its early beginnings in the 1870s until the present day. This will integrate salient educational, health and social policy to identify the origins and development of the service and demonstrate its present-day role in the complex field of public health and health promotion. The chapter itself is based on the belief that children and young people are entitled to a service they can identify with and that meets their needs. Real life case studies from practice will illustrate how their needs may be met with a particular focus on immunization, appropriate sex and relationship education and bullying in school. It will be shown how the school health nurse may effectively involve parents and work collaboratively with children and young people. Likewise, it will be shown how they work with other professionals, and agencies as well as statutory and voluntary bodies.

Introduction

There are clear challenges ahead for school health nursing, which is now high on the political agenda and is supported by a plethora of child public health policy (Department for Children, Schools and Families and Department of Health 2009). In this connection, poverty and social exclusion continue to be a fact of life for many children and young people. The Department for Children, Schools and Families and Department of Health (2009) note the worrying trends in obesity, sexually transmitted infections and increasing alcohol consumption in children and young people while Hall and Elliman (2003) highlight increasing mental health problems. School health nurses need to be forward thinking to meet the changing demands of school-aged children brought about by these challenges to their health and well-being. Through working collaboratively with other agencies school health nurses play a vital role in improving children and young people's life chances (DeBell and Jackson 2000; Day 2009). As this chapter will show it is imperative that the numbers of school health nurses are increased to maintain a proactive and effective service for the school-aged child, and school nurses themselves must work at political and strategic level to achieve this.

The history and development of school health nursing

The role of the school health nurse has seen much development since its birth in the 1870s. The nineteenth century saw the emergence of public health emanating from the industrial revolution and the migration of the masses to the cities to live and work (DeBell 2007). Many children and their families lived in abject poverty and, reflecting present-day policy (Department of Health 2001, 2003), the link between health and education was made by Margaret McMillan and Katherine Bruce Glasier in the 1890s, who in identifying the right of children to healthcare also drew attention to the fact that attention to their health has a positive impact on their educational attainment (Bradburn 1989; Steedman 2000).

The nineteenth century brought about education for all children. Until legislation on the provision of education in the latter half of the 1800s, education did depend on parental ability to pay or on the voluntary and church schools, which were given government grants. Therefore, education was limited despite the need for a literate and numerate workforce because of the industrial revolution. Authors such as Dickens and Kingsley described how the children of the poor had to work to support the whole family during this period. The 1830s saw outbreaks of cholera in many British cities, which led to efforts to improve health, education and social conditions. The first Public Health Act (1848) led to the appointment of the first Medical Officers of Health, who were responsible for, among other things, clean water, disposal of sewage, sanitation of buildings, inspection of food and notification of diseases. This was the start of improvements in public health and eventual educational reforms, both of which were necessary to the health and economic well-being of the country.

Reflection point

★ Consider the impact of social, environmental, economic and political factors on the health of the child at the end of the 1800s.

Compulsory education for children in England and Wales began in 1870 with the Elementary Education Act. This established schools where there had been no previous provision and enforced attendance for children from the age of 5 years. Northern Ireland and Scotland also saw similar legislation such as the Scottish Education Act of 1872. Education legislation continued in rapid succession to improve the plight of the majority of children. The 1876 Education Act saw a duty placed on parents that their children received basic instruction in the 'three R's', i.e. reading, writing and arithmetic. The 1890 Education Act was a landmark in that for the first time it ensured free education for all children. These schools took registers of attendance and noted that absenteeism was mainly due to ill-health in children. In 1892 the Metropolitan and National Nursing Association sent nurses into schools to look at their health. Amy Hughes, a Nightingale nurse, attended Chancery Lane School in London and found many cases of child absenteeism due to ill-health caused by neglect of minor ailments, which often stemmed from a lack of money to pay for medical care. Dr J. Kerr was appointed as the first School Medical Officer in Bradford. His report on the health of school children in Bradford stated that local authorities should improve sanitary conditions for families, such as installing bathrooms in local houses and providing free school meals and milk for all school children to improve health. A stance which once again highlights the link between health and educational welfare.

In response to children requiring specialist help because of conditions such as deafness and blindness, further educational legislation was implemented in 1893 and included the Elementary Education Blind and Deaf Children Act of 1893 and Elementary Education Defective and Epileptic Children Act of 1893. This legislation enabled the education authorities to set up appropriate educational facilities for these children and, by 1895, the school leaving age had been raised to 12 years.

The standard of child health and welfare led to much cause for concern, but it took the Boer War (1899–1902) to galvanize the government into action when a newspaper report of the time highlighted the poor physical health of men enlisting to fight. It noted that 65% of those volunteering were rejected owing to poor health and physique, which led to the government establishing a committee to address the poor health of the British nation. This led to a number of Acts being passed over the next decade in relation to infant and child health as well as education. This began with the 1902 Education Act, which set up Local Education Authorities (LEAs), funded by the rates, that provided free schooling and raised the school leaving age to 14 years. In 1902 the Midwives Act was passed to assist in the reduction of infant and maternal mortality through the registration of midwives and provision of maternity care. In 1904 the Interdepartmental Committee on Physical Deterioration reported grave concerns over children's health and the high rates of infant and child mortality and made the case that good health in children would lead to good health in adults, which was fundamental for the health of the nation. It recommended health checks for school children and the employment of school doctors and nurses, but it was not until further legislation that this became universal. In 1906 the Education Act led to the provision of school meals, and in 1907 further educational legislation stated that it was the duty of the LEAs to provide medical checks. This led to the establishment of the school medical service compulsory medical inspection in elementary schools. Doctors were assisted in their medical inspections by nurses, and Margaret and Rachel McMillan, pioneers of this work, called for all nurses working with children to be specially trained.

> ### Key point
>
> School nurses were first established in the 1890s following the Education Act of 1890, which provided free schooling to all children.

> ### Key points
>
> - Concerns about the poor physical health of men enlisting to fight in the Boer War led to legislation to address the poor health of the nation's children.
> - This resulted in the employment of doctors and nurses to conduct medical inspections in elementary schools.

Health and educational welfare continued apace following the First World War. The 1918 Education Act made school compulsory for children up to the age of 14 years and gave LEAs the duty to provide medical treatments for minor ailments, dental caries, visual defects, enlarged tonsils and adenoids in elementary schools, and medical inspections in secondary schools. The focus of this service was in the main curative but – importantly – it was free. Alongside this there was standardization in the provision of nursing services through the 1919 Nurses Registration Act. The General Nursing Council was established as the regulating body to ensure appropriate standards for education, training and the conduct of nurses. School nursing and health visiting remained the responsibility of LEAs under the supervision of the Medical Officer of Health until 1974 when the 1973 NHS Reorganisation Act was enforced. The Haddon Report (1926) recommended that elementary education should end at 11 years and secondary education at 14 years of age, but this was not fully achieved until the 1944 Education Act.

The 1944 Education Act, also known as the Butler Education Act, changed the focus of education. It highlighted a child-orientated approach, the importance of education and the links between education, the child and his/her family and the community. It established significant developments for both education and the school health service, of which school nursing was a part. It created a Minister and Ministry of Education, which placed a duty on parents to ensure that their children attended school. It set up 'special schools' for children with special educational needs and placed firm responsibility on LEAs to seek advice from the Medical Officer regarding children with disability, regular medical inspections by doctors and nurses and free treatments. In the main, the school nurses' work was curative, but there were opportunities for preventative work with children and their families. The Act also wished to ensure recreational facilities for children and provision of school transport and school meals and milk. Thus, the focus was on the mental well-being of children as well as the physical well-being of children and young people.

The 1945 School Health Regulations recommended that all school nurses should be qualified health visitors, thus cementing a public health focus to the role. In 1948 the NHS was born. The NHS Act 1946 highlighted the importance of the preventative work of the health visitor with the school-aged child. This was a positive step for the public health role but a negative one for school nurses as they were not mentioned by the Act. Although the main work of the health visitor had been with the 0–5 year old child population, they were deemed the appropriate professionals to undertake health education sessions within schools.

In 1959 the School Health Regulations abolished the need for a health visitor qualification for schools. It introduced selective health inspections only because of costs. The school health nurse's role was then interpreted restrictively (Slack 1978) and the belief that school health nurses were capable only of examining heads for lice and known as the 'nit nurse' gave them little scope to fully utilize their skills.

Following the 1973 NHS Reorganisation Act, the school health service became part of an integrated child health service in which school medical, dental and nursing services became the responsibility of the NHS. This emphasized their nursing role as opposed to any public health or health promotion role. The Court Report (1976) emphasized the need for school nursing services and the provision for child health services in schools. It highlighted the importance of the school nursing service and recommended specialist training for school health nurses. To enable them to deliver a more public health-focused service it recommended that there should be one school nurse for every 2500 children. The principles of this report were reiterated by Polnay in 1995 in his report entitled *Health Needs of the School Age Child*. It recommended a ratio of one school nurse to every 1500 school-aged children, and it should be noted that this has yet to be realized across the UK (Royal College of Nursing 2005; Merrell *et al.* 2007). It focused on a child-centred approach, with school health nurses being

Reflection point

Consider the impact of the work of the school nurse in post-war Britain.

Reflection point

Consider why the numbers of school nurses did not increase during the 1970s, 80s and 90s.

responsible for the school-aged population wherever they might be, not only in schools. It emphasized the importance of the interrelationship between school health nurses, children, their families and the community.

The 1970s and 1980s saw the rise of the local health education departments which offered schools support in the provision and delivery of health education. This was welcomed by schools but it had an unforeseen detrimental effect on the role of the school health nurse by emphasizing their clinical skills role. Although health and educational policy drivers and legislation emphasize the importance of the school health service and school nursing they do not recommend any statutory education for them.

The Patients' Charter (Department of Health 1996) established two rights for children and young people. First, the right of parents to know the name of the school nurse for their child and how to contact them and, second, the right to a health check during the first year of primary school. This clearly emphasizes the importance and demand for school health nurses with specialist education. The development of the specialist practitioner qualification and educational changes required for community nursing in 1998 noted school nursing as one of the eight strands that make up the community nursing family. This post-registration degree qualification in community nursing with a specialist pathway for school nursing gave educational recognition for school nurses by the United Kingdom Central Council for Nursing, Midwifery and Health Visiting (UKCC). This significant development was supported by policy drivers from government. These were the beginnings of a major shift in policy for school nurses as, in the decade prior to this, the profession had been in a decline owing to financial cutbacks. The Department of Health (1999b, 2001, 2003) cited the school health nurse as a primary professional in the delivery of public health to the school-aged child. This represents a move from their involvement in screening programmes to a public health role. Public health and health promotion were seen as key factors in the delivery of child health. Therefore, an ability to respond to this new political health climate will enable school health nursing to develop professional leadership with school health services and contribute to the public health agenda for the school-aged child population. This was also highlighted in the work of Hall and Elliman (2003) and DeBell and Jackson (2000).

Although policy and education drivers were highlighting the importance of the public health role for school health nurses this may not be a true reflection of practice at this time. For, as Clark *et al.* (2000) and others (Carlile 2002; DeBell and Tomkins 2006) all noted, school health nursing continued to be regarded as a 'Cinderella service' and to some degree invisible within the NHS. This was regrettable given that school health nurses are the only NHS professional group where the focus is on meeting the health needs of the school-aged child. School health nurses have a variety of employers: the NHS, local authorities or the independent school sector. This has led to Clark *et al.* (2000), the Royal College of Nursing (2005) and Obeid (2002) finding that there was an inequality in the distribution of school nurses and therefore services across various areas.

Reflection point

★ What impact could the inequities in the provision of service have on the school-aged child population?

Present-day demands on the school health nursing service are increasing (Royal College of Nursing 2005; Merrell *et al.* 2007) with changing epidemiological, demographic, social and lifestyle problems adding to the complexity of their role. The school health nurse role has developed and evolved and continues to do so. In 2004, the Department of Health outlined the government's objectives to improve services for school-aged children by increasing the number of school nurses. It noted the government's aim by 2010 that there should be at least one full-time, year-round, qualified school health nurse working with one secondary school and its related cluster of primary schools. The Welsh Assembly Government (2007) also committed to one 'family nurse', now recognized to be a school nurse (Welsh Assembly Government 2009b), being attached to one secondary school by 2011. These commitments are needed to meet the developing policy context. The 2006 publication *Looking for a School Nurse* was aimed at head teachers and others demonstrating the value and effectiveness of school health nurses. This joint publication by the Department for Education and Skills and the Department of Health demonstrated the government's plan to develop services for children and young people supported by the work of health visitors and school health nurses.

Key points

- Since its inception in the 1870s the role of the school health nurse has developed and changed in response to policy, education and legislative drivers.
- The school health nurse is there to meet the needs of the school-aged population working as an autonomous public health practitioner.

School health nursing and the present-day scope of practice

School health nurses (SHNs) are now actively engaged in what has been described as a complex field of practice that has developed into a well defined specialty (Gleeson 2004). They are far removed from the 'panadol and plaster' image of the nurse sited in an obscure area of a secondary school, providing a bolt hole from unpopular lessons in the curriculum, or the caricature 'nit nurse' figure from the primary school days memories of many adults. It has been suggested that their role is to keep the healthy in good health for the future (Bartley 2004) and they have progressed to the point where they are now a distinct and specialist graduate profession registered on the Specialist Community Public Health Nursing, Part 3, of the Nursing and Midwifery Council (NMC).

School nursing in the UK transferred to the NHS in 1974 (DeBell *et al.* 2007) and the majority of SHNs are now NHS employees. Most are based in the community with a caseload of named schools, but many remain contracted to local authority and individual schools, particularly in the independent sector. There is currently a policy push both professionally and politically to bring all SHNs into NHS employment, not least to ensure they are afforded access to development, update and support, and the terms and conditions that many do not currently benefit from (National Board for Nursing, Midwifery and Health Visiting for Scotland 2001; Department of Health 2009: Welsh Assembly Government 2009a,b). From their young clients' perspective, this will facilitate provision of a service that will also be available outside of school premises that can be accessed confidentially and is available in school holidays and outside of school hours. This is essential if SHNs are to meet their young clients' needs as they are not merely school children, but school-aged children who spend the majority of their time in their home and neighbourhood communities rather than their school community setting.

Reflection point

★ Consider how such provision would benefit the young people and what needs to be available to make it a reality.

Despite being identified as key to promoting, improving and protecting the health and well-being of school-aged children and young people (Welsh Assembly Government 2009a) they continue to be a grossly under-resourced service. This was highlighted in the table presented in the government document *Every Child Matters* (Department for Education and Skills 2003, p. 84) which evidenced a workforce of 13 000 health visitors and 6000 speech and language therapists as opposed to a paltry total of 2300 SHNs. Although numerous proposals, consultation documents and workforce reviews have been carried out across most Primary Care and NHS Trust areas, provision has not improved in over a decade (DeBell *et al.* 2007).

Despite this, the reality and stark facts are that school-aged children in the UK equal a total of 11.2 million children and young people, and account for 20% of the population (DeBell 2007, p. 6). These statistics indicate that school-aged children represent a significant group of the population and, as such, deserve not just professional but also political commitment to providing them with long-term, sustainable and robust services.

Key points

School-aged children in the UK account for 20% of the population, but school health nurses (SHNs) are in short supply despite the following recommendations:

- One SHN to every 2500 children (Court Report 1976)
- One SHN to every 1500 children (Polnay 1995)
- One SHN to every secondary school and related cluster of primary schools by 2010 (Department of Health 2004a)
- One SHN to every secondary school by 2011 (Welsh Assembly Government 2007)

The school health service and school nursing have played an important part in preventing childhood diseases and promoting child health and welfare since its beginnings over 140 years ago. It could be argued that considering the levels of poverty and deprivation evident in the population the school health services should have been more proactively developed on a UK basis (Clark *et al.* 2000) given that child health and education have been clearly linked since the nineteenth century. The Department of Health (2001, 2003) have emphasized that children's health is not only a right but attention to their health can also have a positive impact on their educational attainment.

Ensuring a client-focused school health nursing service

Children and young people are entitled to a school health nursing service that they can identify with and which is relevant and appropriate to them. It is not acceptable ethically or professionally to merely provide a service that is informed according to what professionals, politicians and the adult society feel they should be given.

All children's nurses have a duty of advocacy on behalf of their young clients (Nursing and Midwifery Council 2008), and SHNs have tools at their disposal to both lobby and advocate in this respect. These must be utilized to serve the best interests of their young clients, who have enshrined rights to information, education and involvement in all issues that affect them (United Nations 1989; Department of Health 2004b). The ethos of involvement contained in these documents and Acts has been reaffirmed in the national service frameworks (NSFs) relevant to children and young people (Department of Health and Department for Education and Skills 2004; National Assembly for Wales 2004). Of particular significance to all children's nurses are the core aims that children and young people should enjoy the best possible health, be listened to and have their views respected and be provided with a range of learning opportunities and education. The fact that the NSFs identify a need to work more closely with and in support of parents has raised the profile of the SHN. This is because they are acknowledged to be in a unique position of working across the health and education divide while also linking with the family of the children and young people on their caseload (DeBell and Jackson 2000).

All SHNs are involved in health promotion and education. Of particular note is the identified role they now have supporting education colleagues in provision of sex and relationships education (SRE) and providing drop-in venues both inside and outside of school to offer advice on sexual health and contraception. To meet these aims, SHNs in some areas of the UK are also qualified in family planning (Neill *et al.* 2009). SRE has been identified as a contentious area for parents and teachers alike, with both groups valuing SHN input (Jones 2008), and as a result it needs to be included as an explicit role in job descriptions for the future. If the current debate and rhetoric surrounding the need for more SHNs results in more posts being funded, there will be an urgent need to maximize recruitment from nurses who will be comfortable advising in this area after appropriate training has been accessed. This will in turn facilitate retention as the SHN will not have this role thrust upon them once they are in post, but will be aware at an early stage that commitment to this area of public health and health promotion forms an essential and integral part of their role with young people. At this stage it would seem helpful to put into context the dual role that SHNs hold in relation to public health and health promotion. So beginning with public health we will now present an overview of their present-day scope of practice.

SHNs and their scope of practice in relation to public health

Public health may be described as a way of looking at health that takes the population as its starting point. In common with school nursing, it sets out to build relationships with individuals, groups and communities, so that people's health needs can be effectively assessed and agreed priorities identified (Department of

Health 2006a). Neill *et al.* (2009) highlight that recent and successive national government documents that support the SHN role have returned them to their original domain of public health nursing (Department of Health 1997, 2001, 2004a, 2006a) and placed the emphasis of their child-centred role in health promotion (Croghan *et al.* 2004).

There is much discussion about what exactly is meant by the term 'public health', but it is suggested that it includes both public health medicine and health promotion (Naidoo and Wills 2005). The remit of the SHN is certainly involved in both these areas, as well as individual needs for some of their young clients, but public health is further defined as being concerned with population- and not individual-level approaches (DeBell 2007, p. 10). As a result, to meet their young clients' needs within this contradictory stance, a multiprofessional, multidisciplinary and skill mix team approach is a prerequisite for SHNs, and this will be discussed in more detail later.

As graduate specialist community public health practitioners, SHNs need to keep in sharp focus that public health practice has a political dimension. Despite the fact that the four countries of the UK have begun to focus attention on the health implications of the settings in which children live, school-age child health has been under-represented in critical debates that inform public health thinking (DeBell 2007). The emergence of child public health as a concept for the organization of health, social care, public services and voluntary agencies only arrived at the very end of the twentieth century. Encouragingly, however, in just a decade it has become a core part of UK practice and is now embedded in a range of government policy documents (DeBell 2007).

Currently the SHN's public health role is involved with statutory and non-statutory input. The statutory element includes as a minimum school entry screening for height, weight and vision, delivering the new human papilloma virus (HPV) vaccination, and in many (though not all) areas the school leaver's diphtheria, tetanus and polio vaccination. Non-statutory input includes drop-in clinics for advice outside of school premises and school hours, and much of the health promotion and health education work in schools in support of their colleagues in education that will be discussed in more detail later. Being aware of the plethora of policy and documentation that supports the role of the SHN is essential to ensure that, although much of their input is not presently considered to be of statutory nature, this fact does not render it dispensable. They will then be in an informed position to lobby for appropriate interventions and activities to be included within their remit as statutory, resulting in them being sustainably resourced to ensure that they become embedded elements of their practice.

To meet their young clients' needs and documented rights (United Nations 1989; Department for Education and Skills 2003, 2004; Department of Health 2004b, 2009; Department for Education and Employment 2006) and professional standards (Nursing and Midwifery Council 2004, 2008), SHNs also need to be aware of tools provided to assist them in implementing interventions that will enable them to achieve local and national targets for the future. Sharing of best practice, networking at every opportunity via appropriate forums and conference attendance can facilitate this aim being met. Reinventing the wheel is not necessary, and learning what interventions have been successful for colleagues, accessing recommended and evidence-based tools and utilizing specifically designed tools such as the Royal College of Nursing's (2008) *Toolkit* can help ensure that school-aged children in all parts of the UK are receiving a robust, needs-led and constantly evolving service, which leads us naturally on to the scope of practice SHNs also have in relation to health promotion.

Accessing appropriate training and being informed on the latest short intervention programmes sponsored by central and devolved governments will assist SHNs in fulfilling their public health remit. Many of these programmes provide free training to equip professionals with the skills and knowledge necessary to facilitate the intervention sessions. Effective input can then be offered to school-aged children in a variety of settings. Two examples of good practice are described below.

Effective collaboration: an example of good practice

An SHN service not limited to term time coupled with effective collaboration can facilitate negotiated access to local authority premises in shared sessions at youth club or community centre venues. After completing the necessary training, youth workers and SHNs can work together to set up and facilitate short intervention sessions targeting young people's public health issues such as smoking cessation programmes. Advertising such groups can be carried out in the youth club, in school drop-in sessions, during classroom-based health promotion and on local authority school websites.

Obesity and nutrition: an example of good practice

Obesity is a public health issue that is high on the political agenda, and the devolved Welsh government has provided free access to the nutrition course offered by the Open College Network. Many SHNs in Wales have taken the opportunity to attend the course and achieved a recognized qualification. The course content provides current factual information that prepares SHNs to deliver appropriate health education sessions to primary school-aged children. They also acquire knowledge necessary to support them in producing evidence-based lesson plans for secondary school health promotion lessons and ensure that they have up-to-date and accurate advice to impart on an individual basis in drop-in sessions.

Principles for practice

- Children and young people are entitled to a school health nursing service that they can identify with and which is relevant and appropriate to them.
- The Royal College of Nursing (2008) *Toolkit* can help ensure that school-aged children across the UK receive a robust, needs-led and constantly evolving service.

SHNs and their scope of practice in health promotion

Health promotion may be regarded as the 'bread and butter' of public health practice and is centrally concerned with empowering people to take control of and responsibility for their own health (World Health Organization 1986; Department of Health 1999a,b; Wanless 2002). The SHN is nationally identified as a key professional in this area (DeBell and Jackson 2000; Hall and Elliman 2003; Naidoo and Wills 2005; Department of Health 2006a; Neill *et al.* 2009) and the new public health agenda of current policy highlights a lead role for SHNs in promoting and maintaining the health of young people through education and health promotion (Department of Health 2001, 2004a, 2006a; Department for Education and Skills 2004). The *Ottawa Charter* defines health promotion as a process of empowering people to have more control over their own health (World Health Organization 1986), and it has been suggested that the SHN is best placed to link agencies, communities and groups to ensure that tailor-made services are provided to promote this ideal (Coverdale 2005). Despite the evidenced role, the reality is that, currently, SHN involvement in health promotion is at the mercy of the time and resource constraints that have been identified previously in this chapter.

Quality resources now exist to support the SHN in initially profiling a school to identify its particular needs. The Royal College of Nursing's *Toolkit* (2008) provides guidance, suggestions and other useful resources, as well as an overview of the various policies of the four countries of the UK as they apply to SHNs. The *School Nurse: Practice Development Resource Pack* (Department of Health 2006a), aimed at specialist children's public health nurse (SCPHN)-qualified SHNs, aims to inform, support and encourage individual and team approaches to developing practice. It is essential that SHNs keep in sharp focus the fact that they are not the only professional available or capable of supporting education colleagues. In fact, SCPHNs should always be mindful that, as specialist practitioners, they should act as the link professional to other professional- or voluntary-sector colleagues who have more specialized knowledge in areas of health promotion which fall outside their area of expertise (Scottish Executive 2003; Department of Health 2004a, 2006a, 2009; National Assembly for Wales 2004; Welsh Assembly Government 2009b).There will be colleagues locally with a far more in-depth and up-to-date knowledge on several subjects, including, for example, drugs and alcohol or dental health, who would be more appropriate and effective in offering input regarding such issues.

The specialist status that SHNs have achieved has enabled them to move away from being the 'Jack of all trades', in which they, as nurses, were expected to know everything about everything. Working within their limitations and being aware of and linking with appropriate colleagues is a professional responsibility (Nursing and Midwifery Council 2004, 2008) and ensures that the best interests of their young client group is served. Although a plethora of subjects that need to be addressed exists, a realistic approach reflecting what the SHN can sustainably support needs to be negotiated. DeBell *et al.* (2007) suggest that there is a need to determine priorities locally and that currently focus includes:

- nutrition
- physical activity
- child and adolescent mental health
- accidental and non-accidental injury (and therefore includes child protection)
- hygiene
- dental health
- immunizations
- health and teen pregnancies
- risk-taking behaviours
- long-term conditions
- complex health needs
- disabilities.

The wide range of subjects identified in this list evidences the necessity for multidisciplinary and multiprofessional collaboration if all issues are to be effectively addressed.

Health promotion, particularly in primary schools, is largely, though not solely, related to the stated aims of the National Healthy Schools Programme (NHSP) (Department for Education and Employment 1999). All schools are encouraged to participate and achieve recognized standards leading to accreditation as a 'Healthy School'. Each of the countries that constitute the UK has set targets for participation along with locally identified aims and priorities. The national and devolved government websites all have sections dedicated to news and updates on their area's achievements in regard to this programme. Although it was initially teacher led (DeBell *et al.* 2007) the programme is now a multidisciplinary and multiprofessional collaboration, of which the SHN is an integral component (Department of Health 2006a). Topics and subjects covered in the classroom by the SHN in support of their teaching colleagues need to be informed by school profiling (Royal College of Nursing 2008). Ensuring that identified health needs of the local population are being met (DeBell *et al.* 2007) along with the school's stated aims in its individual NHSP plan will result in children benefiting from tailor-made interventions that address local priorities that will benefit the wider community that the school-age child inhabits.

SHN input in health promotion in schools needs to form part of a coherent rolling programme with stated aims agreed by all involved. This will help to ensure that 'one-off' sessions on a subject that serve to merely 'tick the box' when a school inspection is due does not occur. This will also ensure that SHNs can robustly evaluate their input to demonstrate effectiveness and lobby for additional resources as appropriate. Personal health and social education (PHSE) is a key component of the National Curriculum, and the Department for Education and Skills has an internet site dedicated to the subject offering a wealth of information on key stage requirements and resources available to support teaching of the various components that constitute the subject. Working collaboratively with individual class teachers or PHSE coordinators at local authority level, SHNs can identify, access and utilize evidence-based packages that are appropriate to assist them in classroom sessions with pupils.

The current modernization agenda and role redesign impetus at both national and devolved government level provides the opportunity for SHNs to be innovative in approach. The provision of relevant and effective health education that results from multidisciplinary collaboration is an area where skill mix can be used imaginatively to the benefit of children and young people while also meeting recruitment, retention and career progression issues.

The dual role of the SHN in relation to public health and health promotion has now been set out and, as it is outside the scope of this chapter to account for every aspect of their role, it would seem appropriate to expand upon three important issues, namely immunization, sexual health and vulnerable children and young people.

Principles for practice

- School nurses, as graduate specialist community public health practitioners, are aware of the political dimensions of practice.
- SHNs have a dual role in relation to public health and health promotion.

Immunization and the role of the SHN

Immunization programmes are one of the UK's most successful public health measures (Health Protection Agency 2005), and SHNs are the main providers of vaccinations for school-aged children. They have been responsible for organizing, leading and conducting many mass vaccination campaigns successfully. In many areas across the UK they implement the school-leaver's booster dose programme for diphtheria, tetanus and polio, although in some areas this is a GP-led service. More recently, the human papilloma virus (HPV) immunization has been added to the SHN's remit. As already highlighted, SHNs must lobby to ensure that new programmes are appropriately funded and incorporated into their practice. This will help to ensure that new interventions do not have a negative impact on existing practices that have not yet been deemed to be statutory but are not, however, disposable, as shown in the Case study below.

Case study

SHNs in one area were concerned that, as HPV was a new programme, there may be some reluctance for parents to consent to it for their daughters as vaccine safety is currently a hotly debated subject. The SHNs wanted to ensure that the parents and their daughters were accurately informed regarding the HPV programme and as a result empowered to make an informed choice. Working with their named schools the SHNs set up drop-in sessions for parents and daughters and spoke to the young girls in the target age group in school assemblies. This ensured that both parents and daughters had access to accurate and informed advice on which to base their decision.

Minimum standards of training for all professionals who vaccinate were laid down by the Health Protection Agency (2005). As a result, anyone new to the role must undertake a minimum of 2 days' training followed by a period of supervised practice and assessment of competency. There is also a requirement for annual updates, which are usually provided by the National Public Health Service locally.

To meet the school-age child's rights it is not enough for SHNs to be informed regarding the appropriate documents. They must be aware of their young clients' rights with regard to information, input on decisions that affect them and the documented right to consent for themselves under Fraser guidelines, even if their parents disagree (*Gillick v West Norfolk and Wisbech AHA and DoHSS* [1985]; United Nations 1989; Department of Health 2004b). It is, however, best practice to obtain mutual consent from the young person as well as the parent or person who holds parental responsibility for them (Stretch *et al.* 2009). This can only be achieved when both parties have had access to all the necessary information and an opportunity to ask questions about any areas of concern.

In a climate of frequent vaccine controversies, SHNs need to be confident, knowledgeable, up to date and able to explain to young people and their parents why vaccinations are still necessary (Health Protection Agency 2005). As a result, the SHN needs to be well versed on current advice and information on the immunizations that constitute the routine programme from birth to adolescence in the UK. All relevant information is provided in *The Green Book* (Department of Health 2006b). This publication is also available online, where updates are more readily accessible.

Eligible young people should be offered information and a chance to ask questions in sessions provided in their school and offered the opportunity to access individual advice as necessary. Local arrangements and provision for parents and carers to contact their child's named SHN to discuss the issues also need to be in place. This will facilitate informed choice and help ensure that local immunization rates are maintained at the level necessary to achieve 'herd immunity'. Collaborative working with the local education department and individual schools and staff is essential. This will facilitate provision of a mutually agreed protocol to outline the minimum requirements of the SHN team for immunization sessions held on school premises. Such protocols ensure that sessions run smoothly and safely while causing the school as little disruption as possible.

Principles for practice

- SHNs need to be confident, knowledgeable and up to date when advising children and young people as well as their parents.
- Children, young people and their parents should be given the opportunity to ask questions to facilitate informed choice.

Sexual health: promoting appropriate sex and relationships education

SRE was identified as a contentious area which lacked a coherent strategy at national level (Whitehead 2001) and, to date, little has changed. This is evident in the varying approaches and guidance in the countries that constitute the UK, as highlighted by Jones (2008), who also comments that the literature has identified issues for teachers and parents which compromise the delivery of effective SRE. SHNs have been suggested to be key agents of change in this area as they have a significant role in facilitating multidisciplinary collaborative working and coordinating programmes as well as providing a consistent approach to involving the wider community (Day and Lane 1999; Cotton *et al.* 2000; Cooper 2005; Jones 2008; Neill *et al.* 2009). SHNs are also identified to be effective in engaging parents to work in collaboration with them and the schools for the benefit of their children (Harrison 2005; Jones 2008; Neill *et al.* 2009). Facilitation of such collaboration is essential as parents are identified in a plethora of documentation to be a child's first and most important source of information regarding SRE, but their need for help and support in this area is equally well documented (Jones 2008). As the Case study set out below highlights, listening to young people and responding sensitively to their anxieties is important.

Case study

During open question time at the end of a lesson on sex and relationships delivered by the school nurse a teenage boy asked if what his mother had told him was correct. She had advised him that masturbation when practised by young boys results in them 'running out of sperm' by the time they are ready to consider starting a family. The school nurse discussed the appropriate facts regarding the anatomy and physiology of the testicles and sperm production and reassured him that this is not the case. This highlights that even when parents do attempt to educate their children in this subject a lack of knowledge of the correct facts can result in myths being carried through the generations as fact.

Targets set by the World Health Organization and national and devolved government regarding these aims have to date consistently failed to be achieved (Jones 2008). As public health practitioners, SHNs are widely identified to have a role in achieving the desired reduction in unplanned teenage pregnancies and sexually transmitted infections among young people in line with national and devolved government policy (Department for Education and Employment 2000; National Assembly for Wales 2002; Welsh Assembly Government 2009b,c). Working with local education authorities, the school's PHSE coordinator, individual class teachers, parents and governors, SHNs have the opportunity to influence SRE provision to ensure that their young clients' needs in this area are met. Negotiated support for class teachers and provision of agreed sessions within a structured collaborative approach within a robust curriculum can ensure that SRE provides what young people need.

However, it is essential that provision is guided by what pupils themselves identify as necessary and not merely informed by what adults and professionals think they should be taught. Although the ethos of the Children Act (Department of Health 2004b) is to listen to children, it is recognized that failing to hear what young people say can result from adults' unwillingness to listen (Lowden 2002). This is particularly relevant to SHNs, as children are the focus of their practice and, in their advocacy role, a documented responsibility (Nursing and Midwifery Council 2008); they are in a position not only to listen and work in partnership with children, but also to act as their advocate by ensuring their views are heard (Kenney 2002).

Principles for practice

- It is essential to listen to the concerns and anxieties of children and young people.
- SHNs must act as advocates to ensure that the views of children and young people are heard.

Vulnerable children and young people: the role of the SHN

DeBell and Jackson (2000) highlighted vulnerability and child protection as one of the four key areas of SHN work. In Hall and Elliman (2003), vulnerability is viewed as one of the key health and social care issues for children while *Every Child Matters* (Department for Education and Skills 2004) identified five outcomes to ensure the optimal health and well-being of children:

- being healthy
- staying safe
- enjoying and achieving
- making a positive contribution
- achieving economic well-being.

School health nurses, through working with teachers and other professionals, are in an ideal position to identify school-aged children experiencing health difficulties (Hall and Elliman 2003). They are trusted by children and young people and are often the first person with whom they discuss their emotional problems. DeBell and Tomkins (2006) referred to medical distress as the 'largest single source of health need amongst school-aged children in the UK'.

The Department of Health (1999a) defined vulnerable children as 'those disadvantaged children who would benefit from extra help from public agencies in order to make the best of their life chances'; these include:

- homeless young people
- young offenders
- teenage parents
- those being looked after by local authorities
- young carers
- young substance mis-users
- children in public care: hospital or residential
- children with mental health problems
- those living in poverty
- children of refugees or asylum seekers
- children and young people with disabilities
- children and young people excluded from school
- those who have behaviour problems.

The school health nurse works with many of these groups of children through the search for health needs. Health needs assessment of school-aged child populations aims to prioritize the health needs of that population and target interventions. It allows school health nurses to formulate a proactive plan to address the health issues of the school-aged population, including vulnerable children and young people (Department of Health and Department for Education and Skills 2004).

The school health nurse may work with children, their families, professionals or others to target interventions to improve situations such as bullying, peer relationship difficulties or behaviour problems or to refer them to other agencies for services. Bullying, for example, is an increasing problem in schools and, as the following Case study highlights, the SHN may help to resolve this.

Reflection point

Consider where and how school health nurses target and work with vulnerable children and their families.

Case study

During a visit to school a teacher discussed with the named school nurse that she was concerned a young girl who was in local authority care was being bullied by her peers. The girl denied that there was any problem but the teacher was not convinced. As the nurse was carrying out a teaching session on relationships with the group of year 8 pupils, she had the opportunity to raise the issue of bullying and advise the pupils of how to contact her with any problems they were experiencing for support and advice. A few days later, the young girl in question contacted her and stated that she was very unhappy as girls in her class made fun of her and her clothes and the fact that she did not live with her parents. She did not, however, consider it to be bullying as they did not physically assault her. The nurse was able to support her and discuss the concerns with the foster parents and the child's social worker, who then worked to raise the girl's self-esteem so that she was able to recognize the verbal abuse she suffered as bullying and then report it as such in school. Most schools have robust anti-bullying policies in place, and this one was no exception. The nurse and teachers also worked together with the pupils in small interactive interventions to discuss bullying and why it is wrong and should not be tolerated. The situation improved, but, importantly, the girl began to assert herself and formed friendships that resulted in her having the peer support necessary to enable her to enjoy her school life.

As shown above, SHNs may work with other professionals or agencies in assessing risk and health needs of vulnerable children. Inter-agency collaboration and effective communication has been found to have positive outcomes for children. Safeguarding the welfare of children and young people is everyone's business and covers promoting children's welfare through to protection of children from maltreatment (Department for Education and Employment 2006). School health nurses as public health practitioners are at the forefront of the preventative focus in working with vulnerable children to optimize their chances of health and well-being. They highlight significant harm and child protection as an increasing part of their workload (Royal College of Nursing 2005, 2009). Significant harm according to the Children Act (Department of Health 1989) is the threshold at which children are in need of protection, and compulsory intervention in the family through child protection procedures is justified. This can be from an episode or episodes which have a harmful effect on the child's physical or psychological development. This lack of parenting capability for a child may emerge from sources of domestic violence, substance misuse or parental mental illness, as set out in the Case study below.

Case study

A young boy aged 5 was screened in school for height, weight and vision. The school nurse observed that he looked tired and his presentation was poor, although he was in general appropriately dressed. School considered him to be well behaved but the nurse was concerned that he was unusually quiet and reserved for such a young child as they are more often excited when a visitor comes to the school. The school had some concerns about his punctuality and attendance and he had on occasion been picked up late from school by his mother. The nurse contacted the health visitor who had been visiting the family until the child reached school age. It was clear that the situation was very different from the health visitor's experience of the family. As a result the nurse attempted to arrange a home visit to discuss the issues with the mother but she refused, stating that all was well. The nurse discussed the case with social services as she was concerned that he was a 'child in need' and needed assessing in case intervention was necessary. The outcome was that the child was referred to social services for initial assessment, and it was identified that his mother's relationship had broken down and she was drinking heavily, which affected her ability to care for her son. Support was put in place which ensured that the child was able to be cared for at home and his mother received help and support to overcome her alcohol problem.

School health nurses are skilled in working with children and young people and their families and may be the first to identify if the child is at risk of significant harm. Their knowledge, education and training will ensure that they implement the appropriate child protection procedures (Department of Health 1989, 2004b). Shared assessment and working with other agencies are important to ensure appropriate outcomes. The proactive public health role of school health nurses can help identify vulnerable children who are linked to poverty, disadvantage and health inequalities. In addressing or targeting interventions to address the adverse health and well-being of children the school nurse may be required to work with others.

Reflection point

★ Consider the role the school health nurse plays within safeguarding the welfare of children and young people.

★ Working with others is vital if SHNs are to meet the needs of their client group, hence the need for multidisciplinary and multiprofessional working.

Principles for practice

- SHNs can help support vulnerable children and young people and their parents/carers.
- Multidisciplinary and multiprofessional working is essential to meet the needs of the vulnerable group.

PART 3

Multidisciplinary and multiprofessional working: the role of the SHN

Reflection point

Before reading this section consider who and what professions/disciplines may be linked with the SHN.

As qualified public health specialist practitioners it is essential that SHNs keep in focus that the very concept of public health practice resides in a concept of multiprofessional responsibility (Pencheon *et al.* 2006). Added to this, school nursing is acknowledged to be the only professional group whose remit is entirely focused on meeting the health needs of school-aged children, young people and their families (DeBell and Tomkins 2006). This statement does not mean that no other disciplines, professionals or voluntary sector colleagues have a role to play. In fact, the role of the SHN is reliant on the collaboration, expertise and support of all who are involved in the life of their young clients and their families. Their role, which is acknowledged to be unique (DeBell and Jackson 2000), places on them the responsibility to coordinate and collaborate effectively with everyone who can improve outcomes for the children and young people on their case load. The current focus of health promotion discussed earlier (DeBell *et al.* 2007, p. 119) highlights the responsibility to work collaboratively to ensure that the most appropriate and informed colleagues are involved in educating and advising children and young people on all the issues that affect them. This means the SHN must be well informed of who is or could be involved in support of the child or young person on their case load while remaining aware, as professionally guided (Nursing and Midwifery Council 2004, 2008), that this might not be them. This will ensure that the best interests of their young clients are being robustly addressed.

Essential requirements for team working, if a collective goal is to be achieved, include shared vision, effective inter-agency communication and understanding and valuing each other's roles, particularly the recognition of individuals' responsibilities within roles (Freeman *et al.* 2000; Bryar and Griffiths 2003). To be an effective link to ensuring their young clients' needs are addressed by appropriate multidisciplinary and multiprofessional colleagues, SHNs need to be well informed regarding provision in their locality and employ excellent communication skills, professional respect and a collaborative team-working ethos.

This process begins with health visiting colleagues, who, as registered public health specialist nurses, are also on Part 3 of the NMC register. Their degree studies, which are alongside the SHN pathway, begin the process of mutual understanding and professional respect that leads to effective team-working. Handover of care from the health visitor to the SHN when a child achieves school age ensures that any ongoing concerns and issues are seamlessly addressed at this important transition in a child's life.

Although the vast majority of school-aged children enjoy good health and never require hospital admission or even outpatient attendance, it is not the case for all. Children and young people with special needs ranging from mild to complex medical conditions receive their education in appropriate settings. In 'special schools' for children with profound and complex needs, a children's community nurse is usually based in the school on a permanent basis. As registered children's nurses, children's community nurses have the training and expertise to meet the school-age child's needs regarding issues including medication administration and enteral feeding.

In mainstream school, children with less complex but specific needs are supported to lead as normal a life as possible by clinical nurse specialists. These include clinical nurse specialists for asthma, epilepsy, diabetes, dermatological conditions and child and adolescent mental health services nurses (Neill *et al.* 2009). Although mental and emotional health is a specialized area SHNs are identified in *Every Child Matters* (Department for Education and Skills 2004) as being involved at tier 1, and their effectiveness in meeting the aims of this document are reliant on the support and expertise of colleagues in child and adolescent mental health services. Fostering strong links and excellent communication with colleagues who provide essential support to pupils with chronic health and mental and emotional health conditions will help to ensure that these young people achieve their full potential during their school years.

The school-age child with special needs may also receive input from a variety of medical disciplines and professionals, including speech and language therapists, physiotherapists, occupational therapists and paediatricians. Colleagues in education, including class teachers, classroom assistants, one-to-one support workers, education welfare officers, educational psychologists and peripatetic teachers, are often involved with the school-age child whether or not they have identified special needs. An understanding of each other's role, a willingness to share responsibility, robust communication and a mutual respect will ensure that multidisciplinary and multiprofessional teams collaborate effectively and serve the best interests of the child (Kenney 2002).

The SHN's important role in safeguarding (as already discussed in this chapter) places on them a responsibility to work in partnership with all agencies involved and particularly social services. Many outside agencies are involved in providing input in schools, particularly in the PHSE section of the curriculum. Local police and firemen often have strong links with schools, and the SHN should be aware of what they can offer both on and off school premises and in school holidays. Voluntary agencies have a wealth of expertise and are often the most appropriate people to provide up-to-date information to young people with regard to alcohol and drug abuse. Youth workers, who are also available outside school in youth clubs, are usually well accepted as relevant by young people and as a result can be invaluable in helping to engage school-aged children in health promotion activities outside school hours and in their local communities.

Neill *et al.* (2009) discuss that utilizing their unique position, as described by DeBell and Jackson (2000), ideally places the SHN to facilitate the joint working across organizations. This has been identified in the NSFs (Department of Health 2004a; National Assembly for Wales 2004) as crucial to effectively delivering the aims for children and young people and providing a comprehensive range of learning and education opportunities while facilitating informed choice to ensure that their young clients enjoy the best possible health.

Their role as advocate on behalf of their young clients can be effectively applied when engaging with multidisciplinary colleagues to ensure that the child's voice is heard and listened to, especially with regard to service provision (Neill *et al.* 2009). For example, SHNs need to be aware of their local Children and Young People's Partnership (CYPP) plan, which will be available on their local authority website. It is important that they become involved and contribute to discussions regarding local CYPP plans as it will help them to achieve this aim. Sharing the outcomes of school profiles with local authority colleagues and ensuring that young people are appropriately represented on CYPP groups will mean that all their previously highlighted rights to involvement are met.

At this stage, it would seem appropriate to discuss how skill mix within SHN teams is playing an increasingly important role within the service. When appropriately trained and supervised, support workers are integrated into teams and task-orientated work may be delegated to them. This allows SCPHN qualified team leaders to be proactive in approach, and also provides an opportunity for career progression that facilitates recruitment and retention within teams and succession planning for the future. Current modernization agenda documents, exploring the future profile and management structure for both SHN and the broader community nurse roles, are consistent in their ambition to embrace skill mix teams and tackle role design as a means to achieving these aims (Scottish Executive 2003; Department of Health 2006a; Welsh Assembly Government 2009a,b). This innovation, already well established in many areas, affords the specialist SCPHN team leader the ability to delegate task-orientated work to appropriately trained health care support workers or nursery nurses. As a result, SHNs who have not accessed the SCPHN qualification or are consolidating their practice, are freed up to be proactive in addressing locally identified needs as well as meeting the public health agenda specific to their young client group in all the communities they inhabit. Skill mix team-working not only meets the aims of the current modernization agenda but also allows for succession planning within an acknowledged ageing work force and can also facilitate recruitment and retention of staff.

Because of the current focus on school health nursing, for the first time in its history an exciting career pathway exists. To ensure its sustainability, students currently studying to become children's nurses and those recently graduated should consider a career within school nursing. Working with children and their families in their school and local communities to ensure the health of the next generation is a fulfilling, interesting and worthwhile role which offers unrivalled job satisfaction.

Principles for practice

- The SHN is reliant on the collaboration, expertise and support of all who are involved in the life of their young clients and their families.
- The child or young person with special needs may receive input from a variety of disciplines and professionals.
- The SHN may work with outside agencies, such as the police and fire services, as well as voluntary agencies.

Expanding and improving the school nursing service: the role of the SHN

As a population, school-aged children are in need of systematic and coherent attention (DeBell 2007). The political dimension of public health identified above highlights the need for the SHN to be up to date with current thinking and proposals that could affect their young clients. This is essential as the unique position of the SHN in public health, as described by DeBell and Jackson (2000), is becoming highly valued. It is recognized that their role enables them to implement health promotion directly linked to reforming social structures and policies that contribute to the health of individuals in their own community (Whitehead 2003; Neill *et al.* 2009). As a result there is a need for SHNs to be well versed on the latest policy and documents that relate to them at national and devolved government level in the UK. In response to the government pledge to be more open, practitioners have increased opportunities to influence policy as many relevant documents are made available in draft form for consultation (Naidoo and Wills 2005).

SHNs also need to work at a political and strategic level to improve services, and in this connection it is imperative that SHNs are aware of and do respond to all relevant consultations. Recent Welsh Assembly Government (2009a,b) documents were adjusted as a direct result of the consultation process. Notably for SHNs the recognition of the need for a change of name from the 'family nurse' to 'school nurse' identified in the Welsh Assembly Government (2009b) document. Responding enables the process to be utilized as an opportunity to lobby for and advocate on behalf of their young clients' needs in line with their professional responsibilities (Nursing and Midwifery Council 2004, 2008). The constant change endured by SHNs, in common with fellow practitioners, can result in them failing to engage in policy debate, not least because they feel policy-makers have no conception of the reality of the service they are attempting to deliver. However, enthusiastic and committed practitioners who feel that they have achieved a valued input into the formation of policy can go on to have a key role in achieving its intended outcomes (Naidoo and Wills 2005). Accessing appropriate government, devolved government and local government websites and professional journals will facilitate maintenance of an informed stance. The profile of the SHN needs to be raised at local level within the employing NHS organization, local authority and education departments as well as the local community level to ensure that their expertise and remit is fully understood and as a result valued. This can lead to much needed support when lobbying locally and nationally for resources to maintain, strengthen and improve services for the school-age child.

Principles for practice

- SHNs need to work at a political and strategic level to improve services and in this connection it is imperative that SHNs are aware of, and do respond to, all relevant consultations regarding the future of their service.
- Raising the profile of the school nursing service at local and national level is essential to maintain, strengthen and improve services for the school-age child.
- The discussion and analysis of the vitally important role of the SHN and their positive contribution and impact on the health of children and young people highlights key issues for all practitioners across all healthcare settings.

Conclusion

The SHN's role has evolved from its inception as an assistant to the doctor at the turn of the twentieth century to that of a public health practitioner today. The patterns of children and young people's health and illness have also changed from infectious diseases and malnutrition to issues pertaining to their mental health and well-being, sexual health, obesity and substance misuse. SHNs are required to be proactive and creative in the delivery of public health and health promotion to overcome these challenges to children and young people's health (Day 2009). This can be seen in their multidisciplinary team-working role within the delivery of immunizations, promotion of sexual health and safeguarding the vulnerable child. The specialist community public health nurse role places SHNs in a strong position to advocate within local policy-making arenas, including their employing Trust and the local health boards, and nationally by lobbying appropriate government representatives (Jones 2008), as policy and decision-makers must be reminded that investment in public health is sound economic sense (Naidoo and Wills 2005).

Achieving identified child public health aims takes time and SHNs need to utilize their specialist practitioner status to lobby for a long-term vision that is sustainably funded for a minimum of 10 years to allow them to apply a multidisciplinary, skill mixed approach utilizing all the evidence-based interventions that are available to them. Continual robust evaluation will allow them to establish effective programmes that will result in a healthier generation in the future. The outcome for the public and policy-makers will be a well-informed, healthier population that, in line with the Wanless Report (2002), is well enough informed to take responsibility for its own health. To ensure that this is achieved, it is imperative that SHN numbers are increased for equity and effectiveness of provision across the UK.

Summary of principles for practice

- School health nurses play a vital role in providing public health and promoting health for every school child and young person.
- Children and young people are entitled to a school health nursing service that they can identify with and which is relevant and appropriate to them.
- Inter-agency collaboration and effective communication with other professionals and agencies, including those in the voluntary sector, are essential if children and young people are to be safeguarded and receive the help and support they need.
- School health nurses need to work at political and strategic level to increase school health nurse provision.
- School health nursing is another future career opportunity for children and young people's nurses.

References

Bartley JD (2004) Health promotion and school nurses: the potential for change. *Community Practitioner* **77**(2): 61–4.

Bradburn E (1989) *Margaret McMillan: Portrait of a pioneer.* London: Routledge.

Bryar RM, Griffiths JM (2003) *Practice development in community nursing: Principles and processes.* London: Arnold.

Carlile Review (2002) *Too serious a thing. The Review of safeguards for children and young people treated and cared for by the NHS in Wales.* Cardiff: National Assembly of Wales.

Clark J, Buttigieg M, Bodycombe-James M, *et al.* (2000) *A review of health visiting and school nursing in Wales.* Swansea: University of Swansea.

Cooper P (2005) A coordinated school health plan. *Educational Leadership* **63**(1): 32–6.

Cotton L, Brazier J, Hall DMB, *et al.* (2000) School nursing: costs and potential benefits. *Journal of Advanced Nursing* **31**(5): 1063–71.

Court SMD (1976) *Fit for the future. Report on the Committee on the Child Health Service.* London: HMSO.

Coverdale G (2005) School nurses in the spotlight. *Community Practitioner* **78**(2): 48–9.

Day P (2009) School nurses are under-recognized and under-resourced. *British Journal of School Nursing* **4**: 424–7.

Day P, Lane D (1999) Sex education: Lessons to be learnt from going Dutch. *Community Practitioner* **72**(8): 259–60.

DeBell D (ed.) (2007) *Public health practice and the school age population.* London: Hodder Arnold.

DeBell D, Jackson P (2000) *School nursing within the public health agenda: a strategy for practice.* London: MacMillan-Scott.

DeBell D, Tomkins AS (2006) *Discovering the future of school nursing: the evidence base.* London: Amicus/CPHVA.

DeBell D, Buttigieg M, Sherwin S, Lowe K (2007) The school as location for health promotion. In: DeBell D (ed.) *Public health practice and the school age population*, pp. 93–130. London: Hodder Arnold.

Department for Children, Schools and Families and Department of Health (2009) *Healthy lives, brighter futures: the strategy for children and young peoples' health.* London: Department of Health.

Department for Education and Employment (1999) *National healthy school standard.* Nottingham: DfEE.

Department for Education and Employment (2000) *Sex and relationship guidance.* Nottingham: DfEE.

Department for Education and Employment (2006) *Working together to safeguard children: a guide to inter-agency working to safeguard and promote the welfare of children.* London: The Stationery Office.

Department for Education and Skills (2003) *Every child matters.* London: The Stationery Office.

Department for Education and Skills (2004) *Every child matters: change for children.* London: DfES.

Department for Education and Skills and Department of Health (2006) *Looking for a School Nurse.* London: DfES/DoH.

Department of Health (1989) *An introduction to the Children Act 1989.* London: HMSO.

Department of Health (1996) *The patients' charter: services for children and young people.* Norwich: HMSO.

Department of Health (1997) *The New NHS: Modern, Dependable.* London: The Stationery Office.

Department of Health (1999a) *Framework for the assessment of children in need and their families.* Consultation Draft. London: DH.

Department of Health (1999b) *Making a difference.* London: The Stationery Office.

Department of Health (2001) *Public health practice development document for school nurses.* London: DH.

Department of Health (2003) *Tackling health inequalities: a programme for action.* London: DH.

Department of Health (2004a) *Choosing health.* London: DH.

Department of Health (2004b) *Children Act.* London: DH.

Department of Health (2006a) *School nurse: practice development resource pack. Specialist community public health nurse.* London: DH.

Department of Health (2006b) *The green book.* London: DH.

Department of Health (2009) *Healthy child programme from 5 to 19 years.* London: DH.

Department of Health and Department for Education and Skills (2004) *National service framework for children, young people and maternity services.* London: DH.

Freeman M, Miller C, Ross N (2000) The impact of individual philosophies of teamwork on multi-professional practice and the implications for education. *Journal of Interprofessional Care* **14**(3): 237–47.

Gillick vs West Norfolk and Wisbech AHA and DOHSS [1985]. London: House of Lords.

Gleeson C (2004) School health nursing: evidence-based practice. *Primary Health Care* **14**(3): 38–41.

Hall DMB, Elliman D (2003) *Health for all children*, 4th edn. Oxford: Oxford University Press.

Harrison S (2005) Under-12s have sex one night and play with Barbie dolls the next. *Nursing Standard* **19**(39): 14–16.

Health Protection Agency (2005) *National minimum standards for immunisation training.* London: Health Protection Agency.

Jones SA (2008) Provision of sex and relationships education for young people. *Nursing Standard* **23**(14): 35–40.

Kenney G (2002) Children's nursing and interprofessional collaboration: challenges and opportunities. *Journal of Clinical Nursing* **11**: 306–13.

Lowden J (2002) Children's rights: a decade of dispute. *Journal of Advanced Nursing* **37**(1): 100–7.

Maben J, Griffiths P (2008) *Nurses in society: starting the debate.* London: National Nursing Research Unit, Kings College, London. [Q23]

Merrell J, Carnwell R, Williams A, *et al.* (2007) A survey of school nursing provision in the UK. *Journal of Advanced Nursing* **59**(5):463–73.

Naidoo J, Wills J (2005) *Public health and health promotion: developing practice*, 2nd edn. London: Baillière Tindall.

National Assembly for Wales (2001) *A strategic framework for promoting sexual health in Wales.* Cardiff: NAW.

National Assembly for Wales (2002) *Sex and relationships education in schools.* Circular no. 11/02. Cardiff: NAW.

National Assembly for Wales (2004) *National service framework for children, young people and maternity services in Wales.* Full version. Cardiff: NAW.

National Board for Nursing, Midwifery and Health Visiting for Scotland (2001) *Focus on update. School nursing: developing roles in public health.* Edinburgh: NBS.

Neill C, McPake K, Jones SA, *et al.* (2009) National perspectives. In: Moyse K (ed.) *Promoting health in children and young people. The role of the nurse*, pp. 381–97. Chichester: Wiley-Blackwell.

Nursing and Midwifery Council (2004) *Standards of proficiency for specialist community public health nurses.* London: NMC.

Nursing and Midwifery Council (2008) *The code.* London: NMC.

Obeid A (2002) School health nursing and recommendations for the future. *Journal of Community Nursing* **16**(12): 6–15.

Pencheon D, Guest C, Meltzer D, Muir Gray JA (2006) *Oxford handbook of public health practice*, 2nd edn. Oxford: Oxford University Press.

Polnay L (ed.) (1995) *Health needs of the school age child: report of a Joint Working Party of the British Paediatric Association.* London: BPA.

Royal College of Nursing (2005) *School nurses. Results from a census survey of RCN school nurses in 2005.* London: RCN.

Royal College of Nursing (2008) *An RCN toolkit for school nurses.* London: RCN.

Royal College of Nursing (2009) *School nursing in 2009. Results from a survey of RCN members working in schools in 2009.* London: RCN.

Scottish Executive (2003) *A Scottish framework for nursing in schools.* Edinburgh: Scottish Executive.

Slack PA (1978) *School nursing.* London: Ballière Tindall.

Steedman C (2000) Bodies, figures and physiology: Margaret McMillan and the late nineteenth century remaking of working class childhood. In: Cooter R *In the name of the child: Health and welfare 1880–1940. Studies in the social history of medicine.* London: Routledge.

Stretch R, McCann R, Roberts SA, *et al.* (2009) A qualitative study to assess school nurses' views on vaccinating 12–13 year old school girls against human papilloma virus without parental consent. *BMC Public Health* **9**: 254.

United Nations (1989) *Convention on the Rights of the Child.* Geneva: UN.

Wainwright P, Thomas J, Jones M (2000) Health promotion and the role of the school nurse: a systematic review. *Journal of Advanced Nursing* **32**(5): 1083–91.

Wanless D (2002) *Securing our future health: taking a long-term view.* Final Report. London: Department of Health.

Welsh Assembly Government (2005) *Designed for life: creating world class health and social care for Wales in the 21st century.* Cardiff: WAG.[Q23]

Welsh Assembly Government (2007) *One Wales. A progressive agenda for the government of Wales.* Cardiff: WAG.

Welsh Assembly Government (2009a) *A community nursing strategy for Wales.* Consultation Document. Cardiff: WAG.

Welsh Assembly Government (2009b) *A framework for a school nursing service for Wales.* Cardiff: WAG.

Welsh Assembly Government (2009c) *Sexual health and wellbeing for Wales, 2009–2014.* Draft working paper. Cardiff: WAG.

Whitehead D (2003) Health education, behavioural change and social psychology: nursing's contribution to health promotion? *Journal of Advanced Nursing* **34**(6): 822–32.

World Health Organization (1986) *Ottawa charter for health promotion.* Geneva: WHO.

Chapter 9

Community children's nursing

Ruth Davies

Overview

This chapter will begin with a historical overview of the care of sick children to show that care outside of the home is a relatively new development. In doing so, it will trace the early beginnings of community children's nursing, its continuing expansion and present-day scope of practice using real-life exemplars. The underlying theme throughout this chapter is the need to increase the number of community children's nursing teams and community children's nurses, for these can provide practical hands-on care as well as support to the child and family and in effect 'more hands and hearts in the home'. The case for this is put forward with reference to present-day child policy, research with children and their families as well as other empirical findings. It is argued that such a move will reduce hospital admissions, give the child and parents the choice of hospital or home care and in particular support parents who care for a child with long-term complex needs at home. Increasing provision is advocated on humanitarian grounds rather than as a means of saving money for the NHS on expensive hospital care. Suggestions on ways to increase provision are put forward as well as the need for community children's nurses to work at a strategic and political level to achieve this. It is noted that any expansion will have to be matched by an increase in educational places at pre- and post-registration level and in setting out the future opportunities open for children's nurses acknowledges that caring for children and young people in their own homes is in itself a rewarding career.

The care of sick children at home

People have always cared for sick children at home. Prior to the early beginnings of children's nursing in the nineteenth century they would have been cared for by their mothers, female relatives or, as Versluysen (1980) has persuasively argued, 'women healers'. Caring has been seen as a 'virtue' since pre-Christian times, for, as Baly (1987) reminds us, Thucydides writing about the plague that visited Athens in 429 BC refers to the fact that people visited and cared for the sick in their own homes and in doing so lost their own lives. Likewise, Judaism asserted that it was the responsibility of every Jew to visit the sick, while the Prophet Mohammed required his followers to visit sick Muslims as well as non-Muslims. The rise of Christianity across the Mediterranean and Europe and eventual dominance within the Western world saw Christ's teachings on caring for the sick become an accepted Christian duty. Phoebe, commended by St Paul for her visits to the sick and poor, may be regarded as the first Christian role model of a community nurse and one that was emulated by many devout individuals and organizations in the centuries that followed. St Vincent de Paul, in the seventeenth century, with Louse de Marillac set up the Daughters of Charity, an order of French Catholic sisters, who worked outside of the convent caring for abandoned street children as well as the sick poor in their own homes (Purcell 1989). In contrast, in Great Britain no institutionalized discipline focused its work exclusively on the needs of sick children either in hospital or in the community until the nineteenth century (Jolley 2008). By then a small number of religious charities had been set up to care for the sick poor in their own homes. These included the Society of Protestant Sisters set up in 1840 by Elizabeth Fry and her sister, as well as the Sisters of Mercy, a Roman Catholic order, and the Sellonites, an Anglo-Catholic order (Dossey 1999), all of which would have had mixed case loads of children and adults. Aside from these organizations, a system of outdoor relief was provided for the sick poor under the Old Poor Law, which derived from the time of Queen Elizabeth I. This included nursing care in the home, albeit by untrained nurses. The need to reform this antiquated system became apparent as the century progressed and, as will be shown, both government and individual reformers began to take a keen interest in the welfare of the sick poor on utilitarian as well as humanitarian grounds.

> ## Key point 🔑
>
> Throughout history sick children have been cared for at home.

The development of district nursing and home care for the sick poor

By the nineteenth century Britain had evolved from an agrarian society to an industrial one, with a rapidly expanding population which had migrated from the countryside to work in the new industrial cities, towns and conurbations such as Belfast, Manchester, Glasgow, the South Wales Valleys and 'The Potteries'. Between 1751 and 1821 the population of Great Britain had doubled and there were real concerns about overpopulation and the high levels of mortality and morbidity which affected large swathes of the working classes because of overcrowded living conditions, poor sanitation and a general lack of public health. The provision of outdoor relief under the old Poor Law to help people in times of need such as unemployment and sickness came to be regarded as encouraging a form of welfare dependency (Wilson 2005), and so was replaced by a chain of workhouses with their own purpose-built infirmaries across the country. The intention was to discourage entry by making admission a degrading and inhumane experience so only the most needy and desperate would apply. However, the sick poor denied any form of care within their own homes had no other option, and these infirmaries soon became overcrowded with the chronically ill or incurable cases that the voluntary hospitals rejected. This included large numbers of children who were either orphans or from families that were unable or unwilling to care for them. Many had conditions such as tuberculosis, epilepsy, learning disabilities or mental illness and once admitted were left in the 'care' of female able-bodied paupers under the supervision of paid but untrained nurses recruited from the ranks of maids or labourers (Dossey 1999). Workhouses and their infirmaries became places of dread to the working class, and national scandals reported in the public press that detailed the maltreatment of pauper patients probably prevented many a family from seeking admission for their sick child. This meant inevitably that the majority, apart from those able to gain access to a voluntary hospital, had no healthcare with very few having the services of a trained nurse within their homes.

Reflection points

★ Why were the sick children of the poor treated so harshly in Victorian times?

★ Are there any parallels with today's health service? For example, are services still focused on acute and curable conditions rather than chronic and incurable ones?

The precursor to today's community nursing service owes much to the work and vision of two Victorian luminaries, namely Florence Nightingale, who needs no introduction, and William Rathbone, a philanthropist and a member of a wealthy Liverpool shipping dynasty. Rathbone's desire to help the sick poor was based on personal experience when his first wife had been ably nursed at home in her final illness by Mrs Mary Robinson. After his wife's death in 1859, he engaged Mrs Robinson to nurse the sick in some of the poorest areas of Liverpool and it quickly became apparent that more nurses were needed. In 1860, Rathbone wrote to and visited Nightingale to seek her advice on this and sent Elizabeth and Mary Merryweather as observers to the Nightingale School, St Thomas's, London. Four Nightingale nurses returned to Liverpool with the Merryweathers and set up what was in effect the first district nursing service (Stocks 1960).

This system spread to other cities, towns and villages so that by the end of the nineteenth century there was a network of District Nursing Associations supported by various charities across Great Britain. Many of the great and good supported these, including Queen Victoria, and money raised by the women of Great Britain to commemorate her Jubilee in 1887 was used to set up the Queen's Nursing Institute. Admittance to the ranks of a Queen's Nurse was stringent, with applicants having to show they had undergone general hospital training and 3 months of training in a maternity hospital or lying-in hospital plus 6 months of training in the practice of district nursing under the tutelage of a trained district superintendent (Craven 1890; Baly 1987). District nurses, regardless of which association they belonged to or whether they were based in cities, towns or villages, had caseloads which included sick children and adults. Given the high childhood morbidity and mortality during this time their workload would have been considerable. Florence Lees, the first superintendent of district nursing, wrote the first handbook for practitioners under her married name of Mrs Dacre Craven, in which she gave practical advice, based on her own extensive experience as a district nurse. In discussing the care of babies and children with diphtheria, croup and bronchitis, she advised a warm and moist atmosphere and suggested that the child's cradle be brought as near to the side of the fire as possible. Recognizing that many of the children visited lacked even the most basic necessities such as a cradle or individual sick bed she advised 'An extemporary cradle for a sick child can be made out of clothes-basket or a large drawer, and an extemporary bedstead by arranging chairs back and front alternatively tied together by the legs' (Craven 1890, p. 48).

Mrs Craven also gave advice on caring for cases of scarlet fever, typhoid and smallpox, which were endemic at this time. The many pages devoted by her on the best position for the dying patient as well as 'last offices' highlights the fact that the majority of deaths, including those of babies and children, took place in the family home. Thoughtfulness and compassion towards the patient was evident throughout her book and, as she observed, 'A district nurse must have real love for the poor, and a real desire to lessen the misery she may see' (Craven 1890, p. 13). Their work must have lessened this misery not only through their skilled care of the sick and dying but also in their role as health advisors. This was an important aspect of their role in the days before a health visiting or school nursing service, and it is notable that district nursing associations expected them to teach families not only how to care for their sick relative but also how to provide a clean and well-ventilated environment as well as nutritious meals (Craven 1890; Stocks 1960; Baly 1987).

Surgery at home and day surgery for children

District nurses were also involved at all stages of the many surgical cases that took place at home on the kitchen or dining room table and included procedures such as tonsillectomies, adenoidectomies and circumcision as well as emergency operations for appendectomies and tracheostomies. There were many cases that voluntary hospitals would not or could not accept, but the positive aspects of surgery at home were not lost on the Victorians or Edwardians, who noted that it caused less family disruption and was often safer (Baly 1987). That children fared better at home cared for by their own mothers was also recognized by James Nicholl, a surgeon at the Glasgow Hospital for Sick Children (1894–1920) who pioneered the use of day surgery for procedures such as pyloric stenosis, hernia and cleft palate to avoid the hospitalization of young children which he not only considered unnecessary but also harmful, involving as it did separation of the child from his mother (Nicholl 1909). In this he was supported by a 'domiciliary nursing service', which enabled children to be discharged home immediately post-surgery where their progress was monitored by daily visits from a team of nurses. Nicholl not only believed that children fared better at home but cannily identified that the cost of day surgery was one-tenth of inpatient care. Sadly, his innovative scheme was not adopted elsewhere and it was to take nearly another 100 years before this was put into practice again.

Middle and upper class children had access to trained nurses within the home as many voluntary hospitals, including children's hospitals, had a system of providing trained hospital nurses in the home but for a fee. Great Ormond Street Hospital for Sick Children, for example, set up a private domiciliary nursing service to supplement its income that ran successfully from 1888 to 1948 (Hunt and Whiting 1999). Throughout the nineteenth century, with the exception of Wales, voluntary children's hospitals had been built in most of the major cities across Great Britain (Lomax 1996). However, these catered for only a minority of sick children while the majority continued to be housed in workhouse infirmaries. During the 1850s and 1860s Charles Dickens, Florence Nightingale and Louisa Twining campaigned with other reformers against the harsh conditions that prevailed within these which eventually led to the passing of the Metropolitan Poor Act 1867. This was an important landmark, which, as Abel-Smith (1964, p. 82) noted, acknowledged for the first time 'that it is the duty of the state to provide hospitals for the poor' and effectively paved the way for the National Health Service (NHS) that was to follow 80 years later.

Key point

Early district nursing teams, funded by charities, had mixed case loads of children and adults and cared for the sick poor children. Some children's nurses operated outside of children's hospitals but for a fee.

Sick children's care during the first half of the twentieth century

By the twentieth century improvements had been made in workhouse infirmaries, including the employment of trained nurses. Finally, in 1929, responsibility for these was transferred from the Poor Law Board of Guardians to County and County Borough councils. Enlightened councils such as London, Manchester and Birmingham invested in these 'municipal infirmaries' by developing nursing staff and ensuring full-time, salaried medical staff so that, by 1939, these rivalled the elite voluntary hospitals. In the meantime, the majority of children requiring nursing care at home continued to receive this from district nursing teams funded by charitable nursing associations. By the 1930s voluntary hospitals were in serious financial trouble and became fee-charging institutions. The setting up of the Emergency Medical Service for civilians during the Second World War provided a blueprint of what a comprehensive state-funded service could provide. Most nurses, as Baly (1988, p. 44) observed, 'were all too aware of the inequalities of health before the war, particularly the hardship of mothers and children and the everlasting dread of the doctors' bill'. Inevitably, the publication of the Beveridge Report (1942), which outlined a comprehensive NHS, combined with the post-war consensus for a more just and fair society ushered in a Labour Government committed to an NHS funded by general taxation, which was duly set up in 1948. This took over responsibility for the care of children in hospital and the community and in the words of Nye Bevan, first Minister of Health, finally put in place an ethos which recognized that 'rich and poor are treated alike … poverty is not a disability and wealth is not advantaged' (Bevan 1953, p. 77).

The first state-funded 'domiciliary' or community children's nursing teams

Key point 🔑

State-funded community children's nursing teams were only introduced in 1949 following the setting up of the NHS in 1948.

In 1949, the first publicly funded community-based nursing service for children was set up in Rotherham in an attempt to reduce high infant mortality caused by crossinfection in hospital (Gillett 1954). A more ambitious Home Care Programme operated out of St Mary's Hospital, Paddington, and cared for nearly 3000 children, aged 0–10 years, at home during 1954–64. This multidisciplinary team comprised a paediatrician, two children's nurses, a student nurse, a medical student, a part-time secretary, a social worker and a physiotherapist. Between them they carried out what, even today, may be described as fairly sophisticated procedures, including lumbar punctures, subdural taps, duodenal intubations, electrocardiography and intravenous infusions. The case load included newborns with pyloric stenosis, jaundice and prematurity. It also cared for children with acute conditions such as upper respiratory tract infections and gastroenteritis as well as chronic conditions such as cystic fibrosis, asthma and children with cancers. It was concluded that the 'use of the nurse to *support* mothering, rather than take it over, has appeared to have gratifying results in some families' and that the cost of care was roughly one-third the average cost per case of several London children's hospitals (Bergman *et al.* 1965).

Community children's nursing, or 'domiciliary care' as it was referred to in a paper by Professor Smellie in the *British Medical Journal* of 1956, was now perceived as a means of children avoiding hospitals or having earlier discharge. Reporting on the success of the Birmingham Children's Home Nursing Unit, set up in 1954, he noted that over a 1 year period 454 children were cared for at home, totalling 3295 visits. Only 26 of these required hospital admission, and in some of these cases mothers were unwilling to have their child nursed at home, particularly if, as he noted, they had to go out to work, had large families or lived in overcrowded or inadequate housing. The case load included conditions such as respiratory infections, tonsillitis, otitis media, abscesses and gastroenteritis. Reflecting their role as health educators as well as 'hands on nurses', he reported:

> *Often the nurses have been called in initially to give an injection of penicillin etc., but they have always seized this opportunity to teach the mother general nursing care and to advise on diet, clothing, general hygiene, and the like. … In particular, evening visits have been found to be the most important in allaying the fears and worries and anxieties of mothers, so that there have been very few emergency calls during the night.*
>
> *(Smellie 1956, p. 256)*

The publication of the Platt Report (Ministry of Health 1959; Davies 2010a) raised awareness of the adverse emotional effects of hospitalization on children and recommended that they should not be admitted if it could possibly be avoided. Home care was put forward as a better alternative, with both the St Mary's, Paddington, and Birmingham schemes identified as exemplars of good practice (Ministry of Health 1959). Whether children should be cared for at home or in hospital (Essex-Cater 1962) was the subject of much debate within the professions, especially in the light of Illingworth and Knowelden's (1961) study of 22 provincial English hospitals, which showed that paediatric hospital admissions had actually risen from 65 385 in 1950 to 83 184 by 1959. However, despite Platt's recommendation for an increase in home care, which was also reiterated in the Court Report (Court 1976), this did not happen and by 1985 there were still only 17 community children's nursing teams in existence across the whole of the UK (Whiting 1985).

Key point

- Although the Platt Report (Ministry of Health 1959) recommended that children should not be admitted to hospital if it could possibly be avoided, most were, and there were only a few community children's nursing teams across the UK up until the early 1980s.

The expansion of community children's nursing teams from the 1980s onwards

The number of community children's nursing teams provided across the UK accelerated during the 1980s. Research by Whiting (1985) showed that 22 districts in

England provided these, although, as he noted, only two provided a 24 hour, 7 days a week (24/7) service. A decade later, Tatman and Woodruffe (1993), in their postal survey across the UK, identified 62 general and 124 specialist paediatric home care services. However, reflecting Whiting's (1985) findings, they found only a few provided a 24/7 service. For the purposes of their study, a general home care service was defined as that provided by paediatric community nurses based in the community whereas specialist home care was defined as that provided by hospital-based clinical nurses, e.g. paediatric oncology outreach nurses or specialist nurses for conditions such as diabetes. They found that most services lacked a budget within that of the hospital or community where they were based, and identified that the boundary between hospital and community created a barrier to an efficient and effective system of care. In 1997, a House of Commons Select Committee Report (House of Commons 1997) expressed concern that less than 50% of children in the UK had access to community children's nursing services, with less than 10% having access to a 24/7 service. This report was strongly in favour of increasing provision, recommending that all children should have access to a 24/7 community children's nursing service and that every GP should have access to a named community children's nurse. However, as Whiting (1998) noted, it did not make any clear recommendations of how these services might be formulated. This has since resulted in services being developed in an *ad hoc* fashion with a wide range of service models, variation in funding (i.e. through hospital, community or combined hospital/ community trusts) as well as management and location of services.

Nevertheless, expansion continued and a factor, as Bradley (1997) has argued, must have been the realization by childcare professionals that parents were just as capable of meeting their sick child's needs at home as they were in hospital. The end of this decade and century saw the setting up of 10 Diana Community Children's Nursing Teams, to commemorate the life and work of the late Princess of Wales (Davies 1999). These, as well as providing palliative care to children with life-limiting conditions, raised public and political awareness of the need to have dedicated services for children in their homes and communities.

Key point

- Community children's nursing teams started to expand rapidly from the mid-1980s onwards as successive governments aimed to reduce the hospitalization of children on humanitarian and cost grounds.

By 2000, While and Dyson's (2000) postal survey across the UK found that more than half of the current community children's nursing teams had been founded after 1990, and that there were two dominant models of paediatric home care: the community model with strong links to primary care and the hospital outreach model with strong links to the hospital. Again, reflecting previous findings, few provided a 24/7 service. Furthermore, Eaton (2000), in her review of the literature on community children's nursing services, found six models of paediatric home care delivery, which included (1) hospital outreach generalists, (2) hospital outreach specialists, (3) community-based teams, (4) hospital-at-home, (5) district nursing service and

(6) ambulatory assessment unit. These, as Eaton concluded, had been set up in response to local needs or as a result of hero-innovators and so had not been developed strategically, which may, as noted previously, be traced back to the consistent failure at government level to make recommendations on how a comprehensive community children's nursing service may be formulated.

Key point

- Community children's nursing teams have not been developed strategically and so provide different models of care which may have strong links to the hospital or the community. Few provide a 24/7 service.

Developing community children's nursing services to meet the needs of children for the twenty-first century

Today's community children's nursing teams provide support for a diverse range of care needs (Whiting 1998; Royal College of Nursing 2009a), utilizing a range of skills (Box 9.1).

Key point

Community children's nurses and their teams support a diverse range of needs, including hospital-at-home, supporting children and families with chronic conditions, complex needs, continuing care and palliative care including EoLC.

Box 9.1	Care need supported by community children's nursing teams in the twenty-first century

- Care of neonates with complex needs arising from prematurity, facilitating earlier discharge from special care baby units
- Earlier discharge for children and people from hospital with conditions such as febrile convulsions, otitis media and meningitis
- Follow-up and support of children requiring emergency treatment (surgery, trauma and orthopaedics)
- Supporting children and young people undergoing planned surgery
- Supporting children and young people with complex needs and disabilities (most often referred to as 'continuing care')

- Supporting children and young people with long-term chronic conditions such as asthma or diabetes as well as cancer
- Providing children and young people with end-of-life care (EoLC) at home
- Communicating and caring for young adults, including the transition from child to adult services
- Nurse prescribing
- Symptom control
- Modernizing and improving the service for children and young people, including commissioning of specialist and community services
- Management of care packages

At this point it is worth illustrating their work by using a real-life exemplar from practice and, given their *raison d'être* is to prevent hospital admission and/or reduce the length of hospital stay, it would seem appropriate to begin with Lucy's Case study below.

Case study

Lucy aged 6, who has cystic fibrosis, was admitted to the children's ward of her local hospital with a severe chest infection that required intravenous antibiotics. In this Trust, community children's nurses rotate between the hospital and community (e.g. a full-time practitioner would work 3 days on the ward and 2 days in the community), so Lucy and her parents were given the option of continuing with her intravenous regime in hospital or at home. After choosing home, her parents were taught how to administer the drugs and, within 3 days of admission, Lucy was discharged home, where she and her parents were supported by the community children's nursing team Monday to Friday, 9–5 p.m., with open access to the children's ward overnight or at the weekend if required. Lucy successfully completed her course of antibiotics without readmission to hospital. Her parents were happy that she could be treated at home and felt that this was better for her. Lucy accepted her treatment more readily at home and kept to her usual routine, whereas in hospital the same procedures caused her anxiety and her meals and bedtime were disrupted. Hospital-at-home was also less disruptive to them as a family, including Lucy's two older brothers, who also kept to their usual routine of school, after school club and swimming lessons. In all, 11 hospital bed stays were saved for Lucy and the NHS.

As in Lucy's case, research has also shown that children with acute conditions may be cared for at home. Davies and Dale (2003) were able to show that in areas where GPs can refer children with acute conditions such as otitis media and chest infections to the community children's nursing service there was a reduction in the number of hospital beds and lengths of stay. One large randomized controlled trial compared hospital-at-home by community children's nurses with hospital care for a range of conditions, including breathing difficulties, diarrhoea and vomiting as well as fever. Findings showed that there were no significant differences in clinical effectiveness between services and that most parents and children expressed a strong preference for home care (Sartain *et al.* 2002). Care at home has also been promoted for children with complex care needs. Brombley (2008), in her study of seven children with acquired head injury, was able to show how case-managed home care enabled them to be cared for safely and effectively at home. Brombley was also able to show considerable cost savings between hospital and home care. More importantly, it meant the children could return home rather than remain in hospital or be transferred to other institutions. The success of this venture probably owes much to the appointment of a community matron to specifically case manage this group of children and is an excellent example of home care.

Another large group of children who have been variously described as having complex needs, continuing care needs or palliative care needs are those with life-limiting conditions such as severe cerebral palsy and muscular dystrophy. Because of advances in treatment and technologies these children are now surviving longer and making the transition from children's to adults' services (Maunder 2004). The vast majority will be cared for by their parents, most usually their mothers, in the family home. Caring places a heavy responsibility on parents, who run the risk of becoming physically and emotionally exhausted. Community children's nurses can support families by providing practical 'hands-on' care, respite in the home and liaising with health and social services as well as voluntary agencies such as children's hospices. They can also provide a family-centred approach to care and, in doing so, support not only the affected child but also their parents, siblings and grandparents. They may take on the role of an 'informed friend' to the whole family, often over many years (Davies 1999); this is a relationship which, whilst rightly acknowledging parents as the experts in the care of their child, also respects their right to be first and foremost parents rather than just carers. This is a point worth making and is expressed by this single mother of four children who is also a registered nurse; at the time of writing, she was battling to have palliative care at home for her 6 year old terminally ill son:

> *I do not want to be a nurse to my own son …. I just want to be a Mummy to my little boy, I have other children. We need to be at home doing things together and, when my son is well, we need to be living life and having fun.*

(quoted in Dean 2009, p. 13)

Many other families are in a similar position to this mother, hence the campaign by the Royal College of Nursing and WellChild to increase community children's nursing provision as part of their UK Better at Home Campaign (Royal College of Nursing/WellChild 2009). As their report highlights, children with complex needs often experience long-term hospitalization, which means they may:

- do less well than children cared for at home as a result of less stimulation essential for normal development
- are often cared for in inappropriate care settings such as paediatric intensive care units (PICUs)
- miss out on family life, events, school and leisure activities
- are at increased risk of hospital-acquired infections.

Their report argues persuasively on humanitarian as well as cost grounds for increasing community children's nursing provision and, in doing so, identifies that the cost of caring for a child on ventilation in a PICU is £750 455 per annum compared with £100 000–200 000 per annum for those cared for in the community (Murphy 2008). This report also draws attention to a study by Fraser *et al.* (1997), which estimated that 12% of all PICU beds are occupied by those who could be cared for at home. Of particular concern, as Murphy (2008), a clinical development sister, emphasizes, must be the adverse emotional, psychological and social effects of being cared for in PICU on the individual child, who is likely to witness traumatic and distressing events and possibly even the deaths of other children. These adverse effects are probably shared by parents, who, in addition, have other concerns such as loss of earnings, travelling expenses, car parking charges as well as childcare for well siblings while caring for their child in PICU. Providing a 24/7 community children's

Reflection point

Reflect on how family-centred care provided by a children's nurse in hospital may differ from that provided by a community children's nurse in the child's home.

Developing community children's nursing services to meet the needs of children for the twenty-first century   **Page 247**

PART 3

nursing service would ensure that these children could be cared for at home. Indeed, as acknowledged by the Department of Health (2009) and Royal College of Nursing/ WellChild (2009):

Community nurses … are the bedrock of local service provision for children with disabilities, long-term conditions and complex health needs. They are often best placed to take on the role of a lead professional, liaising with other agencies on behalf of, or in collaboration with, the child and family to ensure their wishes, views and choices inform their ongoing care and to explore how best to move towards a multi-disciplinary approach and a more integrated care package in the location of the child and family's choice.

(Department of Health 2009, p. 72)

Key point

- There is a need to increase community children's nursing teams and the number of community children's nurses to provide a 24/7 service and to give children and their families choice with regard to home or hospital care.

As already alluded to, a number of studies point to cost savings for the NHS in providing care at home instead of hospital; therefore, some words of caution would seem necessary. Parker *et al.* (2002), in their systematic review of the costs and effectiveness of different models of home care, question whether it should always be assumed that families necessarily want to provide care at home, especially if it involves 'high technology'. They argue, quite rightly, that just because it may be cheaper for the health service this is not reason in itself for 'pushing as much care as possible into the home, particularly if it imposes both short and longer-term costs on parents and other children in the family' (Parker *et al.* 2002, p. 78). Similarly, Noyes (2006), in a helpful and detailed case study of a 12 year old child with quadriplegia cared for at home on 24/7 ventilation, found the burden of care may well be pushed onto the family, or, in this particular case, a single mother. As Noyes reported, the child in question, Nathan, accessed or used 11 different services and was cared for by five different doctors (GP, community paediatrician attached to the special school and consultants in cardiac, orthopaedic and respiratory care). This, in itself, must have involved many separate appointments for there was no single shared healthcare plan or lead paediatrician. Although Nathan was supposed to receive 24/7 day care at home, major problems had been experienced by his mother at weekends and on nights because of staff sickness. Understandably, she had been prescribed antidepressants as she found it difficult to cope with all these demands. Nathan was also affected and felt that he spent too much time with adults rather than with friends his own age. This case study, which probably reflects many others, shows all too well how an inadequate care package benefits neither the child nor the mother, although it may benefit the NHS by savings on expensive hospital care.

In the final analysis, increasing community children's nursing provision is not just about cost savings but rather about giving children and their families choice about place of care; as research findings show, most would prefer to be cared for in their own homes and communities. It is also about giving them choice with regard to EoLC at home too, if that is their wish. Research across the developed world has shown that most children and young people prefer to die at home and that most parents also prefer this option (Davies 2009). However, despite this, most children continue to die in hospital because of a lack of this provision. As the case study below shows, healthcare professionals in hospital may respect the absolute right of a child to die at home but, to achieve this, they too need access to a community children's nursing team.

Case study

Rhian, aged 13, who had a rare genetic condition, reached the end-of-life stage following a severe bout of pneumonia and was receiving ventilation on the PICU of a children's hospital. A multidisciplinary meeting attended by her parents, physicians, anaesthetists, intensive care nurses and the community nursing team manager was held to discuss her care and management. Her parents wanted her to die at home and, as tests had shown she was not breathing independently or responding to stimuli, it was suggested that she be transferred home and extubated there. Rhian was accompanied home by the consultant anaesthetist and a PICU nurse on full ventilation and, once home, was settled into her own bed. She was then extubated and given 5 litres per minute of oxygen, via nasal prongs, to keep her comfortable. Twenty minutes following extubation she became distressed and agitated, so was commenced on a mixture of diamorphine, haloperidol, midazolam and cyclizine via a syringe driver. Subcutaneous oromorphine was also prescribed for breakthrough pain. Care was transferred to the community children's nursing team, who continued to provide symptom control and support to the family and provide 24 hour cover. Rhian died with her parents at her bedside 51 hours after discharge from hospital.

The close working relationship between the hospital and the community children's nursing team was essential to ensure that Rhian died at home. It was also essential that this team provided 24/7 cover for her parents to prevent any breakdown in care which would have resulted in her readmission, and death, in hospital. In this respect, the Association for Children's Palliative Care and Children's Hospices UK (2009) recommends that commissioners of services should review models of community children's nursing provision to enable 24/7 'hands-on' care, support and advice in situations where community children's nurses act as front-line specialists. This cannot be stated strongly enough, as a recent report in Wales (Palliative Care Planning Group 2008) highlighted the current lack of such a service means unnecessary hospital admissions and unwanted hospital deaths for children and their families.

Reflection points

★ In your present clinical hospital placement/ward, how many children could possibly be cared for at home instead?

★ Does your present clinical hospital placement/ward have access to a local community children's nursing team?

The contribution to care by community children's nurses and the case for expanding provision

Although it is outside the scope of this chapter to describe every role played by community children's nurses it is clear that their contribution is an increasingly important one in the care of sick children, as reflected by their continuing expansion. A major reason for this has, of course, been the desire by successive governments to reduce the number of children admitted to hospital on both humanitarian and cost grounds. Fewer children are now admitted to hospital and those who are will potentially experience early discharge, with day surgery (Calder *et al.* 2001) and ambulatory care (Ogilvie 2005) also reducing the number of hospital admissions and length of stay. Hospital-based children's and young people nurses, including specialist nurses, play a crucial role in transferring care to home by liaising and working closely with community children's nurses teams and individual community children's nurses.

In particular, community children's nurses have a role in supporting children post-surgery and, as the following Case study highlights, their expertise in the assessment and management of child pain can prevent unnecessary suffering to the child and family.

Case study

Ben, aged 6, who has global development delay and lives in complicated social circumstances, underwent an osteotomy. Discharged home from hospital in 'broomsticks' he was referred by the hospital-based children and young people's team to the community children's nursing team for family support and change of dressings. When assessed by the team, it was noted that his hip area was very swollen so he was immediately referred to the Accident and Emergency Department of his local hospital where he was prescribed antibiotics. After a further few days at home, it was noted that his hip area remained swollen and he was also experiencing pain. He was referred once again by the team to hospital, where an X-ray revealed displaced screws on his femur. It is possible that this problem may not have been detected until review by the orthopaedic team if the team had not been involved.

Community children's nurses may also prevent unnecessary and expensive hospital consultations, as follows.

Providing care and support to children with eczema: an example of good practice

One community children's nursing team in Wales receives referrals to review children with eczema from GPs, health visitors and hospital-based nursing and medical staff. The team reviews these children, who are referred to hospital paediatric consultants, before they are seen at outpatient clinics. If the team is able to support and manage the child's eczema satisfactorily, the child is removed from the consultant's list, thereby reducing the waiting list and times for other children. Alternatively, if the child's condition is considered severe, the team can expedite review by the paediatric consultant.

The team offers advice and support to parents/carers of the child for the management of eczema within the home environment, which can help avoid hospital admission, help with earlier discharge from hospital and reduce expensive hospital consultations.

Community children's nursing provision has to take account of the number of children and young people with life-limiting conditions who are surviving longer and making the transition from paediatric to adult services, as exemplified in the Case studies above. At the same time, today's childcare philosophy, based on a rights-centred approach to care, demands that their preferences be taken into account, and this means of course being cared for and even dying within the family home. Taking all these reasons into account, further expansion would seem inevitable and indeed necessary if every child is to have access to a community children's nursing nurse and/or team. However, evaluation of community children's nursing roles, interventions and services may, as Lewis and Noyes (2008) point out, present specific challenges in terms of actual evaluation and cost-effectiveness and not least research.

Principle for practice

- Currently all children, regardless of where they live, have access to a hospital. The ideal would be for all children to also have access to a community children's nursing team and only be hospitalized if absolutely necessary.

However, demand for this service continues to exceed supply with Wales, my own country, providing a typical example of the situation that exists in parts of the other three countries that make up the UK.

Community children's nursing provision in Wales: notes from a small country

Wales is a small country with a child population (0–19 years) of approximately 700 000 plus (Statistics for Wales 2008). Since devolution, and the establishment of a Welsh Assembly Government (WAG), health and social services have differed from the rest of the UK. Wales has its own particular problems with a gross domestic

The role of community children's nurses in expanding provision: educational priorities and professional development   Page 251

PART 3

product well below the European average, and parts of west Wales and former mining communities experiencing high levels of deprivation, social exclusion and health inequalities (Osmond 2004). Set against this background, the National Service Framework for Children, Young People and Maternity Services in Wales (Welsh Assembly Government 2005) identified the need to develop community children's nursing to provide 'a children's community service available to meet the local needs in every local area of Wales' (Welsh Assembly Government 2005, 7.4). This also identified the need to provide 'an appropriate range of outreach services as close to home as possible particularly to meet the need of families living in rural Wales' (Welsh Assembly Government 2005, 7.5). In 2010, in response to the WAG consultation on community nursing in Wales, I, together with the All Wales Community Children's Nursing Forum, conducted a scoping exercise to identify the number of qualified community children's nurses who currently practise in Wales (Davies 2009). This found that, although the number of community children's nursing teams has increased over the last 10 years, there are still only 12 working across the whole of Wales, and these teams vary considerably in size. While older and well-established teams such as Gwent (south Wales) have an effective number of community children's nurses, others are small, with some comprising less than one or two whole-time equivalents (WTEs) covering vast rural areas in north and mid-Wales. Small teams of one or two community children's nurses are a concern, for, as the Royal College of Nursing (2009a) warns, these are vulnerable in times of staff sickness and may lead to 'burn-out' among staff.

In all, outcomes from the scoping exercise found less than a 60 qualified community children's nurses (WTEs) working across Wales, providing hospital-at-home and continuing care to children and young people within their own homes. It highlighted that provision was 'patchy' across Wales with rural areas, in particular, being poorly served. Unsurprisingly, no team was able to provide a 24/7 service, although, anecdotally, some did work outside their contracted hours to meet the wishes of the child and family and provide EoLC at home (as in Rhian's case study). The Royal College of Nursing (2009b) has recommended that for a child population of 50 000 a minimum of 20 WTEs community children's nurses are required to provide a holistic service. Using this formula, the number in Wales would have to increase, i.e. more than quadruple to 280, based on the current child population of 700 000 to provide such a service. In addition, each community children's nursing team would have to consist of six WTEs to provide a 24 hour service (Forys 2001). It should be emphasized that this 'snapshot' of Wales only reflects what is happening elsewhere and, as identified throughout this chapter, there is an urgent need to increase community children's nursing provision to meet the needs of children, young people and their families across all four countries that make up the UK.

The role of community children's nurses in expanding provision: educational priorities and professional development

If the number of community children's nursing teams and qualified community children's nurses is to expand across the UK, those currently in post must work together to make this happen. This calls upon leaders within the profession to demonstrate and, in doing so, publicize the contribution they make already as well as identifying how further expansion will benefit children and their families. This may be difficult for a profession that is perhaps overmodest and more used to getting on with the job rather than self-promotion, but work at a strategic and political level is vital if children and families are to receive the services they so clearly desire and need. The Royal College of Nursing/WellChild (2009) initiative has shown that politically there is cross-party support in England for increasing provision, and the same probably holds true for other countries in the UK, which brings us naturally on to the thorny question of funding. Although there may be some savings in transferring care from hospital to home, it will still require a substantial investment and rebalancing of services to provide a 24/7 service across the whole of the UK. In Scotland (Royal College of Nursing 2009c), it has been proposed that the £28 million set aside for consultants' merit awards should be used to fund a Scottish community children's nursing service instead, but such a redistribution of wealth is unlikely. In the midst of a worldwide recession, seeking funding on the scale put forward may seem overambitious, but we should recall that the setting up of the NHS in 1948 was also at a time when the nation was experiencing economic difficulties but took place because of the post-war desire for a better society. Investment in a nationwide community children's nursing service may strike a similar chord in the nation's collective conscience given that children are usually perceived as the most deserving of causes and how we care for and treat them as the yardstick upon which any civilized country is measured.

Expansion of services on any scale will mean not only looking at future workforce planning but also at how educational places may be increased at pre-registration level, this being the pool from which future community children's nurses are recruited. There are a range of community children's nursing programmes across the UK offering post-registration study at Diploma, Bachelor and Master level, but an increase in capacity is also dependent upon sufficient clinical placements and clinical practice teachers as well as mentors. In parallel with these programmes there must be professional development to support community children's nurses in practice who wish to progress horizontally or vertically. A comprehensive and high-quality community children's nursing service is dependent on a range of roles from staff nurse to advanced practitioner through to consultant (see Table 9.1). The few consultant community children's nurses who presently practice in the UK have already made a contribution, taking on leadership at a strategic level as well as combining excellence in clinical practice with strong links to education and research, but more are needed if community children's nurses are to develop their own evidence base upon which to continuously improve practice. Those who aspire to become a consultant may be well advised to study at doctoral level, for possession of a doctorate is likely to be seen as 'essential' rather than 'desirable' for this role in the future (Rolfe and Davies 2009). To this end, educational and career development opportunities need to be made explicit to those considering a career as a children's nurse and as a future community children's nurse if we are to recruit and retain the 'brightest and best'. In Wales, the predominant programme in preparing community children's nurses is the Specialist Practice Programme (SPQ), which is based on an amalgam of work by the Scottish Government and the Welsh Assembly Government (Welsh Assembly Government 2009). This clearly sets out the career pathways available to nurses and the levels of education required for practice without losing sight of the fact that caring for children and their families in their own homes and communities is reward in itself.

Table 9.1 Skills for health framework and required academic levels of education

Skills for health framework level	Role	Academic level of education required
Level 9	Very senior staff	Professional doctorate/PhD
Level 8	Consultant practitioner	Professional doctorate/PhD
Level 7	Advanced practitioner	Masters degree
Level 6	Senior practitioner/specialist practitioner	Masters or Bachelors degree
Level 5	Practitioner	Bachelors degree
Level 4	Associate practitioner	National vocational qualification
Level 3	Senior healthcare assistant	National vocational qualification
Level 2	Support worker	National vocational qualification
Level 1	Initial entry, e.g. cadet	Not relevant

From Welsh Assembly Government (2009) *A community strategy for Wales: consultation document.* Cardiff: WAG. Crown Copyright.

This chapter has shown how the provision of community children's nurses can prevent hospital admissions and enable earlier discharge. Importantly, this can give children and young people as well as their parents/carers choice between hospital or home care.

Principles for practice

- Community children's nurses must demonstrate their contribution to care at a strategic and political level, and any expansion of service must take into account future educational and professional needs to ensure a comprehensive service that combines practice, education and research.
- Community children's nursing offers another rewarding career opportunity for children and young people's nurses.

Conclusion

This chapter began by showing that throughout most of history the place of care for a sick child was the family home, and that their removal to other institutions, namely hospitals, only began in the nineteenth century and continued unabated until the Platt Report (Ministry of Health 1959) began to question this practice and advocated home care. Likewise, while a few community children's nursing teams resulted following the setting up of the NHS in 1948, these did not catch on immediately, and their expansion only started in earnest in the late 1980s owing to changes in professional attitudes towards parental involvement in their sick child's care as well as the desire by successive governments to shift hospital to home on humanitarian as well as cost grounds.

Throughout the chapter it has been identified how community children's nurses and their teams make a substantial contribution to the care of children in their own homes in a number of roles. At the same time it has been shown that community children's nursing teams have not, in the main, been developed strategically and so, as a consequence, although every child has access to a hospital not every child has access to such a nurse or team. This has led to inequity of provision across the UK, with Wales being a prime example. This is regrettable, for, as research and exemplars from practice highlight, this service can make a real difference in terms of choice between hospital and home for the child and family as well as providing a family-centred and holistic approach to care. All of which is reflected in calls from within and outside the profession to increase provision, with the Royal College of Nursing/ WellChild (2009) initiative being the latest in a string of reports demanding a 24/7 community children's nursing service.

The case for shifting hospital to home has been discussed in relation to children with complex needs with a strong plea being made for this to be for the benefit of the individual child and their family rather than merely a cost-saving exercise for the NHS. The argument put forward throughout this chapter is that community children's nursing provision is in the interests of the child and their family and respects their choice of hospital or home care, ever mindful of the fact that research informs us that the majority of children prefer to be cared for and even die within their own homes and communities. Providing a 24/7 service that is properly funded and underpinned by educational programmes and continuing professional development has also been put forward as the means of ensuring high-quality, evidence-based care. Lastly, in researching this chapter, it is clear that community children's nurses not only have increased in number over the last 10 years but also have made great strides in their practice, education and research, all of which bodes well for their future development and aspiration to provide a comprehensive 24/7 service across the length and breadth of the UK to ensure 'more hands and hearts in the home'.

Summary of principles for practice

- Children and young people should only be admitted to hospital if absolutely necessary. Both they and their parents/carers must have access to community children's nurses to enable choice between hospital or home care.
- Children and young people's nurses, whether based in hospital or in community settings, must work together at political and strategic level to increase community children's nursing provision.
- Any increase in community children's nursing provision must be matched by an increase in educational provision to ensure a safe, effective and high-quality community children's nursing service.

Acknowledgements

I would like to thank the All Wales Community Children's Nursing Forum for their help with this chapter and for donating examples from practice for case studies; pseudonyms have been used in order to protect patient confidentiality.

References

Abel-Smith B (1964) *The hospitals 1800–1948: a study in social administration in England and Wales.* London: Heinemann.

Association for Children's Palliative Care and Children's Hospices UK (2009) *Right people, right place, right time: planning and developing and effective and responsive workforces for children's and young people's palliative care.* London: ACT and Children's Hospices UK.

Baly ME (1987) *A history of the Queen's Nursing Institute: 100 Years 1887–1987.* London: Croom Helm.

Baly ME (1988) NHS thoughts from home and abroad. *International History of Nursing Journal* **3**(3): 44–6.

Bergman AB, Shand MDH, Oppe TE (1965) A pediatric home care program in London: ten years experience. *Pediatrics* **36**(3): 314–21.

Bevan A (1953) *In place of fear.* London: Heinemann.

Beveridge W (1942) *Report on social insurance and allied services.* London: HMSO.

Bradley SF (1997) Better late than never? An evaluation of community nursing service for children in the UK. *Journal of Community Nursing* **6**: 411–18.

Brombley K (2008) Better at home? Benefits of case management for children with complex needs. *Paediatric Nursing* **20**(9): 24–6.

Calder F, Hurley P, Fernandez C (2001) Paediatric day-case surgery in a district general hospital: a safe option in a dedicated unit. *Annals of the Royal College of Surgeons, England* **83**: 54–7.

Court S (1976) *The report of the Committee on Child Health Services: fit for the future.* London: HMSO.

Craven D (1890) *A guide to district nurses and home nursing.* London: Macmillan and Co.

Davies RE (1999) The Diana community nursing team and paediatric palliative care. *British Journal of Nursing* **8**: 506–11.

Davies R (2009) Caring for the child at end of life. In: Price J, McNeilly P (eds) *Palliative care for children and families: an interdisciplinary approach.* Basingstoke: Palgrave MacMillan.

Davies R (2010a) Marking the fiftieth anniversary of the Platt Report: from exclusion, to toleration and parental participation in the care of the hospitalised child. *Journal of Child Health Care* **14**(1): 6–23.

Davies R (2010b) Community Children's Nursing Provision 2010: Position paper and scoping exercise. *Nursing Praxis International* (ISBN 1-903625-20-3).

Davies C, Dale J (2003) Paediatric home care for acute illness. I. GPs and hospital: at-home staff views. *International Journal of Health Care Quality Assurance* **16**(7): 361–6.

Dean E (2009) The bedrock of children's services, so why are there not enough of them? *Nursing Standard* **24**(9): 13–14.

Department of Health (2009) *Healthy lives: brighter futures. The strategy for children and young people's health.* London: HMSO.

Dossey BM (1999) *Florence Nightingale: mystic, visionary, healer.* Springhouse, PA: Springhouse Corporation.

Eaton N (2000) Children's community nursing services: models of care delivery. A review of the United Kingdom literature. *Journal of Advanced Nursing* **32**(1): 49–56.

Essex-Cater AJ (1962) The sick child: home or hospital care. *Public Health* **March**: 157–66.

Forys J (2001) Do children's nurses offer 24 hour care? *Primary Health Care* **11**(6): 31–6.

Fraser J, Mok Q, Tasker R (1997) Survey of occupancy of paediatric intensive care units by children who are dependent on ventilators. *British Medical Journal* **315**: 347–8.

Gillett J (1954) Domiciliary treatment for sick children. *Practitioner* **172**: 281–3.

House of Commons (1997) *Health Committee Session 1996–7: Third report. Health services for children and young people in the community: home and school.* London: HMSO.

Hunt J, Whiting M (1999) A re-examination of the history of children's community nursing. *Paediatric Nursing* **11**(4): 33–6.

Illingworth RS, Knowelden J (1961) The demand on provincial children's hospitals. *Lancet* **1**(7182): 877–9.

Jolley J (2008) The emergence of the 21st century children's nurse. In: Hughes J, Lyte G (eds) *Developing nursing practice with children and young people.* London: Wiley-Blackwell.

Lewis M, Noyes J (2008) The children's community nurse. *Paediatrics and Child Health* **18**(5): 227–32.

Lomax EMR (1996) *Small and special: the development of hospitals for children in Victorian Britain.* London: Wellcome Institute for the History of Medicine.

Maunder EZ (2004) The challenge of transitional care for young people with life-limiting illness. *British Journal of Nursing* **13**(10): 594.

Ministry of Health (1959) *The welfare of children in hospital.* The Platt Report. London: HMSO.

Murphy J (2008) Medically stable children in PICU: better at home. *Paediatric Nursing* **20**(1): 14–16.

Nicholl JH (1909) The surgery of infancy. *British Medical Journal* 753–4.

Noyes J (2006) The key to success: managing children's complex packages of community support. *Archives of Disease in Childhood* **91**: 106–10.

Ogilvie D (2005) Hospital based alternatives to acute paediatric admission: a systematic review. *Archives of Disease in Childhood* **90**: 138–42.

Osmond J (ed.) (2004) *End of the corporate body: monitoring the National Assembly December 2003–2004.* Cardiff: Institute for Welsh Affairs.

Palliative Care Planning Group (2008) *Report to the Minister for Health and Social Services.* Cardiff: Palliative Care Planning Group.

Parker B, Lovett P, Paisley CA, *et al.* (2002) A systematic review of the costs and effectiveness of different models of paediatric home care. *Health Technology Assessment* **6**(35): iii–108.

Purcell M (1989) *Politics, philosophy and religion: the work of Monsieur Vincent, Life of St Vincent de Paul.* Dublin: Veritas Publications.

Rolfe G, Davies R (2009) Second generation professional doctorates in nursing. *International Journal of Nursing Studies* **46**: 1265–73.

Royal College of Nursing (2009a) *Preparing nurses to care for children at home and community settings.* London: RCN. See http://rcn.org.uk

Royal College of Nursing (2009b) *A child's right to care at home.* London: RCN. See http://rcn.org.uk

Royal College of Nursing (2009c) Spend on services – not consultant awards. *RCN Bulletin* 17 June.

Royal College of Nursing/WellChild (2009) *Better At Home Campaign.* Interim Report for MP Reception 10 March 2009 House of Commons, hosted by Tom Clarke MP. See http://wellchild.org.uk

Sartain SA, Maxwell MJ, Todd PJ, *et al.* (2002) Randomised controlled trial comparing an acute paediatric hospital at home service with conventional hospital care. *Archives of Disease in Childhood* **87**: 371–5.

Smellie JM (1956) Domiciliary nursing service for infants and children. *British Medical Journal* (Suppl.): 256.

Statistics for Wales (2008) *Population of 0–19 year olds in Wales.* National Statistics.

Stocks M (1960) *A hundred years of district nursing.* London: George Allen and Unwin Ltd.

Tatman MA, Woodruffe C (1993) Paediatric home care in the UK. *Archives of Disease in Childhood* **69**: 677–80.

Versluysen MC (1980) Old wives' tales: women healers in English history. In: Davies C (ed.) *Rewriting nursing history.* London: Croom Helm.

Welsh Assembly Government (2005) *National Service Framework for Children, Young People and Maternity Services in Wales.* Cardiff: Welsh Assembly Government.

Welsh Assembly Government (2009) *A community nursing strategy for Wales: consultation document.* Cardiff: WAG.

While AE, Dyson L (2000) Characteristics of paediatric home care provision: the two dominant models in England. *Child: Care, Health and Development* **26**(4): 263–76.

Whiting M (1985) Building a nationwide community paediatric nursing service. *Nursing Standard* **17**: 5.

Whiting M (1998) Expanding community children's nursing services. *British Journal of Community Nursing* **3**(4): 183–90.

Wilson AN (2005) *The Victorians.* London: Hutchinson.

Chapter 10

Child and adolescent mental health

Julia Terry and Alyson Davies

Overview

Children and young people's nurses provide a wide range of interventions to children, young people and their families, which include addressing issues pertaining to mental health. Emotional health is part of a child or young person's overall well-being, as neither physical nor mental health exists separately. As most children and young people with mental health problems are managed outside specialized mental health services, all staff who work with them need an understanding of how to assess and address their emotional well-being, identify problems at an early stage and liaise with appropriate services. This chapter is intended as an introduction to the topic of children and young people's mental health issues and begins with a discussion of the role of the children and young people's nurse in relation to mental health. It is widely accepted that a comprehensive, multidisciplinary approach is needed to care for children and young people when they may be at their most vulnerable. While it is recognized that children and young people's nurses often feel they have had little or inadequate training about mental health issues, with support and advice from partner agencies they are often well placed to contribute significantly to the plan of care. It is acknowledged that specialist child and adolescent mental health services (SCAMHS) teams have a limited resource, and therefore focus on serving those with the most severe mental illness. Therefore, children and young people's nurses are key players in assessing, planning, implementing and evaluating the mental health of children and young people in their care.

Introduction

This chapter will set out the risks and protective factors that impact on the mental health of children and young people. The provision of child and adolescent mental health services (CAMHS) will also be discussed, including the roles that are available to support and advise children and young people's nurses in any mental health work they undertake. Emotional literacy and its context will be alluded to as well as the importance of identifying how children and young people learn to understand and manage their feelings, and when a problem may require intervention. This will be followed by a brief discussion of three common mental health problems that they may experience – anxiety, trauma and depression – together with some case study examples. There follows a section addressing the importance of communication, boundaries, managing risk and engaging with children and young people in a therapeutic relationship. The chapter concludes by highlighting the need for increased training and education in children and young people mental health issues for children and young people's nurses and other branches of the nursing profession.

Reflection point

★ During your work as a children's nurse, think about a child or young person with a mental health problem that you have worked with:

   ☆ Did you assess their mental health?
   ☆ Did you leave it to someone else?
   ☆ Who was the person you used if you did 'refer' the child or young person?
   ☆ What were your feelings about caring for this child or young person?

Issues for children and young people's nurses

The foundations for good mental health are laid down in childhood, ensuring that children and young people have the potential to lead positive fulfilling lives and develop resilience and the ability to cope with stressful life events. Their mental health and psychological health are fundamental to their broader health and well-being, as mental health problems significantly compromise the ability to cope, leading to low self-esteem, poor body image, social isolation/exclusion and dysfunctional relationships (Department for Children, Schools and Families and Department of Health 2008; Parry-Langdon 2008; Department of Health 2009).

The incidence of mental health problems among young people, especially those who are looked after, is rising. Emotional and behavioural disorders are the most frequently occurring problems, with boys and children who experience a serious or chronic illness being significantly more at risk (Bone and Knight 2009; Department for Children, Schools and Families and Department of Health 2009). In 2004, 1.1 million children and young people less than 18 years old had a diagnosable mental health disorder that required help from specialist services; of these, 45 000 young people had a severe mental health problem (Green *et al.* 2005; Department for Children, Schools and Families and Department of Health 2009). It is suggested that one in five young people suffer with clinical depression and that the rate of self-harm and suicide among them is still alarmingly high despite initiatives to reduce the incidence (Green *et al.* 2005; World Health Organization 2005). It has been shown that those with mental health problems at age 26 had developed and were showing symptoms of their illness during their childhood and adolescence. The increase is multifactorial and symptomatic of the increasingly complex society in which children and young people live and to which they are expected to contribute (Parry-Langdon 2008; Department for Children, Schools and Families and Department of Health 2009).

Mental health issues are key targets on the health and social agenda and require serious attention by all parties involved in caring for children and young people with mental health problems, including children and young people's nurses. Children and young people with mental health problems may be encountered via routes and settings not traditionally associated with mental healthcare, and it is essential to recognize that those admitted to the acute care setting may also have underlying or accompanying mental health issues (Royal College of Nursing 2004; Department for Children, Schools and Families and Department of Health 2008, 2009). Physical illness has been strongly linked to the onset of emotional disorders, with children who experience a serious or chronic illness being twice as likely to develop an emotional disorder. Such children are a visible group for targeted mental health interventions (Vessey 1999; Immelt 2006; Fuhr and De Silva 2008; Parry-Langdon 2008). Thus, it is vital that children and young people's nurses have knowledge and insight into mental health issues in order to meet the care needs of this vulnerable group.

Perceptions of mental health, publicly and professionally, are important as they influence the care delivered. Mental health problems still carry a stigma which the child or young person will already have experienced among their peer group or in wider society and is a major concern for them (Department for Children, Schools and Families and Department of Health 2008, 2009, 2010; Jorm and Wright 2008). Stigma isolates them and compromises their self-esteem and social competence and excludes them from mainstream society (Department for Children, Schools and Families and Department of Health 2008, 2009; Jorm and Wright 2008). The attitudes of health professionals towards mental health problems determine the ability and willingness of them to seek help, and many feel belittled and denigrated by the professionals they meet at a time when they are most vulnerable and already feel stigmatized. Ironically, they may be seen by a professional who has had little experience or training in the care of those with mental health problems (Jorm and Wright 2008; Department for Children, Schools and Families and Department of Health 2009). This is regrettable for it is imperative that the child or young person and their family are treated with dignity and respect by a competent, experienced children and young people's nurse whose professional interests encompass mental health issues (Royal College of Nursing 2004; Department for Children, Schools and Families and Department of Health 2008, 2009).

However, it has been recorded that children and young people's nurses have had strong reservations about caring for children or young people with mental health problems and have a perception that this is best left to the community/liaison psychiatric nurse (Watson 2006). Some children and young people's nurses feel that they are only trained to care for those with physical healthcare needs and that their knowledge and experience in mental health issues is limited and beyond their professional remit (Watson 2006; Wilson *et al.* 2007). Children and young people's nurses cite lack of experience, confidence and evidence-based knowledge in the care of this client group, and for these reasons feel challenged, inadequate and are sometimes judgemental of their patients. As a result, they are often uncertain of what is required of them and are overwhelmed by the number and complexity of the cases they face, finding it difficult to transfer knowledge into practice (King and Turner 2000; Ramjan 2004; Watson 2006; Wilson *et al.* 2007). This situation is compounded by the slow rate of recovery in that the outcome of care may never be witnessed by the staff and the client never appears to 'get better' (King and Turner 2000; Ramjan 2004). This deficit in knowledge, skills and experience only becomes apparent when children and young people's nurses begin to work with an emotionally distressed child or young person and their families (Jones 2004; Royal College of Nursing 2004; Watson 2006; Wilson *et al.* 2007). As a consequence, it may be seen that mental health nurses should be a part of the nursing team so that they would benefit the staff and clients with their knowledge and expertise (Department for Children, Schools and Families and Department of Health 2010). However, caution must be exercised with regard to this so that such a professional does not assume, or is presumed to have, sole responsibility for the care of those with mental health problems.

The question arises as to whose job it is to care for the mental health of the child or young person. It is apparent that this is not just a mental health or children and young people's nursing issue but a need that can only be met through a wide range of services and professionals. It has to be stated that mental health is everybody's business wherever and whenever children and young people present with needs and is not just the domain of mental health professionals. No one professional has the remit for mental health – it is incumbent upon everyone to meet the needs of the child or young person presenting with mental health problems (Department for Children, Schools and Families and Department of Health 2008, 2010; Royal College of Nursing 2009). All professionals throughout the children and young people's workforce have an invaluable role to play in identifying mental health issues, promoting and maintaining positive mental health as well as providing help or access to support services (Department for Children, Schools and Families and Department of Health 2008, 2009, 2010). If children and young people's nurses claim to care holistically for their patients then mental health issues must be addressed with as much care and attention as physical health needs and without discrimination. Children and young people's nurses are in a prime position to model positive attitudes towards mental health issues, to promote the psychological and emotional well-being of children, young people and their families, to identify mental health problems and to lead by example in coordinating and planning compassionate and non-discriminatory care (Royal College of Nursing 2004, 2009; Wilson *et al.* 2007).

> **Principle for practice**
>
> The mental health of children and young people is everybody's business.

Mental health problems in children and young people

It is recognized that a comprehensive approach is required across and between agencies, in order to deliver effective mental health interventions to all young people (Health Advisory Service 1995; Department for Education and Skills 2003; Department of Health 2004). The demand on SCAMHS is exceeding capacity, with only one in 10 young people reaching this oversubscribed resource (Meltzer *et al.* 2000; Bradley *et al.* 2003), which, therefore, has had a reputation for lengthy waiting lists (Jones and Bhadrinath 1998; Terry 2003). It is therefore essential that children's nurses, and other primary care staff, are able to identify less severe mental health issues (Gale and Vostanis 2003). There is a desperate need for early intervention and recognition of these young people's needs (Lowenhoff 2004), so difficulties do not become more complex. It may be seen that such an approach will result in a reduction in the financial cost of services, as early intervention by one provider may eliminate later intervention by another, with enormous benefits for the mental health of the child or young person (National Assembly for Wales 2001).

The Audit Commission's (1999) report *Children in Mind* identified concern about young people exposed to a range of risk factors, including socioeconomic disadvantage, family breakdown, abuse and neglect, which may predict later mental health problems (Rutter 1985, 1986; Hawkins *et al.* 2000; Callaghan *et al.* 2003) (Box 10.1). Traumatic experiences in childhood affect individuals' core beliefs and are likely to compromise future chances of developing healthy and trusting relationships (Gumley and Schwannauer 2006). Findings from three national studies of the lives of people born in 1946, 1958 and 1970 highlight that mental health problems in children and young people have a significant impact on their chances of success in employment and family life, as well as contact with the criminal justice system (Sainsbury Centre for Mental Health 2009). For example, a young person who is being looked after, and by definition is somewhat separated from his or her family, is far more likely to experience a mental disorder, teenage pregnancy and involvement in crime (Royal College of Paediatrics and Child Health 2003). One of the principal aims of the youth justice system is to provide intervention that tackles family, social, educational and health factors which put the young person at risk of offending, and that helps them to develop a sense of personal responsibility (Department for Children, Schools and Families and Department of Health 2009).

Young people are particularly at risk between the ages of 16 and 18 years, so it is vital that health strategies address their needs particularly in relation to sexual health, substance misuse and accident prevention, which directly relate to their mental health (Royal College of Paediatrics and Child Health 2003). There are particular concerns about young people with mental health problems who require inpatient care and those who make the transition to adult services. In this connection, the inappropriate use of adult inpatient beds for young people is of major concern (Townley and Williams 2009). Likewise, it has been identified that there is frequently a lack of information around transition and that young people have found that adult mental health services may not see them as eligible for a service (Clutton and Thomas 2008).

The scale of the problem is significant: it is estimated that more than 40% of young people have recognizable risk factors (Green *et al.* 2005), further stressing the need for improved inter-agency working and greater clarity of each other's roles in supporting them.

There may be issues within the family setting or context that mean a child is more likely to develop mental health problems (Box 10.2). Additionally, parents who require support may have a sense of guilt and so refrain from seeking help, meaning that their child's mental health problems often increase in severity until crisis point is reached. This frequently leads to further problems, including increased rates of self-harm, alcohol and drug abuse and the long-term risk of developing adult mental health difficulties (Walker 2008). Therefore, early identification of mental health problems is essential.

Box 10.1	**Child risk factors**

- Poverty
- Family breakdown
- Single-parent family
- Parent mental ill health
- Parent criminality, alcoholism or substance abuse
- Overt parental conflict
- Lack of boundaries
- Frequent family moves/being homeless
- Overprotection
- Hostile and rejecting relationships
- Parental failure to adapt to the child's development needs
- Death and loss, including loss of friendships
- Caring for a disabled parent

(Royal College of Nursing 2009)

Box 10.2	Family risk factors

- Learning disability
- Abuse
- Domestic violence
- Prematurity or low birthweight
- Difficult temperament
- Physical illness
- Lack of boundaries

- Looked after children
- Lack of attachment to carer
- Academic failure
- Low self-esteem
- Shy, anxious or difficult temperament
- Young offenders
- Chronic illness

(Department of Health 2004)

We have already highlighted in Boxes 10.1 and 10.2 the risk factors pertaining to the child and his or her environment and how this may affect their mental health, so at this point it is also worth considering the part that brain development plays.

If there is a history of mental illness within the family, the likelihood of a child developing a mental health problem is greatly increased (Maybery *et al.* 2009). The experiences a child has during his or her early years can affect brain development, and therefore a child's mental health. From birth, children develop their abilities to express and experience emotions, as well as the capacity to manage a variety of feelings. Traditionally, motor control, cognition and communication receive a lot of attention, while emotional development may have less focus for health professionals. Certainly, families themselves may be less aware of emotional difficulties initially.

The human brain, formed before birth, continues to develop for another 20 years, constantly receiving information from the sensory nervous system to shape its connections and neuronal pathways (Blows 2003), or, to put it another way, environmental experiences mould the mind. A serious loss of any sensory system or the exposure to severe adverse stimuli can have profound and often permanent effects on the way the brain functions and perceives the world. Sensory deprivation and environmental factors, such as drugs or alcohol at key stages of development, can have a permanent detrimental influence on brain function. Child abuse, be it physical or psychological, has severe implications for brain development, usually with lifelong consequences, and may well threaten the mental capabilities of future generations (Teicher *et al.* 2002; Blows 2003). Hence, the importance of parental bonding, play and positive communication in the early years.

Principle for practice

- Child mental health problems are more likely to develop when a range of social, economic, environmental and familial risk factors are present.

Other external risk factors may impact on children and young people's mental health, such as bullying and peer rejection or peer pressure, or situations where discipline is unclear and they are not recognized as individuals (Royal College of Nursing 2009). It is important for staff working with them to have knowledge about the factors that increase the likelihood of mental health problems developing, in order to increase awareness, especially identification of children most at risk. On a more optimistic note, there are also protective factors that enable children to be more resilient and less likely to develop mental health problems (Box 10.3).

Box 10.3	Protective factors
• Intelligence	• Good parental mental health
• Being loved and feeling secure	• Activities and interests
• Living in a stable home environment	• Positive peer relationships
• Parental employment	• Emotional resilience and positive thinking
• Good parenting	• Sense of humour

(Royal College of Nursing 2009)

The provision of child and adolescent mental health services

Mental health services for children and young people first emerged in the UK in the 1920s in the form of the child guidance clinic model, with most health authorities providing a basic service by the 1940s. After the birth of the NHS, inpatient services began to develop, with medical models of care dominating. It is within the last 20 years that the role of nurses across CAMHS has begun to develop more rapidly, mainly because of changes in roles for social workers and educational psychologists, whose professional time working directly with them has been reduced (Townley and Williams 2009). This has resulted in increased opportunities for nurses, who are now the largest discipline in CAMHS, with many working across the full range of CAMHS.

Access to CAMHS should be available to all children and young people, regardless of age, gender, race, religion, sexuality, class, culture or ability (Department of Health 2007). Both practitioners and commissioners have sought a clear definition of a 'comprehensive CAMHS', which includes clarity as to how services are provided, whether they be for a child with a less severe issue or a young person requiring intensive treatment. Indeed, all staff who work with children and young people work under the CAMHS umbrella. In order to plan care effectively, service delivery and commissioning activity need to be informed by regular audit and multiagency assessment of groups of children and young people with their views sought as well as those of families and stakeholders (Department of Health 2007). This will help meet the mental health needs of children and young people in the most appropriate way.

National frameworks have been instrumental in setting out a tiered approach illustrating how and where children's mental health needs can best be met (Health Advisory Service 1995; National Assembly for Wales 2001; Welsh Assembly Government 2008), and are intended to be flexible and acknowledge the roles that many agencies contribute. This four-tiered approach is aimed at uniting service provision according to the complexity of the child or young person's mental health needs, and highlights the importance of links between the tiers of service (Townley and Williams 2009). This approach is now rooted in the philosophy of service delivery in CAMHS throughout England and Wales (Department for Children, Schools and Families and Department of Health 2008) and has been instrumental in promoting the development of a wide range of services for children and young people.

Framework for child and adolescent mental health services

- Tier 1: non-specialist services provided by professionals whose main role and training is not in mental health. This may be in primary care and the voluntary sector, in which professionals see children and young people with mild mental health issues, identifying problems and providing short-term interventions in a variety of settings (e.g. school health nurses, health visitors, children's nurses, GPs, support workers, voluntary sector staff).

- Tier 2: specialist trained mental health professionals, usually working alone, with children who have more pronounced mental health problems, and may not have responded to intervention at tier 1. Staff working in tier 2 may provide training, consultation and advice to tier 1 (e.g. school counsellors, community mental health nurses, primary mental health workers).

- Tier 3 – specialist child and adolescent mental health services: children and young people who have more severe mental health problems and disorders, which may be more complex, and who need to be seen by members of a multidisciplinary team (e.g. community mental health nurses, psychologists, psychiatrists).

- Tier 4 – very specialized child and adolescent mental health services: children who have very severe mental disorders and require intervention from a very specialist, intensive service, which may include inpatient care (e.g. psychiatrists, psychotherapists, mental health nurses).

(Royal College of Psychiatrists 2005a)

It is worth recognizing that children and young people's mental health problems can change over time, requiring different help from different levels of service. Notably, services have sometimes differentiated which service they provide to reflect the educational and training background of those involved. However, what is fundamental is that children and young people receive the most appropriate, and responsive, care for them as individuals, in the most convenient setting for them and their families.

The government's response to the independent review of CAMHS informs us of a package of support to help Children's Trusts, which will include the rollout of the £60 million Targeted Mental Health in Schools programme, and around £58 million to incorporate mental health provision alongside schools and youth centre settings (Department for Children, Schools and Families and Department of Health 2010). CAMHS commissioners will need to focus on cost-effective services that are offered as locally as possible, and will include:

- universal services, e.g. schools, children's centres and GPs, which will play a pivotal role in promotion, prevention and early detection of emotional well-being and mental health issues, bringing in other professionals as appropriate
- targeted services, which will provide additional help to particular groups such as children in care or those with learning difficulties or disabilities
- specialist services, which will meet the needs of children and young people with complex, severe or persistent problems

with each element essential to effective local provision (Department for Children, Schools and Families and Department of Health 2010).

In terms of referring children and young people to the most appropriate service, it is essential to know the remit of SCAMHS at tiers 2–4 (Box 10.4).

Box 10.4	The remit of specialist child and adolescent mental health services

- Psychosis
- Depressive disorders
- Attention deficit hyperactivity disorder (ADHD)
- Autistic spectrum disorders (ASD)
- Tourette's syndrome and complex tic disorders
- Self-harm and suicide attempts
- Eating disorders
- Obsessive–compulsive disorder (OCD)

- Phobias and anxiety disorders
- Post-traumatic stress disorder (PTSD)
- Mental health problems secondary to abusive experiences
- Mental health problems associated with physical health problems and somatoform disorders
- Behavioural challenges associated with a learning disability

(reproduced from Royal College of Psychiatrists 2006, with permission)

The delivery of CAMHS is fraught with a number of challenges, including the increasing demand on services and prioritizing who receives a service with limited available resources (Williams *et al.* 2005). In addition, there have been frequent reconfigurations of service structures, and the commissioning of CAMHS has been slow to develop.

Key point

- Child and adolescent mental health services are delivered by a range of different services, and are aimed at universal, targeted and specific groups of children.

A helpful role in guiding staff and families around the provision of CAMHS has been that of the primary mental health worker (PMHW). Staff in this role operate at the crucial interface between primary care and SCAMHS (Health Advisory Service 1995), to strengthen and enhance mental health service provision in schools and primary care (Gale and Vostanis 2003). The majority of child mental health problems may be dealt with in primary care with specialist support from PMHWs, through consultation, supervision, training, liaison and joint work to frontline professionals (Gale 2003) (see Case study below). Early identification of mental health problems and intervention may prevent deterioration and referral onto SCAMHS (Health Advisory Service 1995). The PMHW is well placed to bring both agencies, information and specialist mental health knowledge together (Dogra *et al.* 2002), to enable primary care staff to engage in more efficient assessments and to ensure that the needs of children and young people at risk of mental health problems are fully recognized (Department for Education and Skills 2003; Department of Health 2004).

Case study

Matthew is an 11 year old boy who has frequent flare-ups of eczema. He has been visited at home by Sheila, a community children's nurse. She is worried about Matthew as he has appeared down, and would not talk to her much. His mother said he had not been out to play football with his friends for the past week, and seems embarrassed about his skin being so red. Sheila showed Matthew the emollient creams, and gave him advice about looking after his skin. She felt worried by his lack of communication and apparent low self-esteem. On return to the office, she decides to telephone Jim, the PMHW, for advice.

Sheila discusses Matthew with Jim, who says Sheila is right to be concerned, and that it would be a good idea to:

- monitor Matthew's mood over the next few weeks
- suggest to Matthew that he writes down a list of activities he enjoys, and, in discussion with his family, start to engage in some of these again, such as 'Playstation' with his father, cooking with his mother and watching favourite films; these would act as a distraction from the eczema, and may help lift his mood
- suggest to Matthew that he may like to keep a diary of how he is feeling and what he has been doing; this would give Matthew and Sheila something to focus on when she visits
- contact him again if she is concerned that Matthew's emotional health is not improving.

Sheila puts this plan into place when she next visits. After 3 weeks, Matthew's eczema is much improved, and he has been smiling and talking more with Sheila and is engaged in his usual activities. Sheila, although very familiar with eczema and some of the emotional effects on children, was glad to ask a colleague for advice and suggestions regarding interventions to improve Matthew's emotional health.

Although a simple example, this serves to illustrate the importance of early intervention. The community children's nurse was assessing and monitoring Matthew's mental health and providing early intervention, which in this case prevented the situation worsening.

Emotional literacy

Emotional literacy is best defined as the ability to understand, express and manage our own emotions, and respond to the emotions of others in ways that are helpful (Weare 2004). Emotional literacy originates from Goleman's (1995) concept of emotional intelligence. This can be broken down into a combination of five characteristics: self-awareness, managing one's emotions (e.g. handling fear, anxiety, etc.), self-motivation, empathy and handling relationships (e.g. conflict) (Osborne 2004). It has been said that emotional literacy defines emotional development in educational terms (Hoyos 2005), recognizing that emotions are an integral part of cognitive development. As the importance of emotional development of children has been recognized (Liau *et al.* 2003), there has been an increase in emotional literacy programmes, particularly within school settings. Circle time and anger management groups have become common practice in many schools (Hoyos 2005), with a focus on children interpreting emotions in themselves (see the example below).

Example of good practice

'Zippy's Friends' is an international programme now running in 16 countries and is designed to help children with different abilities and backgrounds to expand their range of coping skills. The programme for 6 and 7 year olds helps children to cope with everyday difficulties, to identify and talk about their feelings and to role play ways of dealing with them, and encourages children to help others. Results have shown improved communication and conflict resolution (Bale and Mishara 2004).

Day (2004), a school nurse, noticed that, when children were asked 'how they felt about something', they did not have the language to reply. She facilitated agencies to develop classroom drama (acting to develop emotional literacy) in Sheffield primary schools. During the 10 week programme children expressed their feelings in a positive way in circle time and drama, tackling the impact of bullying and violence, discussing strategies and support, and using stories and characters to discuss feelings, without putting children on the spot. Good knowledge of emotional expression is associated with higher levels of empathy and improved social skills (Day 2004).

Likewise, the Student Assistance Programme (SAP) is an early intervention and prevention model through school-based support groups, facilitated by staff over an 8 week period (Watkins 2009). Each course can be tailored to need, e.g. exploring bereavement, divorce, parents with substance misuse issues. The SAP is designed to have a proactive impact on the entire school community, helping with problems that include physical, drug/alcohol and emotional health issues, and has shown evidence of improved grades, decreased illegal drug use, positive peer relationships and improved attendance (Love 2007). In Caerphilly in south Wales, the SAP is supported through consultation and training by the local primary mental health team. This model was developed in the USA and has now been rolled out in 30 countries worldwide.

Another initiative, 'Scratching the Surface', was developed in response to rising concern by staff working in west Wales with children and adolescents about the increasing number of incidents of self-harm. A successful proposal was made to the Welsh Assembly Government for a part-time project lead for self-harm, as many of those working in education, health and social care had received little or no training in how to respond to self-harm. A generic A5 booklet, 'Scratching the Surface' (Wadman 2007), was developed, and illustrated by CAMHS users, and has been used by a range of multiagency professionals in conjunction with training delivered by the project lead, enabling staff to respond more confidently with incidents of self-harm (self-harm is discussed in more detail in Chapter 11).

Key point

- Emotional literacy programmes can improve children's mental health, as they learn to understand and recognize their feelings and emotions, and how this affects their relationships with other people.

Children's emotional literacy can be improved by encouraging listening, talking and discussing feelings, using books, stories and pictures. Bibliotherapy is the guided use of reading with a therapeutic outcome in mind (Katz and Watt 1992), and can be as simple as reading, looking through or discussing a book with a child. There are many books available that address the issues that children encounter, including death, divorce, siblings who are ill and moving house. Promoting early discussion of these feelings can prevent problems arising later. Further training on emotional development and emotional literacy for people who work with children in all sectors would increase the likelihood of early identification of mental health problems.

Emotional and behavioural problems in children and young people

Although emotional and behavioural problems in young children can be common, it is important to consider the severity and impact of these. Problems such as anxiety, tantrums and poor sleeping patterns may emerge for many reasons, including difficulties with development as well as the parenting the child or young person receives (Thompson 2005). Emotional and behavioural problems may sometimes be mild and short-lived, with no lasting impact, and can be identified by a change in their mood, such as sadness or anger, whereas behavioural problems are usually noticed by a difference in actions, such as sleeping or eating problems. Some problems can be identified by a trigger or precipitant, such as a change or an adjustment reaction (Dogra and Leighton 2009). A child or young person may show a difference in their mood or behaviour after moving school or house, experiencing the death of a family member or pet, experiencing bullying or knowing a family member or friend is ill. Although, as set out in Box 10.5, it is possible to indicate at what point the situation may become a problem, it is not always possible to identify why this has occurred at a particular time.

Box 10.5	When is it a problem?

- When it causes a child or young person significant distress
- When symptoms have an adverse effect on social or educational functioning (i.e. relationships with family and friends are affected, and schoolwork or attending school is more problematic)
- It is important to differentiate between normal and abnormal age-appropriate behaviours and emotions, and parental expectations

(Egeland et al. 1990)

Parents may have difficulties with children who continually cry, have eating problems, have difficulty sleeping, have wetting or soiling problems or have temper tantrums. In the main, these are not considered mental health problems, unless they persist over time, in which case parents and carers are best advised to seek help through primary care or paediatric referral.

The following sections cover three common mental health problems: anxiety, trauma and depression, which may exist on their own or be the basis of a more complex mental disorder (more severe mental health issues, such as eating disorders, self-harm and suicide are discussed in Chapter 11).

Anxiety

Anxiety and fear are powerful emotions that have a strong effect on our minds and bodies (Mental Health Foundation 2009). This can be useful in emergency situations, and is often called the 'fight or flight' response, as the increase in adrenaline helps us to run away or stay and deal with the situation at hand. It is a natural response to a perceived threat, and in small doses can be useful when we are faced with non-dangerous situations, such as examinations, dates or meeting new people. Indeed, children and young people's nurses would expect a child or young person to experience some level of anxiety before an appointment or coming into hospital. Box 10.6 lists common symptoms of anxiety that children may experience.

Box 10.6	**Symptoms of anxiety in children and young people**
• Physical signs: headache, nausea, raised blood pressure, increased heart rate, vomiting, pain, diarrhoea, needing to urinate more often, poor sleep, feeling faint or dizzy, changes to breathing, sweating • Psychological signs: feeling nervous or afraid, sense of apprehension or	distress, having difficulty concentrating, hard to make decisions, feeling tired and irritable • Behavioural signs: avoiding people or situations, isolating self or becoming more clingy, constantly seeking reassurance, pacing around, not being able to settle to an activity

However, feelings of anxiety can last much longer, and commonly occur in school-aged children (see Case study below), sometimes resulting in social isolation, interpersonal difficulties and impaired school adjustment (Messer and Beidel 1994). This can lead to children becoming overwhelmed by fear and wanting to avoid situations that might make them frightened or anxious. Anxiety is at the root of a number of mental health problems, including phobias, panic attacks, generalized anxiety disorder, separation anxiety, social anxiety and obsessive–compulsive disorder. The main aim is for the child or young person to learn to cope with the anxiety so it no longer affects them and prevents them enjoying life. In terms of co-morbidity, depression is eight times more likely to be present in young people who have an anxiety disorder (Costello *et al.* 2004).

Case study

Beth is 7 years old, she has told her school health nurse that she feels sick every morning before coming to school, and has missed many days in the present school term. The school health nurse speaks with Beth's mother, who says this has been a real problem at home on school mornings; she thinks Beth is just seeking attention, but has let her stay at home quite a few times.

Reflection points

★ What could be the cause of Beth's nausea before school?

★ How would you approach this with Beth and her mother?

Parents may be unsure whether their child's behaviour is something to be concerned about or whether it is typical behaviour for a child of that age. For many years it was believed that children did not experience anxiety or depression, and that those who appeared to were just malingering or attention seeking. This has changed and it is now widely accepted that as many as 8–11% of children and adolescents suffer from anxiety that affects their ability to get on with their lives (Mental Health Foundation 1997).

A child's world can be a frightening and unpredictable place, and the same holds for young people, who experience a time of rapid physical and emotional change. Feelings of anxiety, misery and worry are common, and they can be particularly sensitive to what happens around them, sometimes feeling things that happen are their fault (such as rows or parents becoming ill). These feelings can lead to further anxiety and guilt, as not all children's emotions are logical. It is usual for small children to have fears about the dark, insects, ghosts, kidnappers and getting lost; usually children grow out of these, but they can persist as the child gets older (Mental Health Foundation 1997).

Anxious children can be irritable and demanding, and a real worry for parents. In addition to this, it often takes a lot of patience for parents to see that behind the difficult behaviour there is anxiety and uncertainty. It is common for parents to respond angrily to their children's behaviour, when what the children need is for their parents to be calm and to know exactly how they are feeling and why (Huberty 2009). If parents appear not to understand, children can feel ignored, which may exacerbate their difficult behaviour. During the period of adolescence there is much uncertainty, which can produce anxiety in both children and their families. Anxiety symptoms may include overeating or undereating, excessive sleepiness and overconcern with appearance, and some will experience phobias and panic attacks. Although the majority will experience feelings of unhappiness at times that are all part of adolescence, there will be a minority who go on to develop more serious problems (Sma'ri *et al.* 2001).

Panic can happen even when there is no immediate threat, and these are often called 'panic attacks' (Black *et al.* 2005). Panic attacks are one of the most common psychological problems in the Western world, affecting 2–3% of the population in any one year. Many people get over this with no need for treatment; when treatment is required, it is usually short and often successful (Hands on Scotland 2009). A child or young person experiencing these distressing feelings and thoughts is often not really aware why they feel so frightened. If panic attacks happen regularly they can start to interfere with normal daily activities such as school and social life. This can add to distress and lead to the child avoiding things or places that they may associate with a time when they experienced panic. This avoidance might be called agoraphobia, school phobia or social phobia, depending on which area of the child's life is affected.

Agoraphobia, as with adults, is when a child or young person fears open space, queues and public places, which may affect their school attendance. Social phobia can mean that people fear talking or eating in public or just being looked at, which can result in the young person not being able to face other people at all. School phobia is when the individual develops a powerful fear of attending school, and finds themselves unable to leave home and go to school, which highlights the question of whether the child or young person is refusing to attend school as opposed to refusing to leave home, or whether both these factors are interacting (Rethink 2009). How this problem is resolved is significant, as to whether treatment should be directed primarily towards returning the individual to school and/or resolving parent–child relationships in the home. After a significant absence from school, e.g. after a lengthy illness, it is understandable that a child or young person may fear returning to school. However, they can also develop more irrational phobias which appear to have no trigger or source. Generalized anxiety disorder is present in about 3% of children (World Federation for Mental Health 2008), who experience persistent anxieties and worries that are unrelated to any particular event or situation.

A third of adults who have obsessive–compulsive disorder find that it started when they were in childhood (Basu and Padmore 2009). Obsessions are repetitive thoughts that crowd the mind and are difficult to get rid of (even though the person knows they may make no sense). These obsessions prompt compulsive rituals such as counting, hand-washing or cleaning, which are intended to ward off such thoughts or deal with the anxieties (Adams *et al.* 1994). For instance, children may feel they have to say goodnight to their toys nine times or they might die in their sleep. While child development and learning theory often encourages parents to develop routines with children, e.g. dinner time, followed by a bath, a story, then saying goodnight, these are simply patterns of living that promote safety and security. Obsessive rituals can be unpleasant and much more distressing.

Principle for practice

- Anxiety in children that is persistent can be debilitating, and can have a profound effect on family and peer relationships, education and day-to-day functioning.

Treatment for children and young people with anxiety problems

The most important intervention when working with an anxious child or young person is to encourage them to be calm and to explain what is happening and why their body has 'gone into overdrive'. Simple explanations can help the child realize that things may feel overwhelming, but that they will soon feel better and are not alone in experiencing these symptoms. It is common for people with anxiety or panic to feel that they may faint or die, and simple deep-breathing techniques can help the child or young person regain control.

During the past two decades, much progress has been made in treating those experiencing anxiety; cognitive–behaviour therapy (CBT) has emerged as the treatment of choice (Kendall 1994), whether in individual or group format (Flannery-Schroeder and Kendall 2000). During CBT children are taught to cope with anxious feelings and thoughts, and to learn increased positive self-talk and relaxation techniques (Muris *et al.* 2009).

Children and young people who experience trauma

Children and young people experience events that are unplanned and significant, which may include traumatic experiences such as sexual, physical or emotional abuse, violent crime, suicide, assault or even natural disasters such as floods or fires as well as medical procedures. Non-fatal injuries occur in 10–30 million children each year (World Health Organization 2008), and research suggests that 14–43% of these have experienced at least one traumatic event in their lifetime that can have lasting effects on their mental health. Indeed, children and young people's nurses will encounter children and young people all the time who have experienced trauma, in the form of illness or accident, and this will have a different impact on each individual, according to their own situation.

Some children and young people may experience short-term anxieties after a trauma that improve quickly, whereas others experience long-term problems such as depression, anger, haunting memories and regressive behaviour (Armsworth and Holaday 1993). Reactions can occur immediately after the event or weeks later (International Society for Traumatic Stress Studies 2009) (Box 10.7). They may play in ways that repeat something from their traumatic experiences (e.g. hiding from an attacker or escaping from a threat) and recreate aspects of the traumatic experience in their behaviour, which can be important to help them process and think about what has happened. Children and young people may display sadness, have less emotion or feel guilty about things they did or did not do related to the traumatic experience. These thoughts may not be verbalized, and it is important that distress is identified by parents and carers.

The greater the severity of the trauma, the greater the likelihood of the child or young person developing problems. They may go on to develop post-traumatic stress disorder, and this can be screened for using the Child Trauma Screening Questionnaire (Kenardy *et al.* 2006). If close family members were extremely distressed after the trauma, this may have an impact on them. Additionally, risk increases if the event is an interpersonal trauma (caused by another person), such as rape or assault, or if the child or young person has been exposed to numerous stressful life events in the past or has a pre-existing mental health problem. For all these reasons, it is crucial to support them at this time, as set out in Box 10.8.

Box 10.7	How children and young people respond to trauma

- Young children (age 5 years and younger): may experience new fears such as separation anxiety or fear of strangers or animals. They can become more clingy, or may act like a younger child
- School-aged children (6–11 years): may get parts of the traumatic experience confused or out of order when recalling the memory. They may complain of body symptoms that have no medical cause (e.g. stomach aches). They may stare into space or startle easily

- Adolescents (12–18 years): may experience visual, auditory or bodily flashbacks of the events, have unwanted distressing thoughts or images of the events, demonstrate impulsive and aggressive behaviours, or use alcohol or drugs to try to feel better. They may feel depressed or have suicidal thoughts

(International Society for Traumatic Stress Studies 2009)

Box 10.8	Coping with trauma in children and young people

- Create a safe environment
- Provide children with reassurance and extra emotional support
- Be honest with children about what happened

- Monitor exposure to the media (if the event was publicized)
- Try to put the event into perspective

(Cardiff Council 2009)

Children and young people's nurses at some time in their career may care for a child or young person who has experienced trauma and can support both them and their family during this difficult time, as shown in the case study below.

Case study

After a road traffic accident, Clare (aged 4) was admitted to the paediatric ward after experiencing concussion and injuries to both legs. Her father was also admitted to the acute medical ward with serious injuries to his right arm. Clare's mother had asked the nursing staff for advice regarding how to talk to Clare about the accident. She had noticed that Clare was starting to play crash games with the toy cars on the ward.

Naomi, one of the children and young people's nurses, set aside time to talk with Clare's mother about this while Clare was playing with another nurse in the playroom. Naomi encouraged Clare's mother to talk about the accident, how she felt about it and what changes she had noticed in Clare. Naomi then talked with Clare's mother about how children can react after a traumatic event. Clare's mother was reassured to hear that experiencing nightmares, talking a lot about the incident and re-enacting the trauma were behaviours often necessary to help children start to come to terms with what had happened.

Naomi encouraged Clare's mother to:

- talk with Clare about what had happened in the car accident, in a way that Clare could understand
- invite Clare to play or draw what had happened if Clare wanted to
- seek support for herself as a parent, to ensure she had others to support her

- ensure Clare knew where her father was, and arrange a visit when suitable
- notice any concerns or changes in Clare's behaviour that may be present after a few weeks, and to seek further advice if she was concerned.

While it is often said that children are resilient and cope with change, traumas will occur in all families, and it can be hard to predict how children will respond to them. Children and young people's nurses need to consider the thoughts, feelings and potential anxieties of children at all times. How trauma is talked about and managed will affect the child's current and future mental health (Box 10.8). As nurses we are in a primary position to encourage family discussion, provide age-appropriate information and provide support to children and their families.

Principle for practice

- Children who have experienced trauma need to feel safe, supported and have age-appropriate information about their traumatic experience.

Depression

The majority of children and young people will feel low or blue at times, as this is a normal reaction to stressful experiences. If these feelings continue or begin to interfere with the child's day-to-day activities this can deteriorate into depression. In the early 1980s, many psychiatrists believed children did not experience depression because they lacked the emotional maturity to feel hopeless. Depression probably affects one in every 200 children under 12 years old and two or three in every 100 teenagers (Royal College of Psychiatrists 2005b). Although figures are variable for young people experiencing depression, with reports of between 4% and 20%, there is evidence that there is an increase in children and young people experiencing depression in the last three decades (Green *et al.* 2005).

A higher incidence of depression has been found in children and young people whose parents are not working or have no educational qualifications, or are in a lone-parent family (Green *et al.* 2005). While no direct causes have been found in children and young people who come from homes where families have separated, research has shown that there does appear to be a link, as the incidence of emotional problems in this group is significantly higher (Office for National Statistics 2008). This suggests that sociological factors do have an impact and link with the causes of depression (Walsh 2009). Depression occurs usually as a result of a mixture of genes and familial factors. The concept of learned hopelessness has been influential in childhood research, as a child may learn an expectation of hopelessness or helplessness within the family, leading to negative thinking and ultimately depression (Thompson and Nelson 2005). Signs and symptoms of depression are set out in Box 10.9.

Depression is still not understood clearly, but we do know that some children and young people are more at risk, particularly those who have a physical illness, have experienced abuse or come from a home where there is family breakdown or refugee status. Depression can lead to academic difficulties and social isolation, and can create relationship problems with family and friends. Depression in children is also associated with an increased risk of suicide. It has been estimated that more than

Box 10.9   What are the signs of depression?

- Having a depressed mood most of the day, nearly every day (children and young people are often irritable rather than sad)
- Having no interest in activities that used to be fun
- Losing weight, gaining weight or having a change in appetite

- Having problems sleeping or needing too much sleep
- Feeling restless or sluggish
- Being tired and having no energy
- Feeling worthless or guilty for no reason
- Having trouble concentrating or making decisions
- Thinking about death or suicide

90% of children and young people who complete suicide had a depressive illness. The risk is greatest among young men if accompanied by alcohol or substance misuse (Rethink 2009). Suicide is discussed in greater detail in Chapter 11.

What causes depression?

Depression can occur for many reasons, with events or personal experiences often acting as a trigger, such as bereavement or loss, bullying, neglect or a physical illness. Depression may also be triggered if too many changes happen in a child or young person's life too quickly. They are also more at risk if they have no one to share their worries with and lack practical support (see Box 10.10 for further risk factors). Depression seems to be linked with chemical changes in the part of the brain that controls mood. These changes prevent normal functioning of the brain and cause many of the symptoms of depression shown in Box 10.9.

Box 10.10   Risk factors for children

- Past psychosocial risk factors, such as age, gender, family discord, bullying, physical, sexual or emotional abuse
- Co-morbid disorders, including drug and alcohol use

- A history of parental depression, significant loss, multiple risks, e.g. homelessness, refugee status and living in institutions

Treatment for depression

The National Institute for Health and Clinical Excellence (2005) guidelines on depression in children and young people are a useful template in identifying the steps in treating this. The guidelines cover assessment and identifying risk, through to recognition and treating mild, moderate and severe depression. There is clear guidance as to when the child or young person should be referred on to specialist services (National Institute for Health and Clinical Excellence 2005).

For those with moderate to severe depression, as a first-line treatment, a specific psychological therapy should be offered, such as individual CBT or family therapy, for at least 3 months. Antidepressant medication should only be offered in conjunction with current psychological therapy, and monitoring arrangements must be made to observe for adverse drug reactions and to review the child's mental state (National Institute for Health and Clinical Excellence 2005) and progress.

Principle for practice

- Depression in children may arise from a number of risk factors or triggers, and requires prompt assessment and treatment.

Communication, boundaries and managing risk

Communicating with children and young people

It is important that all children and young people's nurses have the ability to talk with, and engage, children and young people and, although this may be something that you do on a daily basis, it needs careful thought and skill. Whether in a community or hospital environment, there may be certain staff who are employed to work with children and young people for a specific purpose with regards to mental health, such as play therapists or psychologists. However, we all have the ability to engage with them and need to build on these essential skills, while recognizing that there are times we need to engage services of other staff.

All children and young people's nurses engage in work with children and young people that has therapeutic value, which may be as simple as talking with them about favourite toys and hobbies, depending on their age and their health condition (Box 10.11). The ease with which we engage with each child or young person will vary enormously.

Box 10.11	Important points when engaging in therapeutic work with children and young people
• Know how to create appropriate boundaries • Consider different ways of working through the use of play and the creative arts	• Remember that therapeutic work can help children and young people make sense of current and past experiences • Contemplate how therapeutic work can add to the actual assessment • Understand that this can be a valuable part of their care

Using play media and art means the child and young person can explore their own thoughts and stories, which helps them understand their experiences and gain greater resilience.

Play media with children may include sand tray work, water, puppets, clay, books and soft toys, which can help them learn about feelings and increase their emotional literacy. In addition to talking with children and spending time with them, using play therapeutically can be one of the most important interventions in preparing children for painful or invasive procedures, as demonstrated in the example of good practice below. Play therapy provides developmentally appropriate ways to facilitate children's coping strategies when faced with the stresses of being in hospital (Goymour *et al.* 2000). There are a number of useful activities that children and young people's nurses can use to get to know children and encourage them to help explore their feelings, such as 'the feelings pie' as described by Sori and Biank (2006). For this, a child is asked to draw a circle and make six or eight sections, and then label these happy, sad, angry, proud, worried, etc., thus leaving the child or yourself space to include other relevant feelings. The child can then name, write or draw in the sections in response to, for example, 'tell me a time when you feel happy'. This leads to the child discussing a wide variety of situations and relationships within their life, is of great therapeutic value and helps to identify areas where there may be problems.

Improving communication between children and young people and hospital staff: an example of good practice

In Leicester, third-year medical students (the 'teddy doctors') work alongside children to 'look after' poorly or injured teddy bears. This play with a purpose provides a chance to reduce the fear and anxiety that children may feel on either being admitted to hospital themselves or visiting a sick relative. Each child has an appointment with the teddy doctor and, through role play, they have treatments for teddy and get a certificate and teddy gets a sticker. The doctors answer questions, as this is also a learning experience which has an impact on emotional development as fear is reduced. By familiarizing children with the hospital through fun, it helps them to clarify and demystify their worries; to know what the instruments are and how they may be used; who the staff are; and how they would help. Likewise, the scheme helps medical students to improve their communication skills with children. Such a scheme could be easily adapted across a range of settings where children and young people's nurses work.

Boundaries and managing risk

It is essential that all people working with children and young people do so in a way that is appropriate to the child or young person's age, ability, level of development and understanding. It should also be in a way that is consistent with organizational policies, practices and procedures, and within regulatory and legislative frameworks. The Nursing and Midwifery Council Code (Nursing and Midwifery Council 2008) states that nurses must make the care of people our first concern, treating them as individuals and respecting their dignity; this includes maintaining clear professional boundaries.

A child-centred approach is vital, and a values-based approach must be demonstrated in terms of equality of opportunity and inclusivity and which demonstrates respect for children, young people and their families. Core nursing values include human dignity, integrity, autonomy, altruism and social justice (Fahrenwald *et al.* 2005). It is important for us as nurses to have an awareness of our own underlying values, beliefs and principles. This can help us to identify, reflect on, review and apply personal and professional boundaries in relation to our care of children and young people.

At times you may need to set achievable goals and boundaries with or for children and young people, and it is important that they and their families understand them. For example, this may relate to behaviour that is challenging, where it is important that boundaries are consistently applied. You can act as a good role model by ensuring that your own actions and behaviour are appropriate. Children and young people need to know what behaviour is acceptable, and learn to recognize and understand their own behaviour and its consequences.

As nurses we too must know our limitations, and not overstretch ourselves. Engaging with a child or young person about emotional health can be challenging at times. However, if we keep in mind good child protection practices, we will serve to keep the child safe, observe confidentiality and liaise with other members of the multidisciplinary team, who are best placed to work with the child or young person and their family.

It is vital that children and young people's nurses are aware of those who are most at risk of harm, and those who may develop mental health problems, in order to safeguard them and plan the most appropriate care. Agreed protocols are essential in order to effectively manage the interface between CAMHS and other agencies, which will clearly set out the respective roles and responsibilities of those involved in a child or young person's care (Department of Health, Social Services and Public Safety 2008), thus strengthening joint working. In order to protect and promote their health and well-being this must also include managing risk (Nursing and Midwifery Council 2008).

Principles for practice

- Communicating and developing therapeutic relationships is the key to finding out more about children and young people's emotional well-being.
- Identifying and managing risk is fundamental for mental health practice.

In order to address the mental health needs of children and young people nurses need increased pre- and post-registration training opportunities to assist them to develop skills and expertise in this area and across all healthcare settings (Townley and Williams 2009).

The need for increased training and education about mental health issues in children and young people for all nurses

The need for robust and rigorous CAMHS education is a recurrent theme addressed in a number of policy and research documents (Department for Children, Schools and Families and Department of Health 2008; Royal College of Nursing 2009). What emerges with distinct clarity is that children and young people's nurses perceive their training and education with regard to this as inadequate and preventing them from caring effectively for children and young people with mental health problems (Jones 2004; Watson 2006). This would appear to emanate from pre-registration nursing education, resulting in a lack of confidence, evidence-based knowledge, experience and the necessary skills and abilities to deal with complex issues in order to effectively support the children, young people and their families (Jones 2004; Watson 2006; Wilson *et al.* 2007). Such research highlights the need for ongoing multidisciplinary education at all levels (Department of Health 2009; Welsh Assembly Government 2009; Department for Children, Schools and Families and Department of Health 2010). This must be addressed in pre-registration nursing programmes and the curricula should address this highly pertinent issue throughout the course for all students and not just during specialized placements (National Assembly for Wales 2001; Royal College of Nursing 2004; Department for

Children, Schools and Families and Department of Health 2008). Several educational initiatives have demonstrated the value of interdisciplinary teaching, illustrating that, where students are exposed to intensive, interactive, experiential learning about mental health issues, they develop positive attitudes (Curtis 2007; Happell *et al.* 2008; Happell 2009; Terry *et al.* 2009). Such an approach facilitates the sharing of evidence-based knowledge and experience which can be honed and developed.

It is essential that the skills and competencies of the CAMHS workforce at all levels of service provision meet the mental health needs of children and young people (Jones 2004; Department for Children, Schools and Families and Department of Health 2009; Royal College of Nursing 2009). The children and young people's nurse has a vital role in ensuring a multidisciplinary approach to care is adopted so that professional boundaries are broken down enabling practitioners to communicate effectively across all sectors (Mental Health Foundation 2006; Department for Children, Schools and Families and Department of Health 2008; Department of Health 2009; Welsh Assembly Government 2009). Professional roles, responsibilities and access to services must be transparent to the child, young person and their families. Children and young people's mental healthcare is an integral part of the role of all children's nurses across the diverse settings in which they work; it is every nurse's business (National Assembly for Wales 2001; Department for Children, Schools and Families and Department of Health 2008; Nursing and Midwifery Council 2008).

Conclusion

This chapter began by highlighting that the mental health of children and young people is everybody's business and it has been shown that even though children and young people's nurses may feel unprepared for this they may, through a collaborative approach with other agencies, contribute positively towards this. This chapter has also drawn attention to the individual, familial and environmental risk factors that may be present in children's and young people's lives and the need to have an understanding of the way CAMHS are structured to ensure that the individual child or young person and their family can access the most appropriate help. A number of interventions, such as advice from the primary mental health worker, parent support groups and emotional literacy programmes, have demonstrated that these can make a real difference to a child's mental health and that it is essential to take opportunities to promote the resilience of vulnerable children and their families.

This chapter has also discussed how anxiety, trauma and depression are common mental health problems which may require short-term support or referral on to a more specialist service. In this respect, the importance of engaging and communicating with children cannot be overstated, as this forms the basis of a therapeutic relationship, and is central to the work of the children and young people's nurse. Identifying problems at an early stage and managing risk may be viewed as safeguarding children and young people as this has the potential to prevent problems escalating. On reflection, it may be stated that all children and young people's nurses are engaged in supporting the mental health needs of children and young people in whatever setting they may practise, and how we engage with them has a great bearing on their overall emotional and mental well-being and is integral to our care and practice.

Summary of principles for practice

- Everyone who works with children and young people in whatever setting has a responsibility for their mental health. Child and adolescent mental health is everybody's business.

- Emotional literacy programmes offer a range of opportunities for children to recognize and understand their feelings and relationships, increase their self-esteem and reduce the stigma associated with mental health problems.

- Early identification of a child's or young person's mental health problem leads to early intervention and may prevent problems becoming worse for both them and their family at a later stage.

- Children and young people who experience mental health problems need to feel safe and supported and to have age-appropriate information which may help them and their families understand the situation. Professionals need to identify and manage risk effectively when working with the individual child or young person.

- The training and education of all nurses, particularly children and young people's nurses, in the mental health issues that affect children and young people is essential if the individual child or young person is to receive the compassionate and informed care they are entitled to.

References

Adams G, Waas G, March J, Smith M (1994) Obsessive compulsive disorder in children and adolescents: the role of the school psychologist in identification, assessment, and treatment. *School Psychology Quarterly* **9**(4): 274–94.

Armsworth M, Holaday M (1993) The effects of psychological trauma on children and adolescents. *Journal of Counseling & Development* **72**: 49–56.

Audit Commission (1999) *Children in mind.* London: Audit Commission.

Bale C, Mishara B (2004) Developing an international mental health promotion programme for young children. *International Journal of Mental Health Promotion* **6**(2): 12–16.

Basu R, Padmore J (2009) Mental health problems in childhood and adolescence. In: Norman I, Ryrie I (eds) *The art and science of mental health nursing,* 2nd edn. Milton Keynes: Open University Press.

Black S, Donald R, Henderson M (2005) *What is a panic attack?* See http://www.scotland.gov.uk/Resource/Doc/98780/0023930.pdf

Blows W (2003) Child brain development. *Nursing Times* **99**(17): 28–31.

Bone D, Knight D (2009) The mental health of children and young people: the EMHA role. *Community Practitioner* **82**: 27–30.

Bradley S, Kramer T, Garralda E, *et al.* (2003) Child and adolescent mental health interface with primary care services: a survey of NHS provider trusts. *Child and Adolescent Mental Health* **8**(4): 170–6.

Callaghan J, Pace F, Young B, Vostanis P (2003) Primary mental health workers within youth offending teams: a new service model. *Journal of Adolescence* **26**: 185–99.

Cardiff Council (2009) Coping with trauma in children: some practical advice. Cardiff: The Cardiff and Vale Traumatic Stress Initiative. See http://www.cardiff.gov.uk/ObjView.asp?Object_ID=5558

Clutton S, Thomas M (2008) Mental health provision for 16 and 17 year olds in Wales: policy and practice briefing. Cardiff: Barnardo's Cymru.

Costello E, Egger H, Angold A (2004) Developmental epidemiology of anxiety disorders. In: Ollendicdk T, March J (eds) *Phobic and anxiety disorders in children and adolescents: a clinician's guide to effective psychosocial and pharmacological interventions.* New York: Oxford University Press.

Curtis J (2007) Working together: a joint initiative between academics and clinicians to prepare undergraduate nursing students to work in mental health settings. *International Journal of Mental Health Nursing* **16**(4): 285–93.

Day P (2004) Classroom drama: acting for emotional literacy. *Youngminds,* p. 61.

Department for Children, Schools and Families and Department of Health (2008) *Children and young people in mind: the final report of the National CAMHS Review.* London: DCSF/DH.

Department for Children, Schools and Families and Department of Health (2009) *Healthy lives, brighter futures: the strategy for children and young people's health.* London: DCSF/DH.

Department for Children, Schools and Families and Department of Health (2010) *Keeping children and young people in mind: full government response to the CAMHS Review.* London: DCSF/DH.

Department for Education and Skills (2003) *Every child matters.* Nottingham: DfES.

Department of Health (2004) *The National Service Framework for children, young people and maternity services.* Standard 9. *The mental health and psychological well being of children and young people.* London: DH.

Department of Health (2007) *The National Service Framework for children, young people and maternity services: the mental health and psychological wellbeing of children and young people: Standard 9.* London: DH.

Department of Health (2009) *New horizons: towards a shared vision for mental health – consultation.* London: DH.

Department of Health, Social Services and Public Safety (2008) *Standards for child protection services.* London: DHSSPSNI.

Dogra N, Leighton S (2009) *Nursing in child and adolescent mental health.* Milton Keynes: Open University Press.

Dogra N, Parkin A, Gale F, Frake C (2002) *A multidisciplinary handbook of child and adolescent mental health for front-line professionals.* London: Jessica Kingsley.

Egeland B, Kalkoseke M, Gottesman N (1990) Pre-school behaviour problem: stability and factors accounting for change. *Journal of Child Psychology and Psychiatry* **31**(6): 891–909.

Fahrenwald N, Bassett S, Tschetter L, *et al.* (2005) Teaching core nursing values. *Journal of Professional Nursing* **21**: 46–51.

Flannery-Schroeder E, Kendall P (2000) Group and individual cognitive-behavioural treatments for youth with anxiety disorders: a randomized clinical trial. *Cognitive Therapy Research* **24**: 251–78.

Fuhr D, De Silva M (2008) Physical long-term health problems and mental comorbidity: evidence from Vietnam. *Archives of Diseases in Childhood* **93**: 686–9.

Gale F (2003) When tiers are not enough: the developing role of the primary child mental health worker. *Child and Adolescent Mental Health in Primary Care* **1**: 5–8.

Gale F, Vostanis P (2003) The primary mental health worker within child and adolescent mental health services. *Clinical Child Psychology and Psychiatry* **8**(2): 227–40.

Goleman D (1995) *Emotional intelligence.* New York: Bantam Books.

Goymour K, Stephenson C, Goodenough B, Boulton C (2000) Evaluating the role of play therapy in the paediatric emergency department. *Australian Emergency Nursing Journal* **3**(2): 10–12.

Green H, McGinnity A, Meltzer H, *et al.* (2005) *Mental health of children and young people in Great Britain 2004.* London: Palgrave Macmillan.

Gumley A, Schwannauer M (2006) *Staying well after psychosis: a cognitive interpersonal approach to recovery and relapse prevention.* Chichester: John Wiley.

Hands on Scotland (2009) Anxiety. See http://www.handsonscotland.co.uk/topics/anxiety/panic.html

Happell B (2009) Influencing undergraduate nursing students attitudes towards mental health nursing: acknowledging a role for theory. *Issues in Mental Health Nursing* **30**: 39–46.

Happell B, Robins A, Gough K (2008) Developing more positive attitudes towards mental health nursing in undergraduate students part 3: the impact of theory and clinical experience. *Journal of Psychiatric Mental Health Nursing* **15**(7): 527–36.

Hawkins JD, Herrenkohl TI, Farrington DP, *et al.* (2000) *Predictors of youth violence.* Washington, DC: Office of Justice Programs, Office of Juvenile Justice and Delinquency Prevention.

Health Advisory Service (1995) *Together we stand.* London: HMSO.

Hoyos C (2005) Emotional development and emotional literacy. In: Cooper M, Hooper C, Thompson M (eds) *Child and adolescent mental health: theory and practice,* pp. 21–7. London: Hodder Arnold.

Huberty T (2009) *Anxiety and anxiety disorders in children: information for parents.* See http://www.nasponline.org/resources/intonline/anxiety_huberty.pdf

Immelt S (2006) Psychological adjustment in young children with chronic medical conditions. *Journal of Pediatric Nursing* **21**(5): 362–77.

International Society for Traumatic Stress Studies (2009) *Children and trauma.* See http://www.istss.org/resources/children_and_trauma.cfm

Jones J (2004) *The post registration education and training needs of nurses working with children and young people with mental health problems in the UK.* London: Royal College of Nursing.

Jones S, Bhadrinath B (1998) GPs' views on prioritisation of child and adolescent mental health problems. *Psychiatric Bulletin* **22**: 484–6.

Jorm AF, Wright A (2008) Influences on young people's stigmatising attitudes towards peers with mental disorders: national survey of young Australians and their parents. *British Journal of Psychiatry* **192**: 144–9.

Katz G, Watt J (1992) Bibliotherapy: the use of self help books in psychiatric treatment. *Canadian Journal of Psychiatry* **37**: 1730–8.

Kenardy JA, Spence SH, Macleod AC (2006) Screening for posttraumatic stress disorder in children after accidental injury. *Pediatrics* **118**: 1002–9.

Kendall P (1994) Treating anxiety disorders in children: results of a randomized clinical trial. *Journal of Consulting Clinical Psychology* **62**: 100–10.

King SJ, Turner DS (2000) Caring for adolescent females with anorexia nervosa: registered nurses' perspective. *Journal of Advanced Nursing* **32**: 139–47.

Liau A, Liau A, Teoh G, Liau M (2003) The case for emotional literacy: the influence of emotional intelligence on problem behaviours in Malaysian secondary school students. *Journal of Moral Education* **32**: 51–66.

Love N (2007) *Open eyes, closing gaps and rising tides.* See http://www.edwardsville.merthyr.sch.uk/SAP/Untitled_1/SAP%20Presentation%20Texas.pdf

Lowenhoff C (2004) Emotional and behavioural problems in children: the benefits of training professionals in primary care to identify relationships at risk. *Work Based Learning in Primary Care* **2**: 18–25.

Maybery D, Reupert A, Patrick K (2009) Prevalence of parental mental illness in Australian families. *Psychiatric Bulletin* **33**(22): 26.

Meltzer H, Gatwood R, Goodman R, Ford T (2000) *Mental health of children and adolescents in Great Britain.* London: HMSO.

Mental Health Foundation (1997) *The anxious child: a booklet for parents.* London: MHF.

Mental Health Foundation (2006) *Truth hurts.* London: MHF.

Mental Health Foundation (2009) *What is fear and anxiety.* London: MHF. See http://www.mentalhealth.org.uk/information/mental-health-a-z/fear-and-anxiety/what-is-fear-and-anxiety/

Messer S, Beidel D (1994) Psychosocial correlates of childhood anxiety disorders. *Journal of the American Academy of Child and Adolescent Psychiatry* **33**: 974–83.

Muris P, Mayer B, den Adel M, *et al.* (2009) Predictors of change following cognitive-behavioural treatment of children with anxiety problems: a preliminary investigation on negative automatic thought and anxiety control. *Child Psychiatry Human Development* **40**: 139–51.

National Assembly for Wales (2001) *Child and adolescent mental health services: everybody's business.* Cardiff: NAW.

National Institute for Health and Clinical Excellence (2005) *Depression in children and young people: identification and management in primary, community and secondary care.* London: NICE. See http://www.nice.org.uk/nicemedia/pdf/cg028fullguideline.pdf

Nursing and Midwifery Council (2008) *The Code: standards of conduct, performance and ethics for nurses and midwives.* London: NMC.

Office for National Statistics (2008) *Childhood stress linked to emotional disorders.* See http://www.statistics.gov.uk/pdfdir/cpm1008.pdf

Osborne S (2004) Can we teach emotional literacy? *Mental Health Nursing* **24**(2): 20.

Parry-Langdon N (2008) *Three years on: survey of the emotional development and well-being of children and young people.* Newport: Office for National Statistics.

Ramjan LM (2004) Nurses and the 'therapeutic relationship': caring for adolescents with anorexia nervosa. *Journal of Advanced Nursing* **45**(5): 495–503.

Rethink (2009) *Depression in children.* See http://www.rethink.org/about_mental_illness/who_does_it_affect/children_and_mental_illness/anxiety_disorders_in.html

Royal College of Nursing (2004) *Children and young people's mental health: every nurse's business.* London: RCN. See http://tinyurl.com/d3xk3r

Royal College of Nursing (2009) *Mental health in children and young people: an RCN toolkit for nurses who are not mental health specialists.* London: RCN.

Royal College of Paediatrics and Child Health (2003) *Bridging the gaps: healthcare for adolescents.* Royal College of Psychiatrists Council Report CR114. London: RCPCH.

Royal College of Psychiatrists (2005a) *Building and sustaining specialist CAMHS: workforce, capacity and functions of tiers 2, 3 and 4 specialist child and adolescent mental health services across England, Ireland, Northern Ireland, Scotland and Wales.* London: RCP.

Royal College of Psychiatrists (2005b) *Depression in children and young people: Factsheet 34.* London: RCP.

Royal College of Psychiatrists (2006) *Building and sustaining specialist child and adolescent mental health services.* Council report CR137. London: RCP.

Rutter M (1985) Resilience in the face of adversity: protective factors and resistance to psychiatric disorders. *British Journal of Psychiatry* **147**: 598–611.

Rutter M (1986) Meyerian psychobiology, personality, development, and the role of life experiences. *Am J Psychiatry* **143**(9): 1077–87.

Sainsbury Centre for Mental Health (2009) *Childhood mental health and life chances in post-war Britain.* London: Sainsbury Centre for Mental Health.

Smari J, Petursdottir G, Portsteindottir V (2001) Social anxiety and depression in adolescents in relation to perceived competence and situational appraisal: panic attacks, phobias, and obsessive compulsive disorder (OCD). *Journal of Adolescence* **24**: 199–207.

Sori C, Biank N (2006) Counselling children and families experiencing serious illness. In: Sori C (ed.) *Engaging children in family therapy: creative approaches to integrating theory and research in clinical practice.* Abingdon: Routledge.

Teicher M, Andersen S, Polcari A, *et al.* (2002) Developmental neurobiology of childhood stress and trauma. *Psychiatric Clinics of North America* **25**(2): 397–426.

Terry J (2003) Brief intervention: a pilot initiative in a child and adolescent mental health service. *Mental Health Practice* **6**(5): 18–19.

Terry J, Maunder EZ, Bowler N, Williams D (2009) Interbranch initiative to improve children's mental health. *British Journal of Nursing* **18**(5): 282–7.

Thompson M (2005) Problems in young children. In: Cooper M, Hooper C, Thompson M (eds) *Child and adolescent mental health: theory and practice*, pp. 73–109. London: Hodder Arnold.

Thompson M, Nelson R (2005) Mood disorders. In: Cooper M, Hooper C, Thompson M (eds) *Child and adolescent mental health: theory and practice*, pp. 120–5. London: Hodder Arnold.

Townley M, Williams R (2009) Developing mental health service for children and adolescents. In: Dogra N, Leighton S (eds) *Nursing in child and adolescent mental health*, pp. 181–92. Milton Keynes: Open University Press.

Vessey JA (1999) Psychological co morbidity in children with chronic conditions. In: *RCN Mental health in children and young people: an RCN toolkit for nurses who are not mental health professionals.* London: Royal College of Nursing.

Wadman S (2007) Scratching the surface. *Mental Health Practice* **10**(8): 18–19.

Walker S (2008) The challenge of child and adolescent mental health. *British Journal of School Nursing* **3**(7): 349–52.

Walsh L (2009) *Depression care across the lifespan.* Chichester: Wiley-Blackwell.

Watkins C (2009) Student assistance program. See http://www.cherylwatkins-studentassistanceprogram.com

Watson E (2006) CAMHS liaison: supporting care in general paediatric settings. *Paediatric Nursing* **18**: 30–3.

Weare K (2004) *Developing the emotionally literate school.* London: Sage.

Welsh Assembly Government (2008) *Annual operating framework CAMHS targets 2008–2009.* Cardiff: WAG.

Welsh Assembly Government (2009) *A national action plan to reduce suicide and self harm in Wales 2009–2014.* Cardiff: WAG.

Williams R, Rawlinson S, Davies O, Barber W (2005) Demand for and use of public sector child and adolescent mental health services. In: Williams R, Kerfoot M (eds) *Child and adolescent mental health services: strategy, planning, delivery and evaluation*, pp. 445–70. Oxford: Oxford University Press.

Wilson P, Furnivall J, Barbour RS, *et al.* (2007) The work of the health visitor and school nurse with children with psychological and behavioural problems. *Journal of Advanced Nursing* **61**(4): 445–55.

World Federation for Mental Health (2008) *Understanding generalised anxiety disorder. An international mental health awareness packet.* See http://www.wfmh.org/PDF/GAD%20Body-Toc%20cx.pdf

World Health Organization (2005) *Child and adolescent injury prevention: a global call to action.* Geneva: WHO. World Health Organization (2008) Preventable injuries kill 2000 children every day. See http://www.who.int/mediacentre/news/releases/2008/pr46/en/index.html

Chapter 11

Caring for children and young people with complex mental health problems

Alyson Davies and Julia Terry

Overview

This chapter will discuss a number of complex mental health problems which the children and young people's nurse may encounter among the children and young people who attend healthcare settings. The topics include suicide, self-harm, anorexia nervosa, autistic spectrum disorders and attention deficit hyperactivity disorder. The incidence and causative and contributory factors will be discussed, highlighting the role of the children and young people's nurse within the therapeutic relationship that should occur between the nurse and patient. The discussion draws on the relevant research and policy to inform the debate and provide further reading material for practice. This chapter should be read in conjunction with Child and adolescent mental health (Chapter 10) as complex mental health problems are influenced significantly by the issues raised in this chapter. Depression, anxiety and emotional disorders are contributory factors in more complex problems. Also, the role of the children and young people's nurse and his or her knowledge and expertise are interwoven with the issues raised in this chapter, as it is often the quality of their education and skills concerning mental health issues which influences the care delivered to the patient with complex mental health problems.

Introduction

It is widely recognized that the incidence of complex mental health problems is increasing among children and young people (Department for Children, Schools and Families and Department of Health 2008, 2009; Welsh Assembly Government 2009a). It can be argued that psychological pressures on young people have increased, with high value being placed on academic achievement, personal success and material acquisition; all of these can oppress children and young people, affecting their mental health as they strive to cope with their development and fit into a modern society which can appear toxic to their well-being. Health professionals have a heightened awareness and knowledge of such issues and so diagnosis, support and interventions can be offered at an earlier stage than was done so previously. This is pertinent to the diagnosis of neurodevelopmental disorders such as autistic spectrum disorders (ASDs) and attention deficit hyperactivity disorder (ADHD), in which early diagnosis and intervention ensures that timely support is offered to the child, young person and their family. It is this early recognition and support which is a key issue for all children's nurses and those working with children and young people who have mental health problems. It is imperative that children and young people's nurses have insight and knowledge of complex mental health problems and their causative and contributory factors so that sensitive care can be delivered and the appropriate support offered to enable the child and young person to cope and develop positive mental health.

Suicide in young people

Suicide is one of the leading causes of non-natural death in young people and is a matter of national and global concern (Pearson 2008; Cheung 2009). Between 1997 and 2003 in the UK, suicide was the cause of 1722 deaths of young people in the 10–19 year age range. Of these, 1598 cases were 15–19 years old and 124 were 10–14 years old (Cheung 2009). These figures are supported by the World Health Organization (2009), which reported that, in 2007, 309 young men and 70 young women aged 15–24 years as well as 14 children aged 5–14 years committed suicide in the UK. It is suggested that the figures may be significantly higher owing to underreporting or the death being classified as misadventure or open verdict (Department for Children, Schools and Families and Department of Health 2008; Welsh Assembly Government 2009a). This is reflected across Europe, especially in the east, where rates of youth suicide are alarmingly high and it is suggested are underpinned by the rapid social, political and economic changes which have taken place (World Health Organization 2009). Young men are two to three times more at risk of completing suicide than young women. This is undoubtedly because of the fatal methods employed (Brent 2001; National Public Health Service for Wales 2008; World Health Organization 2009). Young women, however, have been found to favour alcohol and both licit and illicit drugs (Toero et al. 2001; Agritmis et al. 2004). It is suggested that teenagers remain a particularly vulnerable group who require specific attention (National Mental Health Development Unit 2009).

Several strategic documents have been published in response to public and professional concerns about the youth suicide rate. They discuss the specific issues affecting young people in their own countries. The documents outline a number of common objectives to be reviewed annually; these include reducing risk, developing research and knowledge of youth suicide and promoting well-being using targeted interventions (Department of Health 2002; Scottish Executive 2002; National Mental Health Development Unit 2009; Welsh Assembly Government 2009a). They discuss the responsibilities of the voluntary and statutory sectors and the multidisciplinary collaboration and communication which must occur in order to reach those young people who are in crisis; these include delivering early intervention, responding to crisis and managing the consequences of suicide (Welsh Assembly Government 2009a). A 10–20% reduction in suicide rates across the constituent countries of the UK by 2010–13 is proposed and is appearing to be achievable (Department of Health 2002; Scottish Executive 2002; National Mental Health Development Unit 2009; Welsh Assembly Government 2009a).

The strategies are published some years apart in areas which are diverse both culturally and demographically (Department of Health 2002; Scottish Executive 2002; National Institute for Mental Health in England 2007; Welsh Assembly Government 2009a). This would suggest that there is social and political concern that the underlying contributory factors have not been addressed in sufficient detail or with enough funding to ensure that the need to reiterate the objectives is not required (National Mental Health Development Unit 2009; Welsh Assembly Government

2009a). Conversely, it can be argued that there is an imperative to reiterate and address the specific cultural and socioeconomic issues which abide in each of the UK countries since devolved government. The policy documents focus public and professional attention onto the specific issues which affect young people in their own countries (Department of Health 2002; Scottish Executive 2002; National Mental Health Development Unit 2009; Welsh Assembly Government 2009a).

Why do young people commit suicide?

Reflection point

Make a list of reasons why a young person would contemplate suicide.

Suicide is a complex, highly individual, multifactorial event in which it is difficult to unravel a single contributory factor. There is usually an escalation of life events and other stressors which occur simultaneously, oppressing the individual whose resources to cope are compromised by deteriorating mental health. The young person feels they have no control over events and little support is available to them. It is an explosive, impulsive act (Department of Health 2002; Spender 2007; Welsh Assembly Government 2009a).

Case study

Mike is 15 years old and was diagnosed with insulin-dependent diabetes 4 months ago. He has been brought into his local Accident and Emergency Department semiconscious, with breathing difficulties. He was found by his best friend hanging from a tree in the local woods. Mike is well liked among his few close friends but has recently been picked on at school for being different. He has been called names by one group of boys. He has been unable to play rugby for several weeks because of a sore on his heel which is not healing. His blood sugar levels have not been stable over the last few months. Mike had a girlfriend but they have split up. His friend says he has been 'down' for a while about things and had given him some of his favourite CDs, DVDs and a signed photo of his favourite footballer.

Reflection points

★ What may have prompted this suicide attempt?

★ Think about the factors/issues involved in this attempt and reflect on why they would affect Mike.

Developmental issues

Adolescence is a time of rapid physical and psychological development when the capacity to problem solve and to deal with multiple problems is not sophisticated and emotions are experienced on a more heightened level, leading to stress (Coleman and Henry 1999; Bee and Boyd 2004). Thus, the adolescent may have fewer resources for resolving difficulties. These issues, coupled with significant life events, conflict within the family about behaviour/development or mental health issues, leave the young person extremely isolated, vulnerable and disenfranchised. Parents may be perceived to be controlling and blocking the developmental needs, leading to conflict, anger, aggression and increased impulsivity (Pillay and Wassenar 1997; National Mental Health Development Unit 2009; Welsh Assembly Government 2009a).

Self-esteem and social desirability are particularly important in adolescence and are reinforced through belonging to the 'correct' peer group that provides an arena to refine social skills, behaviour, values and beliefs (Bee and Boyd 2004; Miotto and Preti 2008). 'Failure' to gain entry or be accepted leads to a loss of self-esteem and distress that is often not disclosed. Miotto and Preti (2008) suggested that adolescents with high social desirability scores would be less likely to report suicidal ideation. They found in a study of Italian high school students that there is an inverse relationship between social desirability and psychological distress. High school students who were acutely distressed had low social desirability but concealed their negative feelings by appearing outwardly positive. They were unable to deal with sadness and frustration, they felt isolated, with negative self-regard which motivated a search to end the psychological pain through suicide. Self-esteem and confidence is underpinned by a sound body image. A negative or dysfunctional body image in young people can lead to self-hatred and is a predictor of suicidal ideation. At times of distress, harming oneself – the 'object' of hatred and disgust – is a feasible option to eradicate self-hatred, depression and hopelessness (Brausch and Muehlenkamp 2007).

Mental health issues

Poor mental health is a contributory factor in youth suicide. Anxiety and depression are implicated in and contribute significantly to suicidal behaviour (Ghaziuddin *et al.* 2000; Goldstein *et al.* 2005). Also having a conduct disorder and emotional problems exacerbates the distress experienced as these young people can be socially and educationally excluded, as well as becoming involved with the police (Green *et al.* 2005). Boys with a conduct disorder and alcohol misuse have a ninefold risk of suicide and girls a threefold risk of attempting suicide. Alcohol may be used to palliate the psychological distress but in fact exacerbates deteriorating mental health (Windle 2004; Green *et al.* 2005; Ilomaki *et al.* 2007).

This has implications for parents, who need to be able to respond to their children's needs; however, if their mental health is compromised, the risk of suicide increases as they may be emotionally unavailable to their children and may not observe the indicators of suicidal intent. The young person can feel they have no confidante to assist in dealing with complex emotions (Green *et al.* 2005; Fortune *et al.* 2007; Department for Children, Schools and Families and Department of Health 2010). Stanley (2005) found parents bereaved by the suicide of their children were unaware of the signals and wished they had been more accessible to their children. When the mother has a history of mood disorders, there is increased conflict, less cohesiveness and emotional expression (Green *et al.* 2005; Spender 2007). Parenting styles may also be compromised with hostility, increased criticism and a high level of negativity. This leaves the young person feeling vulnerable, isolated and unable to communicate their distress, which becomes internalized to avoid exacerbating a difficult situation at home. There is substantial evidence to suggest that suicidal behaviour is transmitted through families; thus, the young person may copy this believing it to be an appropriate means by which to deal with the distress and psychological turmoil they are experiencing (Fortune *et al.* 2007; Spender 2007; Welsh Assembly Government 2009a).

Ethnicity

Traditionally, ethnic groups within a different culture have provided a protective influence over young people, ensuring access to support and help specific to their personal and cultural needs (Hallet *et al.* 2007; Silviken and Kvernmo 2007). It is suggested that as social change occurs and prompts changes within our social structure so traditional/ethnic communities struggle to preserve their identity and heritage. The communities are expected to integrate into the dominant society. Thus, as integration occurs young people find themselves becoming distanced from their traditional ethnic groupings, leaving them feeling isolated, displaced and disenfranchised and without a focus as they try to integrate with a different culture. Traditional values, support networks, ways of living and viewing the world are eroded (Hallet *et al.* 2007; Silviken and Kvernmo 2007; Khan and Waheed 2009).

Beautrais (2000, 2001) examined youth suicide below the age of 15 years in New Zealand and found differences in rates between ethnic groups. Maori youths accounted for the highest number of suicides (57%) compared with Caucasian youths (26%). Higher rates of suicidal ideation, planning and attempts were found in the Maori and Pacific Islander youths than in Caucasian youths. Also, Pacific Islander youths had higher rates of suicide attempts than Maori youths. Silviken and Kvernmo (2007) examined the stressors on and incidence of suicide for Sami and Norwegian youths living in urban settings. The study showed that, although the rates of suicide ideation and attempts were comparable between groups, there was a difference in the risk factors. Sami youth were diverging from cultural and traditional norms; alcohol use, single-parent homes and paternal overprotection were all associated with increased suicide attempts.

Language and customs are a tangible symbol of the culture and are of immense importance. It is postulated that, when distressed, the use of their original language enables the speaker to fully express their emotions and to access support within traditional communities. Hallet *et al.* (2007) found that as aboriginal Canadian young people began to move away from their traditional groups and lost their language through integration so the rate of suicide increased. Where over half the community spoke and used their indigenous language the suicide rate was six times lower than in communities who had lost their language (13/100 000 and 96.55/100 000 respectively). Thus, without this link, young people are faced with the challenge of constructing a new identity in a modern world while witnessing the disintegration of a way of life, leaving them isolated, unsure, depressed and vulnerable.

Family structure

Increasing divorce rates and the nature of modern relationships mean that family life is now more dynamic and unpredictable. As families change so they disintegrate and reconstitute themselves, leading to a loss of roles, support networks, confidantes and friends (Ayyash-Abdo 2002). Children and young people from non-intact families reported lower levels of self-esteem, increased anxiety and loneliness, depression and suicidal ideation and attempts (Garnefski and Diekstra 1997; Tulloch *et al.* 1997). A closer analysis found that boys within step-parent families reported increased negative feelings but reported less anxiety when part of a lone-parent family. It was suggested that within the lone-parent family boys found a role as 'head' of the house, they had responsibility and a sense of contributing and being independent. This is eroded when a new partner and other children arrive. Roles and functions are realigned and the young person is expected to compromise and conform to a new regime that may corrode their sense of self and independence (Green *et al.* 2005; Parry-Langdon 2008). However, girls fared better in step-parent families, having higher levels of self-esteem. For the young girls, being in a lone-parent family was stressful as expectations to be involved in the domestic load were high, whereas being in a step-family meant they could share the burden and take on new roles from choice, develop their sense of self and gain support and confidantes by being part of a family. Emotionally they felt safe (Parry-Langdon 2008; Welsh Assembly Government 2009a).

Substance misuse

Substance misuse in young people has increased and is implicated as a risk factor in suicidal behaviour (Rowan 2001; Fortune and Hawton 2007). The young person who misuses drugs becomes integrated with their fellow users but becomes isolated and disenfranchised from mainstream society, leading to stigma and increased vulnerability. Garnefski and De Wilde (1998) examined the role of drugs as a predictor of youth suicide in the Netherlands. They found that suicidal ideation was five to seven times higher in chemically dependent youths. They found the highest rate of suicide attempts was in boys who reported hard-drug use. Where poly-drug misuse occurred, girls were 40% more likely to report suicide attempts than boys at 15%. Alcohol is strongly linked with suicidal ideation, attempts and completion. Binge drinking is certainly a specific predictor of attempted and completed suicide (Windle 2004; Ilomaki *et al.* 2007; Swahn and Bossarte 2007). What is suggested is that substance and alcohol misuse may be associated with risk factors that contribute to stressful events, leading to higher levels of depression and isolation, which results in alcohol being misused to palliate the psychological pain and turmoil experienced (Windle 2004). The substances appear to be a part of a larger more chaotic picture in which several other risk factors are implicated, with the young person unable to identify or access sources of help.

Other risk factors

- Poor school performance
- Marital discord
- Poor health
- High parental expectation
- Socioeconomic deprivation
- Unemployment
- Homelessness

- Domestic violence
- Sexuality issues
- Death of relative/close friend

(Fortune and Hawton 2007; National Mental Health Development Unit 2009; Department for Children, Schools and Families and Department of Health 2010)

PART 3

Red flag indicators

These are the cardinal signs that suicide is being contemplated and help must be provided in order to support and retrieve the young person.

Reflection points

★ Look again at the Case study on p. 286. What are the red flag indicators for Mike?

★ Reflect on why these are so important to a young person.

Red flag indicators

- History of sexual abuse
- Death of a parent
- Previous suicide in family
- Depression
- Change in appearance – poor hygiene
- Giving away cherished possessions
- Preoccupation with death
- Repeated visits to GP
- Antisocial behaviour

- Describing oneself as worthless
- Changes in school performance
- Social withdrawal
- Dramatic changes in appetite
- Impaired concentration
- Deliberate self-harm – increased frequency and severity

(Fortune and Hawton 2007; Gledhill and Hodes 2008; Welsh Assembly Government 2009a)

Protective factors

These focus on the provision of a warm, caring environment with access to emotional support, building self-esteem and developing resilience. Resilience is:

A person's capacity for adapting psychologically, emotionally and physically reasonably well and without lasting detriment to self, relationships or personal development in the face of adversity, threat or challenge.

(Williams 2007, in Welsh Assembly Government 2008a, p. 8)

Resilience is not static, but is a dynamic range of personal characteristics, experiences and relationships that provide protection in the face of stress. Thus, it is about enabling sound problem-solving, good communication skills, the ability to tolerate negative affect and frustration, skills to seek out support, development of good self-esteem and development of social skills, strong locus of control and developing supportive networks (Miotto and Preti 2008; Kerfoot 2009; Welsh Assembly Government 2009a).

Reflection point

★ Think again about the scenario in the Case study on p. 286. What measures could you suggest that would have protected Mike?

Protective factors

- Warm and caring family environment
- Self-esteem, locus of control, self-confidence, social skills
- Belonging to a faith or religious group
- Someone who will listen to them

- Realistic parental expectation
- Supportive friendships
- Ability to tolerate negative affect, frustration

(Spender 2007; Gledhill and Hodes 2008; Miotto and Preti 2008; Welsh Assembly Government 2009a)

The onus lies with the children and young people's nurse to assess the young person's development, lifestyle and exposure to risk factors, and to acquire skills in suicide prevention. It requires a multidisciplinary approach to care which demands liaison with the Child and Adolescent Mental Health Services so that a care package which transcends professional boundaries is put in place as well as providing ongoing access to support services (Department for Children, Schools and Families and Department of Health 2008, 2010; National Mental Health Development Unit 2009; Welsh Assembly Government 2009a).

Reflection points

- ★ What are your personal feelings about a young person attempting suicide?
- ★ Do your feelings influence your practice/attitudes towards patients admitted following a suicide attempt?

Principles for practice

- Suicide is a multifactorial event.
- Poor mental health and resiliency disable the ability to cope.
- The ability to cope with multiple events is compromised.
- It is an impulsive act in response to crisis.

Self-harm

Self-harm is complex multifactorial behaviour which is underpinned by profound psychological issues and is defined as:

Self poisoning or injury, irrespective of the apparent purpose of the act.

(National Institute for Health and Clinical Excellence 2004a, p. 16)

It is important to point out that, although self-harm does not always lead to suicide and those who self-harm are not always suicidal, there is a shared continuum of self-harm behaviour (Van Heeringen *et al.* 2000, cited in Webb 2002). Suicide is an impulsive, final, aggressive act that has a decreased escape potential, whereas self-harm is carried out in response to stress as a coping mechanism in order to carry on living (Mental Health Foundation 2006; Spender 2007). It is an impulsive, but not final, act with many individuals thinking about it for just minutes before acting.

Self-harm is becoming increasingly common in young people – almost a cultural norm in which self-injury and self-harm have become acceptable behaviours in order to relieve and cope with emotional pain and great sadness (Wadman 2007). However, self-harm is a major public health issue (Mental Health Foundation 2006). It affects one in 15 adolescents and is three times more prevalent among young females. It is thought to be responsible for 25 000 adolescents presenting at Accident and Emergency Departments following non-fatal self-harm, yet this may not be an accurate figure as it is estimated that only one in 10 young people who self-harm present themselves at hospital following an incident (National Institute for Health and Clinical Excellence 2004a; Fortune and Hawton 2007). Indeed, in the general population of 11–15 year olds, 6.5% of girls and 5% of boys report self-harming (Spender 2007; Gledhill and Hodes 2008). The rates of repetition are high, as 10–15% will repeat the self-harm within 2–3 months and 3.6% will die within 5 years (Fortune and Hawton 2007; Gledhill and Hodes 2008).

Reflection points

★ What do you understand by the term self-harm?

★ What do you feel/think about young people who self-harm?

Categories of self-harm

- Self-poisoning: overdose of drugs, alcohol
- Self-injury: cutting, mutilation, burning, scalding
- Self-mutilation: head-banging, pulling hair
- Suicide attempts: hanging, jumping, overdose

(National Institute for Health and Clinical Excellence 2004a; Mental Health Foundation 2006; Spender 2007; Welsh Assembly Government 2009a)

Why do young people self-harm?

The National Inquiry into self-harm (the *Truth Hurts* report; Mental Health Foundation 2006) states:

> *Self-harm is a response to profound emotional pain. It is a way of dealing with distress and of getting release from feelings of self-hatred, anger, sadness, depression. By engaging in self-harm people may alter their state of mind so that they feel better able to cope with the other pain they are feeling.*

(Mental Health Foundation 2006, p. 15)

Self-harm is characterized by depression, feelings of hopelessness and worthlessness. The pain of self-harm ends the emotional numbness, pain and dissociative feelings, transforming them into manageable physical pain (Spender 2007; Gledhill and Hodes 2008). Self-harm reflects serious, distressing personal,

Reflection point

What might cause a young person to self-harm?

emotional, behavioural and mental health problems (Evans *et al.* 2005). The young person feels guilty and will often go to great lengths to conceal their behaviour, which can lead to difficulties in accessing support. Spender (2007) suggests self-harm is an avoidant strategy indicative of an inability to solve problems and deal with frustration, anger and aggression in an externalized manner. The development of alternative coping strategies requires significant help (Evans *et al.* 2005; Spender 2007; Gledhill and Hodes 2008).

Depression and hopelessness

Feelings of hopelessness and depression are major psychological features strongly associated with self-harm. In this context, low self-esteem, poor self-concept, despair and self-blame are key emotions (Fortune and Hawton 2007; Spender 2007; Gledhill and Hodes 2008). A survey of young females found that they felt overwhelmed by a number of issues, such as bullying, teasing, exclusion, academic pressures, family problems, media portrayal of young people and peer pressure to 'be cool'. These left the girls feeling frustrated, isolated and lonely as they felt their independence and autonomy was eroded (Girlguiding UK/Mental Health Foundation 2008).

The young person who self-harms finds it difficult to handle the complex emotions they are experiencing and is uncertain where to seek help or feels guilty about what they do (National Institute for Health and Clinical Excellence 2004a; Mental Health Foundation 2006). Their problem-solving capacity is inhibited by the depression and hopelessness and dissociation they experience. It is challenging to deal with frustration, problems and life events (National Institute for Health and Clinical Excellence 2004a; Spender 2007). Thus, they become socially and emotionally isolated, and self-harm becomes the way to relieve the distress.

Life events

The incidence of self-harm increases substantially in relation to the number of life events which occur within families, e.g. marital breakdown, trouble with police, death and serious illness (Meltzer *et al.* 2001; Department for Children, Schools and Families and Department of Health 2010). The individual loses sight of their own worth and value and so avoids further emotional pain and rejection through self-harm.

The incidence and repetition of self-harm also rises in response to chronic illness or ongoing health issues (Meltzer 2001; National Institute for Health and Clinical Excellence 2004a; Mental Health Foundation 2006). Meltzer *et al.* (2001) found that those who had tried to harm or kill themselves were more likely to have a physical problem/impairment such as speech and language problems, coordination problems, epilepsy and soiling. In the 5–10 year old groups, two-thirds of the children who had tried to harm themselves had special educational needs and were visiting the GP and outpatient clinics more frequently than those children who did not self-harm. One-third of the group had been involved with specialist mental healthcare services.

In the older age group around 40% of the 11–15 year old cohort who had tried to harm themselves had special educational needs and/or a mental health problem and were at an increased risk of self-harming. This was particularly true of those with anxiety disorders, depression, conduct disorder and hyperkinetic disorder (Meltzer *et al.* 2001; Mental Health Foundation 2006; Welsh Assembly Government 2009a). Thus, anger about their situation is internalized and may only be expressed through self-harming, including neglecting to take essential prescribed treatment (Mental Health Foundation 2006; Spender 2007).

Family

The parent–child relationship is vitally important in protecting the young person from self-harm. Cohesive families with open communication are more supportive and protective of the young person (Tulloch *et al.* 1997). Young people who self-harmed were found to belong to families who were dysfunctional, experiencing some form of breakdown and in some cases were living with relatives (Tulloch *et al.* 1997; Hawton *et al.* 2002). Parental mental health and significant life events disrupt interactions and the parent's availability as a confidante, which is strongly associated with self-harm (Evans *et al.* 2005; Spender 2007).

The socioeconomic and demographic data strongly suggest that those from poorer socioeconomically deprived backgrounds are more at risk of self-harming because of poverty, which affects them economically, psychologically and socially (National Institute for Health and Clinical Excellence 2004a; Welsh Assembly Government 2009a). Consequently, the emotional climate in the house is heightened owing to anxieties and worries concerning day-to-day survival and the burden of care. Expectations of the young person may increase substantially, and materially they are disadvantaged compared with the more affluent members of their peer group. This oppresses the young person, lowering their self-esteem and resilience to cope (National Mental Health Development Unit 2009; Welsh Assembly Government 2009a). Young people who have an internal locus of control experience feelings of self-blame and worthlessness. Those with an external locus of control are less distressed by negative events and can cope in more appropriate ways (Tulloch *et al.* 1997; Meltzer *et al.* 2001; Green *et al.* 2005).

Young people who self-harmed were less likely to seek support from family, teachers or friends than their peers who did not self-harm. They concealed the self-harm, feeling that even if they spoke out their concerns and fears would be dismissed (Evans *et al.* 2005; Spender 2007). Evans *et al.* (2005) found that the adolescents in their study had fewer categories of people to talk to than their peers, and in 40% of cases no one else was aware of the self-harm. It is suggested that these adolescents may not seek help but, if help is proffered, their responses may have driven that help away (Evans *et al.* 2005).

Where parents are aware of the self-harm they may be distressed and anxious about how to provide support. Parents need advice on dealing with this complex and frightening situation (Mental Health Foundation 2006; Department for Children, Schools and Families and Department of Health 2010). If support is not forthcoming, ultimately the young person is left isolated and unsupported within the family; the young person thus seeks help externally through friends or conceals their behaviour, leading to a worsening of the issues they are experiencing (National Institute for Health and Clinical Excellence 2004a; Mental Health Foundation 2006). Roles may become blurred as the young person may feel compelled to protect their parents/ friends from further stress as their mental health and coping skills deteriorate (Mental Health Foundation 2006).

Socioeconomic and demographic factors

- Lone parent
- Single-child families (5–10 year olds)
- Families with stepchildren (11–15 year olds)
- Families with 5+ children (11–15 year olds)

- Unskilled occupation
- Unemployment
- Housing type: terraced/maisonettes
- Social sector housing

(Meltzer et al. 2001; Green et al. 2005)

Abuse

Abuse, both physical and sexual, is highly correlated with suicide and self-harm in young people (Hawton *et al.* 2002; National Institute for Health and Clinical Excellence 2004a; Mental Health Foundation 2006). Where there is frequent use of physical chastisement, the incidence of reported self-harm increases (Meltzer *et al.* 2001). It is suggested that physical abuse increases the risk of self-harm fivefold, and emotional abuse increases the risk 12-fold. Sexual abuse is a risk factor regardless of socioeconomic and demographic factors (Zoroglu *et al.* 2003; Green *et al.* 2005). Zoroglu *et al.* (2003) found that, where abuse occurred, the rate of self-mutilation increased 2.7-fold compared with those who were not abused. Dissociation was a key feature exhibited by the young people who felt disconnected from the world and emotionally numbed. The study revealed that students engaged in destructive, mutilating behaviours which enabled the psychological distress to be managed as physical pain and the student to 'reconnect' with their feelings (Solomon and Farrand 1996; Zoroglu *et al.* 2003).

Psychosocial risk factors

- Family/friends/school
- Unable to problem solve
- Bullying
- Cycles of hopelessness
- Depression
- Sexuality
- Illness

- Personal loss
- Family dysfunction
- Suicides in close friends/family member
- Substance misuse

(Fortune and Hawton 2007; National Mental Health Development Unit 2009; Welsh Assembly Government 2009a)

Reflection point

What do you say to a young person who has self-harmed?

Thus there is no one single factor which can identify which child or young person is at risk of self-harming. What is clear is that there is a complex combination and interplay of factors which predispose the individual to self-harm.

Principles for practice

- Self-harm is a multifactorial event in response to feelings of dissociation.
- Self-harm and suicide are different but have the same trajectory.
- It is a maladaptive coping mechanism to crisis events.
- It is often concealed, leading to feelings of guilt and self-disgust.

PART 3

Eating disorders: anorexia nervosa

Eating disorders are among the commonest of all psychiatric disorders and, in the case of anorexia nervosa, carry the highest mortality rate (Morris and Twaddle 2007; Royal College of Psychiatrists 2009a; Welsh Assembly Government 2009b). They are highly complex, multifaceted disorders which encompass physical, psychological and social features and are affecting young people with increasing frequency (National Institute for Health and Clinical Excellence 2004b). The most commonly known disorders are anorexia nervosa and bulimia nervosa, which can significantly affect long-term health and psychosocial functioning. The impact on the family cannot be underestimated as everyone is profoundly affected by this disorder (Honey and Halse 2006, 2007).

Anorexia nervosa literally means a 'loss of appetite'; however, this is too simplistic in describing a highly complex eating disorder with a multifaceted aetiology and with varying approaches to treatment (Finelli 2001). The World Health Organization (2007) defines anorexia nervosa as:

> *A disorder characterized by deliberate weight loss, induced and sustained by the patient … whereby … a dread of fatness and flabbiness of body contour persists as an intrusive overvalued idea, and the patients impose a low weight threshold on themselves*

Sufferers are deemed to wilfully induce starvation because of a fear of eating and gaining weight. They become obsessed with three forms of control: their eating pattern, body weight and food consumed (Ramjan 2004; National Institute for Health and Clinical Excellence 2004b). The fundamental causes remain elusive, but the behaviours are symptomatic of underlying complex and intersecting biological, psychosocial and cultural issues which have an impact on a vulnerable personality (National Institute for Health and Clinical Excellence 2004b; Royal College of Psychiatrists 2009a).

Prevalence

Anorexia nervosa commonly starts in adolescence, with the risk of onset highest at the ages of 14–18 years. It is suggested that, of those aged 15 years, one in 150 girls and one in 1000 boys are affected by anorexia nervosa. Anorexia nervosa is 8–11 times more common in females, although it has been found that 25% of boys aged 7–14 years have anorexia nervosa (Royal College of Psychiatrists 2009a). The chance of recovery is less than 50% in 10 years, 25% remain ill and the mortality rate can be up to 25% of sufferers (Morris and Twaddle 2007; Zandian et al. 2007).

It has been asserted that anorexia nervosa is becoming almost an epidemic (van't Hof and Nicolson 1996). However, Bruch (1985, cited in van't Hof and Nicolson 1996) states that the reconceptualization of anorexia nervosa as a disorder with underlying psychological issues means that it is recognized, diagnosed and treated with specialist interventions much earlier than had been the case previously. Also, perspectives have now shifted to cast a critical eye across modern society and the potential contributing factors which affect young girls and boys, e.g. the media, celebrity-oriented culture as well as academic expectation. However, it can be argued that the majority of adolescents are subjected to these factors, yet not all develop anorexia nervosa; thus, these factors are only a part of the picture, which illustrates the complexity of the disorder (Orbach 1986, cited in Surgenor *et al.* 2002; Bryant-Waugh 2006).

Case study

Jade is 15 years old and has anorexia nervosa. She has been admitted to the ward for stabilization and refeeding. Jade is part of a close-knit family who are very proud of her achievements and have high expectations for her future. Jade is doing well academically and in her hobbies. However, she has become depressed since the death of her grandmother, to whom she was close, and the loss of a close friend through a house move. She is losing interest in her work and hobbies.

Reflection points

★ Why might Jade have developed anorexia nervosa?

★ What are the potential risk factors?

Theories of anorexia nervosa

Bruch (1962) proposed a psychodynamic perspective of anorexia nervosa, identifying that control issues were central to the disorder at a familial and interpersonal level (Bruch 1973). The sufferer struggles for control, a sense of identity, competence and effectiveness. Control is exerted in response to a situation whereby the child/young person's development of autonomy is inhibited, yet, once reaching adolescence, they need and are expected to function independently at both a familial and a social level. They are, however, ill prepared to do so and experience low self-esteem, deficits in self-regulation and a sense of inadequacy. The fear of having no control is overwhelming. The control is gained through withstanding hunger; the denial of food and the resultant low weight is the proof (Bruch 1973). Bruch suggests that it is an adaptive mechanism to achieve autonomy, competence and effectiveness. Three perceptual and conceptual disturbances occur. These include body size/image, personal control, and interpretation of hunger and satiation signals (Bruch 1973).

Orbach (1978, 1986), in her seminal work, has proposed that anorexia nervosa is a flight from growth. The individual fails to master his or her biological and psychological experiences accompanying the attainment of adult weight. These require mastery and integration, which the young person cannot achieve or for which they are psychologically unprepared, and so the young person adapts by avoiding puberty, thus gaining control over their development and a sense of safety (Crisp 1997). However, in order to maintain this control over a changing self, it becomes necessary to exert control over the environment and others through 'dominating' the relationship with them.

Orbach (cited in Surgenor *et al.* 2002) locates anorexia nervosa within a gendered culture and political system. She argues that young women are subject to changes, of both a predetermined biological and culturally determined social nature, which are oppressive, leaving them with a sense of fear, powerlessness and confusion. Orbach (cited in Surgenor *et al.* 2002) argues that anorexia nervosa restores control and allows the individual to resist the 'controls' placed on them by the external world, thus enabling the self and autonomy to be reasserted.

Disturbed body image

Disturbed body image occurs when an individual has body dysmorphia. Sufferers see their emaciated body as normal or even fat. They fear being fat and view any attempt to nourish them as an attempt to 'fatten them up'. This distorted image is a cardinal feature of anorexia nervosa (National Institute for Health and Clinical Excellence 2004b) and is a cognitive distortion in which appearance stimuli are given priority and amplified. Sufferers focus on the negative aspects of their appearance that are deemed to be 'ugly' (Jansen *et al.* 2005). Great value is placed upon the ideal body image, which is transmitted via peers, the media and societal influences. The idea that appearance provides confidence, self-esteem and self-worth pervades the social environment, and becomes an overvalued ideal (Benninghoven *et al.* 2007a). Such social messages have a strong impact on young women with low levels of self-esteem and confidence, who may compare themselves unfavourably with the images they are presented with, yet feel the images are those to aspire to in order to be truly successful. There is a problem with processing self-referential information regarding body image (Benninghoven *et al.* 2007a).

Benninghoven *et al.* (2007b) postulated that distorted body image and body dissatisfaction are associated with family dysfunction in relation to control, communication and cohesion. It is suggested that a controlling family with negative communication styles, negative expression and involvement, together with discrepancies in values and norms, may be a risk factor for the development of body image problems. Thus, if the mother is dissatisfied with her body image within this heightened climate, this could then be relayed to the daughter, who would then develop similar ideas leading to an eating disorder to achieve body satisfaction. The dissatisfaction with one's emotional environment and body is mistakenly projected onto weight, which can be easily changed (Jansen *et al.* 2005; Benninghoven *et al.* 2007b).

Food perception and hunger

Inaccurate and confused perception about food is present. The young person is preoccupied with eating, food preparation and food-related activity, yet derives pleasure from refusing food and partaking in family meals. Fasting and food refusal is viewed as a means to gain control – it is empowering (Dingemans *et al.* 2006). Hunger awareness is pronounced, yet the individual does not recognize nutritional need and is, it is suggested, unable to assess the amount of food taken or to be consumed (Vinai *et al.* 2007). However, Vinai *et al.* (2007) found that their patients with anorexia nervosa did not assess food amounts differently from control subjects. Both groups were incapable of assessing food amounts accurately. Vinai *et al.* (2007) concluded that this inability to accurately assess food amounts may play a role in the multidimensional nature of the onset and maintenance of anorexia nervosa.

Personal control

The young person experiences a profound paralysing sense of effectiveness; the individual is convinced that they can only function in response to the wishes and demands of others, rather than making their own choices (Bruch 1973). Potential trigger events can be significant life events seemingly outside the control of the individual, who is overwhelmed by a number of developmental, familial, academic and social pressures (National Institute for Health and Clinical Excellence 2004b; Pike *et al.* 2008). Depression and anxiety are frequently diagnosed in young people with an eating disorder, who are more at risk of suicidal ideation, attempts and completion (Unikel *et al.* 2006; Spindler and Milos 2007; Holm-Denoma *et al.* 2008). This would suggest a spiralling into hopelessness, low self-esteem and an increasing sense of worthlessness, leading to increasing control over eating while contending with the ongoing pressures, which are perceived as threatening and eroding autonomy and a sense of self (Colton and Pistrang 2004; Holm-Denoma *et al.* 2008).

Family functioning has an impact. It is thought that a negative, conflictual relationship leads to a controlling parent, and verbal and physical abuse lead to interpersonal problems; these, when linked with other life events, have the potential to lead to eating disorders and suicidal behaviour (Unikel *et al.* 2006; Pike *et al.* 2008). Individuals with an eating disorder have recounted a disturbed father–daughter relationship, lower paternal care and empathy and overprotection (Unikel *et al.* 2006; Fernández-Aranda *et al.* 2007). Also, living in a large family with grandparents at home was related to an increase in eating disorders. Eating patterns became chaotic, with grandparents perhaps adopting authoritarian styles of eating, resulting in conflict and a heightened emotional climate around food and its consumption (Fernández-Aranda *et al.* 2007). Protective factors would appear to be open, honest communication; warm, empathetic parents; and the development of autonomy with less oppressive parental control (Unikel *et al.* 2006).

Attitudes to treatment

Attitudes towards treatment are complex. Young people reported that being with other sufferers was beneficial as they had access to understanding, support and empathy. However, although they understood the value of being an inpatient on the eating disorders unit, which in some respects provided a sense of belonging and kinship, the treatment exacerbated their loss of individuality, the arresting of their development and the rejection they perceived from their families (Colton and Pistrang 2004; Cottee-Lane *et al.* 2004; Offord *et al.* 2006). The autonomy which patients wanted was removed and they sensed they were being manipulated. Enforced treatment equalled punishment and, for some, prolonged the inevitable outcome which they wanted. Parents were placed in the invidious position of having to consent to and watch their child undergo enforced life-saving treatment, which they felt further damaged their trust and relationship with their child (Tan *et al.* 2003). Aspects of treatment served to prolong or exacerbate the symptoms and feelings underpinning the anorexia nervosa (Offord *et al.* 2006). Not all found the inpatient units a negative experience; the positive aspects meant the adolescents had contact with peers, a sense of community and the opportunity to learn from others in terms of coping (Colton and Pistrang 2004; Offord *et al.* 2006).

Family issues

Parental involvement is widely recognized as being important to the success of the treatment interventions. However, parents do need support in order to present a consistent approach to interventions and managing the disorder at home (Tan *et al.* 2003; Unikel *et al.* 2006; Benninghoven *et al.* 2007a,b). Parents said they were slow to recognize the impact of the anorexia nervosa, initially thinking the change in their daughter's eating habits was a developmental issue (Cottee-Lane *et al.* 2004). As a result, they felt guilty and angry with the GP who had failed to recognize the condition despite their concerns. Parents wanted to develop knowledge, but also tried to pinpoint the cause in order to rationalize its appearance (Cottee-Lane *et al.* 2004). They felt their child had been taken over, they had become 'devious' and life had changed profoundly for the whole family, which they described as a living nightmare. Parents needed support to cope with their own emotions, maintain their partnerships and support their children, which drained them emotionally (Cottee-Lane *et al.* 2004; Honey and Halse 2006, 2007; Honey *et al.* 2006).

The impact on the siblings was profound as they encountered the conflict, heightened emotions and disrupted routines in the household. Parents made great efforts to compensate for the disruption, struggling to maintain some normality by protecting those children from the conflict and distress as well as giving dedicated time to them. They were vigilant for similar symptoms in their well children (Cottee-Lane *et al.* 2004; Honey and Halse 2006, 2007; Honey *et al.* 2006).

The research illustrates vividly the complexity of parenting a young person who has anorexia nervosa. If, as the research and the National Institute for Health and Clinical Excellence (NICE) (2004b) guidelines postulate, parents are central to the process of recovery and support, the body of research into families and the type of support given must be extended and services provided (Department for Children, Schools and Families and Department of Health 2010). Policy documents may be eloquent in describing their vision for services, yet it is mere rhetoric if the reality is not realized. The children and young people's nurse has a pivotal role to play in developing services, liaison roles and therapeutic relationships with the patient while empowering them to take control in their initial care (National Institute for Health and Clinical Excellence 2004b; Welsh Assembly Government 2009b).

Nurse attitudes

Although anorexia nervosa is conceptualized as a mental health problem, it affects the physical health of the adolescent, who may require admission to hospital for medical care and stabilization before further interventions or treatments are carried out (Colton and Pistrang 2004; National Institute for Health and Clinical Excellence 2004b). Such an admission will bring the young person into contact with nurses who are trained in the acute care of sick children and young people – nurses who may not have a mental health background and whose experience with mental health issues is limited. King and Turner (2000) found that nurses did not like caring for young people with anorexia nervosa, believing that, over time, they challenged their core values as nurses. They found the patients challenging and found themselves making judgements and resenting their patients. Nurses felt they were in emotional turmoil, feeling angry, disheartened and inadequate. The study found that they reached a point of not being able to cope and 'turned off', distancing themselves from the patients. This is a bleak scenario that erodes the therapeutic relationship the nurse can develop with the young person to begin the process of recovery (Colton and Pistrang 2004; National Institute for Health and Clinical Excellence 2004b). Some nurses did begin to view the situation from the patient's perspective, which refreshed their attitudes and care delivery.

Ramjan (2004) also found nurses struggled to understand the situation. Their knowledge base was poor, and they struggled to understand a complex disorder. They described the care in militaristic terms as a 'battle', in which the young people fought 'tooth and claw'. The difficulty in forming a therapeutic relationship was highlighted. Nurses wanted control rather than to work in partnership, patients were labelled and emotive language was used. However, it should be borne in mind that the young person with anorexia nervosa who is admitted to an acute children's ward may be critically ill and require life-saving treatment. Thus, for staff the physical needs, care and treatment may have overwhelmed and taken precedence over considerations of psychological care. However, what emerges with distinct clarity is that the nurses had had no education or training in caring psychologically for these patients and so felt the care they delivered was compromised. Such research throws into sharp relief the need for cross-branch education in these issues and the urgent need to provide ongoing multidisciplinary education at post-registration level (National Assembly for Wales 2001; Department for Children, Schools and Families and Department of Health 2008; Department of Health 2009; Welsh Assembly Government 2009b).

Anorexia nervosa is a highly complex disorder – it is not just a refusal to eat. Many pressures have an impact on the adolescent who is vulnerable, and the role of psychological factors is paramount in the development of anorexia nervosa. The children and young people's nurse is a linchpin in coordinating and delivering compassionate care via a multidisciplinary approach.

Principles for practice

- Anorexia nervosa occurs in response to a lack of perceived control in the individual's life.
- Body image and perception is distorted, leading to body dysmorphia.
- Hunger perception is altered.
- It is multifactorial, but may be triggered in response to a traumatic event.

Neurodevelopmental disorders

Autistic spectrum disorder

Autistic spectrum disorder is the term used to describe children who have particular characteristics in common, and may have difficulties:

- understanding and using non-verbal and verbal communication
- interpreting social behaviour, which affects their ability to relate to others
- thinking and behaving flexibly.

The autistic spectrum of disorders come under the umbrella term of pervasive developmental disorders (World Health Organization 2007), with ASD first being described by Wing (1976), who defined the triad of impairments that are experienced (National Autistic Society 2008):

- *social interaction* (difficulty with social relationships, e.g. appearing aloof and indifferent to other people)
- *social communication* (difficulty with verbal and non-verbal communication, e.g. not really understanding the meaning of gestures, facial expressions or tone of voice)
- *flexibility in thinking and behaving* (difficulty in the development of play and imagination, e.g. having a limited range of imaginative activities, possibly copied and pursued rigidly and repetitively).

There has been confusion around the different diagnostic criteria and terminology that define ASDs. Autistic spectrum disorder is a complex developmental disability, which can make diagnosis difficult, but families do greatly benefit from a timely diagnosis and access to appropriate services and support. Children with ASD may be quite different from each other in terms of their abilities and their areas of strength and weakness.

There are a number of categories within the spectrum. In the 1940s, autism was first described in the USA by Kanner (1944), with Asperger's syndrome identified by the Austrian physician Hans Asperger (Frith 1991). Children of all levels of ability can have an ASD, and it can occur in conjunction with other disorders, including sensory loss, language impairment and Down's syndrome. Children with an ASD have a different perspective and experience of the world from ours. It is important to value and develop their particular interests and activities and not to focus solely on trying to change them (Mental Health Foundation 2001).

In practice, a diagnosis of an ASD might be given by a paediatrician, a psychiatrist, a speech and language therapist, a clinical or educational psychologist, or a GP. Others who see the child and family regularly, such as pre-school staff and teachers, may already have suspected that the child has an ASD and referred them for further assessment. The *National Service Framework for Children, Young People and Maternity Services* (Department of Health 2004) includes an exemplar on the care pathway for a child with autism from early childhood through to the transition phase, and serves as a template for quality care, and as a multidisciplinary training tool.

Wales was the first country in the world to develop a cross-cutting national strategic action plan for people with autism, and has put £1.8 million into driving forward its key actions (Welsh Assembly Government 2008b). The action plan aims to give all children and adults with autism every opportunity to fulfil their potential, by putting a plan in place to address the needs of all ages, involving individuals and their families and carers in the decision-making process (Welsh Assembly Government 2008b). The key actions will commence with country-wide mapping of needs and services, setting up systems to record populations with ASD to estimate the current and future demand for services, and identifying an ASD champion to work with key stakeholders to promote the plan. ASD coordination groups, which include service users and carers, will be established in each area, and there will be increased awareness training for commissioners and those working in education, leisure, careers and youth offending services. These actions will go a long way to address the omissions of the past, as care of children with ASD has been a much neglected area, with families often isolated and unsupported.

Behaviours that professionals look for in diagnosing an autistic spectrum disorder

- Delay or absence of spoken language
- Unusual uses of language (e.g. pronoun reversal – saying 'you' instead of 'I')
- Repeating others' words beyond the usual age
- Difficulties in playing with other children or sharing interest with others

- Inappropriate eye contact with others
- Unusual play activities and interests
- Failure to point with their index finger to communicate
- Resistance to changes in familiar routines

(Blamires 2006)

Supportive interventions for children with autistic spectrum disorder

- Behavioural interventions: designed to change behaviour
- Diets and supplements: based on the deliberate selection of foods and supplements
- Medical interventions: the use of prescribed drugs and other medical treatments
- Physiological interventions: based on the mechanical, physical and biochemical functions of the body

- Relationship-based interventions: seeking to encourage attachment, bonding
- Service-based interventions: including education and parental support services
- Skills-based interventions: aiming to develop, maintain or support specific skills

(National Autistic Society 2009)

In order to communicate effectively, observation is the key to the autistic child's world, and is not something that can be learned quickly, as it takes time to anticipate and interpret the meaning of the slightest gesture (Brown 2006). Considering how you approach a child is important, as it is no use demanding that they do this or that, as in most instances you will get a negative response. It is important to speak slowly, clearly and to keep language simple. Tell the child what to do ('Put your knife and fork down please'), as it is easier for a child to do something than to stop doing something (Brown 2006). Give the child time to work out what it is you have said, what it means and what you want him or her to do. Be prepared to wait, and wait a little longer, which can be very effective (Brown 2006). Further information can be obtained from the world's first national website resource for autism (Autism Cymru

2009), which provides information on autism services, treatments and therapies including an online library.

Children and young people's nurses can play a key role by problem-solving with families and negotiating healthcare, education and a range of resources to improve the life of the child and his or her family, and are ideally placed to help families access resources (Giarelli *et al.* 2005).

Principles for practice

- Children with autistic spectrum disorders have difficulties with social interaction, social communication and flexibility in thinking and behaving.
- Think carefully when you communicate with a child who has autism, speak slowly, clearly and be specific.
- Value the child's interests and activities to promote their self-esteem.

Attention deficit hyperactivity disorder

Attention deficit hyperactivity disorder is the most common behavioural disorder that starts in childhood. In the UK, ADHD affects 6% of children (Schachar 1991) whereas in the USA 3–7% are affected (Salmeron 2009). It is referred to as both a neurodevelopmental disorder and a heterogeneous behavioural syndrome that is characterized by core symptoms of inattention, hyperactivity and impulsivity (Biederman and Faraone 2005). It should not be confused with normal childhood behaviour that is excitable or boisterous. Although it was initially thought that children outgrow ADHD, it is now known that 60% of children continue to have significant symptoms as adults (Harpin 2005).

Children with attention deficit hyperactivity disorder/hyperkinetic disorder

These children

- are restless, fidgety and overactive
- continuously chatter and interrupt people
- are easily distracted and do not finish things
- are inattentive and cannot concentrate on tasks

- are impulsive, suddenly doing things without thinking first
- have difficulty waiting their turn in games, in conversation or in a queue.

(Royal College of Psychiatrists 2009b)

References to children with ADHD-type symptoms date back to the nineteenth and early twentieth century, initially with Hoffman, a German physician, who in 1865 described 'fidgety Philip' (cited in Barkley 2006) as one who 'won't sit still, wriggles, giggles, swings backwards and forwards, tilts up his chair – growing rude and wild'. This was shortly followed by others who described children with similar behaviours (Still 1902; Tredgold 1908, cited in Barkley 2006), who they said could not sit still, maintain attention or learn from consequences of their actions.

While symptoms may appear irritating, if they are ignored or left untreated, the persistent effects of ADHD can have a negative impact. Children with ADHD have an increased risk of academic failure, social isolation and involvement with deviant peer groups (Harpin 2005). Research suggests ADHD occurs as a result of a combination of environmental and genetic factors (Furman 2005) that have an impact on brain chemistry. The current theory that tries to explain ADHD implicates the frontal cortex and its importance in response inhibition, as ADHD sufferers have difficulty in suppressing impulse (Myttas 2001). Such children respond to all impulses, being unable to exclude those unnecessary for a situation. Rather than failing to pay attention, they pay attention to everything, meaning they become overwhelmed with information that they cannot process. Children then find it difficult to think about a situation, to 'put the brakes on' and think through possible consequences before they act.

Children will show different symptoms of ADHD, and may have limited control over what they do or say (as they tend to act impulsively). ADHD does not always have a negative impact upon academic ability. However, half of all children with ADHD also have a learning difficulty, such as dyslexia. ADHD may have an impact on speech, language and coordination. Children and adults with ADHD are also more likely to experience depression, anxiety and obsessive thoughts or behaviours. Children with ADHD have been shown to prompt negative parenting, which becomes reinforced in a vicious circle, as parents and children maintain each others' negative patterns of interaction, highlighting the need for parenting programmes to be a key part of treatment.

A diagnosis of ADHD may be given by a paediatrician or a psychiatrist, after a period of comprehensive assessment. There needs to be clear evidence of a significant impairment in the child's functioning in social or school settings. New developments in brain-imaging technology are assisting with diagnosis in the USA, as professionals have a clearer picture of the underlying physiology of the brain (Amen 2010). There has been much debate around the role of diet in children with ADHD, and although high-protein, low-carbohydrate diets are being discussed in the USA (Amen 1998), in the UK, the NICE guidelines simply stress the value of healthcare professionals promoting a balanced diet, good nutrition and regular exercise for children and young people with ADHD (National Institute for Health and Clinical Excellence 2009). Benefits found in omega-3 fatty acids and the elimination of artificial colouring and additives from the diet are, at the time of writing, still to be subject to large scale trials.

Managing the main symptoms of ADHD

Attention deficit hyperactivity disorder cannot be cured, but a variety of treatments are available to support the child and his or her family. Although the ethical issues associated with long-term stimulant medication use in children have been much debated (Daley 2006), there is further debate around parents' motivations for the use or non-use of such medication (Taylor *et al.* 2006). The rationale for medication is that it can improve children's concentration, but emotional and educational support are essential care components too. A treatment plan should be developed according to the individual needs of each child. Usually, a specialist will decide initial treatment, liaise with the GP and regularly review progress. Current UK guidelines recommend that everyone diagnosed with ADHD should receive information and advice about all aspects of ADHD, so informed choices about the treatment options can be made. In the USA, 60% of children receive medication for ADHD, while in Finland less than 1% are prescribed medication and fare similarly both socially and academically to peers without ADHD (Smalley *et al.* 2007).

The NICE guidelines for treatment of children with ADHD (National Institute for Health and Clinical Excellence 2009) recommend a comprehensive needs assessment, including parents'/carers' mental health, and that parents/carers are referred to a parent-training programme as first-line treatment. Drug treatment should always form part of a comprehensive treatment plan that includes psychological, behavioural and educational advice and interventions.

When working with families, it is essential to understand what parents know and believe about their child's ADHD, and, because there is no cure, parents often seek a magic intervention, rather than realizing that successful treatment involves a variety of educational, behavioural and parenting interventions (Cormier and Harrison Elder 2007). As children's self-esteem is shaped by their thinking, their expectations and their experiences of how others think and feel about them (in terms of how they are treated), ADHD can have an enormous impact. Many children with ADHD have problems in school, including relationships with teachers and peers. Children with ADHD find people often do not understand their behaviour and judge them. They may experience punishments for being disruptive, but find it easier not to bother trying to fit in, and do not engage in schoolwork. This can mean that children with ADHD feel they are a failure and have low self-esteem. Engaging with such children to find out how they feel about themselves is a vital skill.

Principles for practice

- Children with ADHD are usually restless, easily distracted, are impulsive and find concentration difficult.
- Children with ADHD are at risk of academic failure, social isolation and further mental health problems.
- Current UK guidelines recommend a comprehensive needs assessment, and a treatment plan that includes psychological, behavioural and educational advice and interventions.

Conclusion

This chapter has reviewed a number of complex mental health problems with which children and young people may present within a variety of healthcare settings. There is no one single predisposing factor which precipitates the development of these problems. It would appear that there is a complex interplay of social, psychological and biological factors/issues which contribute to the development of complex mental health problems at a time when the child or young person is vulnerable and in need of positive easily accessible support.

It is imperative that, while children and young people may be assessed for physical health problems, mental health must also be assessed and considered (Vessey 1999;

Welsh Assembly Government 2005; Immelt 2006). It is essential that truly holistic care takes place because, as has been pointed out in Chapter 10, physical health is closely linked with mental health and well-being. This chapter has sought to reiterate this point in relation to the problems reviewed. The children's nurse needs to have well-honed knowledge of the potential risk factors which may precipitate the development of suicidal thinking and behaviour, self-harm and anorexia nervosa, and can play a pivotal role in educating fellow practitioners about mental health issues. Such insight is also required with regard to ASD and ADHD, for which families require support and help to cope with problems that can often take time to diagnose and to receive the appropriate support.

Personal and professional attitudes must also be examined in relation to care delivery so that collaborative working with the mental health professionals, the multidisciplinary team and voluntary agencies can be strengthened in order to deliver high-quality care and support to the child and young person in distress.

This chapter has discussed and highlighted the research evidence underpinning care delivery as well as addressing the key issues that children and young people's nurses need to critically consider for practice when caring for children and young people with complex mental health problems.

Summary of principles for practice

- Children and young people's nurses need to value and support their patients who present with complex mental health problems so that children and young people feel their problems are being taken seriously.
- Children and young people's nurses must develop knowledge of complex mental health issues and their contributory factors to inform the care they deliver.
- Children and young people's nurses need to develop insight into their own knowledge, skills and attitudes regarding complex mental health issues through ongoing education and training in the care of children and young people with complex mental health problems.
- Children and young people's nurses are in a prime position to provide support, care, reassurance and access to helping services for children, young people and their families.
- Care needs to be collaborative and multidisciplinary in nature and all members of the multidisciplinary team need to liaise clearly with one another.

References

Agritmis H, Yaci N, Colak B, Aksoy E (2004) Suicidal deaths in childhood and adolescence. *Forensic Science International* **142**, 25–31.

Amen D (1998) *Change your brain, change your life: the breakthrough program for conquering anxiety, depression, obsessiveness, anger and impulsiveness.* New York: Three Rivers Press, 1998.

Amen D (2010) *Images of attention deficit disorder.* See http://www.amenclinics.com/brain-science/spect-image-gallery/spect-atlas/images-of-attention-deficit-disorder-addadhd/

Autism Cymru (2009) *AWARES.* See http://www.awares.org/homepage.asp?languageID=0

Ayyash-Abdo H (2002) Adolescent suicide: an ecological perspective. *Psychology in the Schools* **39**: 459–75.

Barkley R (2006) *Attention-deficit hyperactivity disorder: a handbook for diagnosis and treatment,* 3rd edn. New York: Guildford Press.

Beautrais AL (2000) Methods of youth suicide in New Zealand: trends and implications for prevention. *Australian and New Zealand Journal of Psychiatry* **34**: 413–19.

Beautrais AL (2001) Child and young adolescent suicide in New Zealand. *Australian and New Zealand Journal of Psychiatry* **35**: 647–53.

Bee H, Boyd H (2004) *The developing child*. London: Allyn and Bacon.

Benninghoven D, Raykowski L, Solzbacher S, *et al.* (2007a) Body images of patients with anorexia nervosa, bulimia nervosa and female control subjects: a comparison with male ideals of female attractiveness. *Body Image* **4**: 51–9.

Benninghoven D, Tetsch N, Kunzendorf S, Jantschek G (2007b) Body image in patients with eating disorders and their mothers, and the role of family functioning. *Comprehensive Psychiatry* **48**: 118–23.

Biederman J, Faraone S (2005) Attention-deficit hyperactivity disorder. *Lancet* **366**(9481): 237–48.

Blamires M (2006) *Autism and the autistic spectrum*. See http://www.ttrb.ac.uk/ViewArticle2.aspx?menu=11774andContentId=11811

Brausch AM, Muehlenkamp JJ (2007) Body image and suicidal ideation in adolescents. *Body Image* **4**: 207–12.

Brent DA (2001) Firearms and suicide. *Annals of the New York Academy of Sciences* **932**: 225–40.

Brown M (2006) Communicating with the child who has autistic spectrum disorder: a practical introduction. *Paediatric Nursing* **18**: 14–17.

Bruch H (1962) Perceptual and cognitive disturbances in anorexia nervosa. *Psychosomatic Medicine* **24**: 187–94.

Bruch H (1973) *Eating disorders*. London: Routledge and Kegan Paul.

Bryant-Waugh R (2006) Recent developments in anorexia nervosa. *Child and Adolescent Mental Health* **11**(2): 76–81.

Cheung AH (2009) Suicide rate in young people in the UK declined from 1997 to 2003. *Evidence-Based Mental Health* **12**: 96.

Coleman JC, Henry L (1999) *The nature of adolescence*, 3rd edn. London: Routledge.

Colton A, Pistrang N (2004) Adolescents' experiences of inpatient treatment for anorexia nervosa. *European Eating Disorders Review* **12**: 307–16.

Cormier E, Harrison Elder J (2007) Diet and child behaviour problems: fact or fiction? *Pediatric Nursing* **33**: 2.

Cottee-Lane D, Pistrang N, Bryant-Waugh R (2004) Childhood onset of anorexia nervosa. *European Eating Disorders Review* **12**: 307–16.

Crisp AH (1997) Anorexia as a flight from growth: assessment and treatment based on the model. In: Garner DM, Garfinkel PE (eds) *Handbook of treatment for eating disorders*, 2nd edn, pp. 248–77. New York: Guildford Press.

Daley D (2006) Attention deficit hyperactivity disorder: a review of the essential facts. *Child: Care, Health and Development* **32**: 193–204.

Department for Children, Schools and Families and Department of Health (2008) *Children and young people in mind: the final report of the National CAMHS Review*. London: DCSF/DH.

Department for Children, Schools and Families and Department of Health (2009) *Healthy lives, brighter futures: the strategy for children and young people's health*. London: DCSF/DH.

Department for Children, Schools and Families and Department of Health (2010) *Keeping children and young people in mind: the government's full response to the independent review of CAMHS*. London: DCSF/DH.

Department of Health (2002) *The national suicide prevention strategy for England*. London: DH.

Department of Health (2004) *The National Service Framework for Children, Young People and Maternity Services: autistic spectrum disorders*. London: DH.

Department of Health (2009) *New Horizons: towards a shared vision for mental health – consultation*. London: DH.

Dingemans A, Spinhoven P, Furth EF (2006) Maladaptive core beliefs and eating disorder symptoms. *Eating Behaviours* **7**: 258–65.

Evans E, Hawton K, Rodham K (2005) In what way are adolescents who engage in self harm or experience thoughts of self harm different in terms of help-seeking, communication and coping strategies? *Journal of Adolescence* **28**: 573–87.

Fernández-Aranda F, Krug I, Granero R, *et al.* (2007) Individual and family eating patterns during childhood and early adolescence: an analysis of associated eating disorders factors. *Appetite* **49**: 476–85.

Finelli L (2001) Revisiting the identity issue in anorexia. *Journal of Psychosocial Nursing* **39**: 23–9.

Fortune S, Hawton K (2007) Suicide and deliberate self harm in children and adolescents. *Pediatrics and Child Health* **17**: 443–7.

Fortune S, Stewart A, Vikram Y, Hawton K (2007) Suicide in adolescents: using life charts to understand the suicidal process. *Journal of Affective Disorders* **100**: 199–210.

Frith U (ed.) (1991) *Autism and Asperger syndrome*, pp. 37–92. Cambridge: Cambridge University Press.

Furman L (2005) What is attention-deficit hyperactivity disorder (ADHD)? *Journal of Child Neurology* **20**: 994–1002.

Garnefski N, De Wilde EJ (1998) Addiction risk behaviours and suicide attempts in adolescents. *Journal of Adolescence* **21**: 135–42.

Garnefski N, Diekstra RF (1997) Adolescents from one parent, stepparent and intact families: emotional problems and suicide attempts. *Journal of Adolescence* **20**(2): 201–8.

Ghaziuddin N, King CA, Naylor M, Ghaziuddin M (2000) Anxiety contributes to suicidality in depressed adolescents *Depression and Anxiety* **11**: 134–8.

Giarelli E, Souders M, Pinto-Martin, *et al.* (2005) Intervention pilot for parents of children with autistic spectrum disorder. *Pediatric Nursing* **31**(5): 389–99.

Girlguiding UK/Mental Health Foundation (2008) *A generation under stress.* London: MHF. See http://www.mentalhealth.org.uk/

Gledhill J, Hodes M (2008) Depression and suicidal behaviour in children and adolescents. *Psychiatry* **7**(8): 335–9.

Goldstein TR, Birmaher B, Axelson D, *et al.* (2005) History of suicide attempts in pediatric bipolar disorder: factors associated with increased risk. *Bipolar Disorders* **7**: 525–35.

Green H, McGinnity A, Meltzer H, *et al.* (2005) *Mental health of children and young people in Great Britain 2004 (a survey for the Office for National Statistics).* London: Palgrave Macmillan.

Hallet D, Chandler M, Lalonde C (2007) Aboriginal language knowledge and youth suicide. *Cognitive Development* **22**: 392–9.

Harpin V (2005) The effect of ADHD on the life of an individual, their family, and community from preschool to adult life. *Archives of Disease in Childhood* **90**: 12–17.

Hawton K, Rodham AK, Evans E, Weatherall R (2002) Deliberate self harm in adolescents: self report survey in schools in England. *British Medical Journal* **325**(7374): 1207–11.

Holm-Denoma JM, Witte TK, Gordon KH, *et al.* (2008) Deaths by suicide among individuals with anorexia as arbiters between competing explanations of the anorexia-suicide link. *Journal of Affective Disorders* **107**(1–3): 231–6.

Honey A, Halse C (2006) The specifics of coping: parents of daughters with anorexia nervosa. *Qualitative Health Research* **16**: 1611.

Honey A, Halse C (2007) Looking after well siblings of adolescent girls with anorexia: an important parental role. *Child: Care, Health and Development* **33**: 52–8.

Honey A, Clarke S, Halse C, *et al.* (2006) The influence of siblings on the experience of anorexia nervosa for adolescent girls. *European Eating Disorders Review* **14**: 315–22.

Ilomaki E, Rasanen P, Viilo K, Hakko H (2007) Suicidal behaviour among adolescents with conduct disorder: the role of alcohol dependence. *Psychiatry Research* **150**: 305–11.

Immelt S (2006) Psychological adjustment in young children with chronic medical conditions. *Journal of Pediatric Nursing* **21**(5): 362–77.

Jansen A, Nederkoorn C, Mulkens S (2005) Selective visual attention for ugly and beautiful body parts in eating disorders. *Behaviour Research and Therapy* **43**: 183–96.

Kanner L (1944) Early infantile autism. *The Journal of Pediatrics* **25**(3): 211–17.

Khan F, Waheed W (2009) Suicide and self harm in South Asian immigrants. *Psychiatry* **8**(7): 261–4.

Kerfoot M (2009) Managing suicidal behaviour in adolescents. *Psychiatry* **8**(7): 252–6.

King SJ, Turner DS (2000) Caring for adolescent females with anorexia nervosa: registered nurses' perspective. *Journal of Advanced Nursing* **32**: 139–47.

Meltzer H, Harrington R, Goodman R, Jenkins R (2001) *Children and adolescents who try to harm, hurt or kill themselves: a report of further analysis from the National Survey of the Mental Health of Children and Adolescents in Great Britain in 1999.* London: Office of National Statistics.

Mental Health Foundation (2001) *All about autistic spectrum disorders: a booklet for parents and carers.* London: MHF.

Mental Health Foundation (2006) *Truth hurts.* London: MHF.

Miotto P, Preti A (2008) Suicide ideation and social desirability among school aged young people. *Journal of Adolescence* **31**: 519–33.

Morris J, Twaddle S (2007) Anorexia nervosa. *British Medical Journal* **334**: 894–8.

Myttas N (2001) Understanding and recognising ADHD. *Practice Nursing* **12**(7): 278–80.

National Assembly For Wales (2001) *Everybody's business: strategy document*. Cardiff: NAW.

National Autistic Society (2008) *Diagnosis of autism spectrum disorders: a brief guide for health professionals*. See http://www.autism.org.uk/working-with/health/screening-and-diagnosis/diagnosis-of-autism-spectrum-disorders-a-guide-for-health-professionals.aspx

National Autistic Society (2009) See http://www.nas.org.uk/nas/jsp/polopoly.jsp?d=297

National Institute for Health and Clinical Excellence (2004a) *Self harm: the short term physical and psychological management and secondary prevention of self harm in primary and secondary care*. Clinical guidelines CG16. London: NICE. See http://www.nice.org.uk/nicemedia/live/10946/29424/29424.pdf

National Institute for Health and Clinical Excellence (2004b) *Eating disorders*. Clinical guidelines CG9. London: NICE. See http://guidance.nice.org.uk/CG9/Guidance/pdf/English

National Institute for Health and Clinical Excellence (2009) *Attention deficit hyperactivity disorder: diagnosis and management of ADHD in children, young people and adults*. Clinical guidelines CG72. London: NICE. See http://www.nice.org.uk/nicemedia/live/12061/42060/42060.pdf

National Institute for Mental Health in England (2007) *National suicide prevention strategy for England: annual report on progress 2006*. Leeds: NIMHE.

National Mental Health Development Unit (2009) *National suicide prevention strategy for England: annual report on progress 2008*. London: NMHDU.

National Public Health Service For Wales (2008) *Suicide in Wales: data to support implementation of the national action plan to reduce suicide and self harm in Wales*. Cardiff: NPHS.

Offord A, Turner H, Cooper M (2006) Adolescent inpatient treatment for anorexia nervosa: a qualitative study exploring young adults' retrospective views of treatment and discharge. *European Eating Disorders Review* **14**: 377–87.

Orbach S (1978) *Fat is a feminist issue*. London: Hamlyn.

Orbach S (1986) *Hunger strike: the anorectic's struggle as a metaphor for our age*. London: Faber and Faber.

Parry-Langdon N (2008) *Three years on: survey of the emotional development and well-being of children and young people*. Newport: Office for National Statistics.

Pearson G (ed.) (2008) *Why children die: a pilot study 2006*. London: Confidential Enquiry into Maternal and Child Health.

Pike KM, Hilbert A, Wilfley DE, *et al.* (2008) Toward an understanding of risk factors for anorexia nervosa: a case-control study. *Psychological Medicine* **38**: 1443–53.

Pillay AL, Wassenaar DR (1997) Recent stressors and family satisfaction in suicidal adolescents in South Africa. *Journal of Adolescence* **20**(2):155–62.

Ramjan LM (2004) Nurses and the 'therapeutic relationship': caring for adolescents with anorexia nervosa. *Journal of Advanced Nursing* **45**(5): 495–503.

Rowan AB (2001) Adolescent substance misuse and suicide. *Depression and Anxiety* **14**: 186–91.

Royal College of Psychiatrists (2009a) *Eating disorders*. London: RCP. See http://www.rcpsych.ac.uk/mentalhealthinfoforall/problems/eatingdisorders/eatingdisorders.aspx

Royal College of Psychiatrists (2009b) *Mental health and growing up: attention deficit hyperactivity disorder and hyperkinetic disorder*. London: RCP. See http://www.rcpsych.ac.uk/mentalhealthinformation/mentalhealthandgrowingup/adhdandhyperkineticdisorder.aspx

Salmeron P (2009) Childhood and adolescent attention-deficit hyperactivity disorder: diagnosis, clinical practice guidelines, and social implications. *Journal of the American Academy of Nurse Practitioners* **21**: 488–97.

Schachar R (1991) Childhood hyperactivity. *Journal of Child Psychology and Psychiatry* **132**: 155–91.

Scottish Executive (2002) *Choose life: the National Strategy and Action Plan to Prevent Suicide in Scotland*. Edinburgh: Scottish Executive. See http://www.scotland.gov.uk/Publications/2006/09/06094657/6

Silviken A, Kvernmo S (2007) Suicide attempts among indigenous Sami adolescents and majority peers in Arctic Norway: prevalence and associated risk factors. *Journal of Adolescence* **30**(4): 613–26.

Smalley S, McGough J, Moilanen I, *et al.* (2007) Prevalence and psychiatric comorbidity of attention-deficit/hyperactivity disorder in an adolescent Finnish population. *Journal of the American Academy of Child and Adolescent Psychiatry* **46**: 1575–83.

Solomon Y, Farrand J (1996) Why don't you do it properly? Young women who self injure. *Journal of Adolescence* **19**: 111–19.

Spender Q (2007) Assessment of adolescent self harm. *Pediatrics and Child Health* **17**(11): 448–53.

Spindler A, Milos G (2007) Links between eating disorder symptom severity and psychiatric comorbidity. *Eating Behaviors* **8**: 364–73.

Stanley N (2005) Parents' perspectives on young suicide. *Children and Society* **19**: 304–15.

Still GF (1902) Some abnormal psychical conditions in children. *Lancet* **1**: 1008–12, 1077–82, 1163–8.

Surgenor LJ, Horn J, Plumridge EW, Hudson SM (2002) Anorexia nervosa and psychological control: a reexamination of selected theoretical accounts. *European Eating Disorders Review* **10**: 85–101.

Swahn MH, Bossarte RM (2007) Gender, early alcohol use and suicide ideation and attempts: findings from the 2005 Youth Risk Behaviour Survey. *Journal of Adolescent Health* **41**: 175–81.

Tan JO, Hope T, Stewart A, Fitzpatrick R (2003) Control and compulsory treatment in anorexia nervosa: the views of patients and parents. *International Journal of Law and Psychiatry* **26**: 627–645.

Taylor M, O'Donoghue T, Houghton S (2006) To medicate or not to medicate? The decision-making process of Western Australian parents following their child's diagnosis with an attention deficit hyperactivity disorder. *International Journal of Disability, Development and Education* **53**: 111–28.

Toero K, Nagy A, Sawaguchi T, *et al.* (2001) Characteristics of suicide among children and adolescents in Budapest. *Pediatrics International* **43**: 368–71.

Tulloch AL, Blizzard L, Pinkus Z (1997) Adolescent-parent communication in self harm. *Journal of Adolescent Health* **21**: 267–75.

Unikel C, Gomez-Peresmitre G, Gonzalez-Forteza C (2006) Suicidal behaviour, risky eating behaviours and psychosocial correlates in Mexican female students. *European Eating Disorders Review* **14**: 414–21.

van't Hof SE, Nicolson M (1996) The rise and fall of a fact: the increase in anorexia nervosa. *Sociology of Health and Illness* **18**(5): 581–608.

Vessey JA (1999) Psychological comorbidity in children with chronic conditions. In: *Mental health in children and young people: an RCN toolkit for nurses who are not mental health professionals.* London: RCN.

Vinai P, Cardetti S, Ferrato N, *et al.* (2007) Visual evaluation of food amount in patients affected by anorexia nervosa. *Eating Behaviours* **8**: 291–5.

Wadman S (2007) Scratching the surface. *Mental Health Practice* **10**(8): 18–19.

Webb L (2002) Deliberate self harm in adolescence: a systematic review of psychological and psychosocial factors. *Journal of Advanced Nursing* **38**(3): 235–44.

Welsh Assembly Government (2005) *The National Service Framework for children, young people and maternity services in Wales.* Cardiff: WAG.

Welsh Assembly Government (2008a) *A National Action Plan to reduce suicide and self harm in Wales 2008–2013: consultation document.* Cardiff: WAG.

Welsh Assembly Government (2008b) *The Autistic Spectrum Disorder (ASD) Strategic Action Plan for Wales.* Cardiff: WAG.

Welsh Assembly Government (2009a) *A National Action Plan to reduce suicide and self harm in Wales 2009–2014.* Cardiff: WAG.

Welsh Assembly Government (2009b) *Eating disorders: a framework for Wales.* Cardiff: WAG.

Windle M (2004) Suicidal behaviours and alcohol use among adolescents: a developmental psychopathology perspective. *Alcoholism: Clinical and Experimental Research* **28**(5): 29s–37s.

Wing L (1976) Diagnosis, clinical description and prognosis. In: Wing L (ed.) *Early childhood autism*, pp. 15–48. Oxford: Pergamon.

World Health Organization (2007) *International Statistical Classification of Diseases and Related Health Problems,* 10th edn, vol. 2. Geneva: WHO. See http://apps.who.int/classifications/apps/icd/icd10online/

World Health Organization (2009) *Suicide rates: country reports and charts.* Geneva: WHO. See http://www.who.int/mental_health/prevention/suicide/country_reports/en/index.html

Zandian M, Ioakimidis I, Bergh C, Sodersten P (2007) Cause and treatment of anorexia nervosa. *Physiology and Behaviour* **92**: 283–90.

Zoroglu SS, Tuzun U, Sar V, *et al.* (2003) Suicide attempt and self mutilation among Turkish high school students in relation with abuse, neglect and dissociation. *Psychiatry and Clinical Neurosciences* **57**: 119–26.

Chapter 12

Transitional care for children and young people with life-threatening or life-limiting conditions

Katrina McNamara-Goodger

Overview

This chapter will cover the need for nurses to work with young people who have a life-threatening or life-limiting condition and their families; to develop an integrated person-centred approach; to guide and support young people, their families and professionals through the transition maze; and to help services to better support young people to adjust to, prepare for, and move on to adult services.

Introduction

An increasing number of young people live with a life-threatening or life-limiting condition, and many know that they will face a premature death during their teenage years or early adulthood. These young people have a wide range of conditions, some congenital or genetic and apparent from a young age, others developed later in childhood or adolescence. Their journey through adolescence into adulthood is compounded by facing a complex and often bewildering transition from children's palliative care to adult services. Young people with palliative care needs should be recognized as a distinct care group as they have physical, psychological and developmental needs that are significantly different from those experienced by children and adults.

The person-centred approach aims to ensure that young people, their families and carers experience a coordinated approach to person-centred care throughout their care journey. It requires clear and open communication and support to enable the young person to build up and maintain access to an appropriate network of support, wherever they are cared for – whether that is in their own home, in their family home or in alternative residential placements such as supported or communal housing or educational settings. Services for young people with palliative care needs should be multidisciplinary and multiagency and should provide a flexible approach to service and care provision, recognizing individual needs. This chapter will explore the complex and challenging issues in relation to this and, in doing so, demonstrate how use of an integrated care pathway (ICP) can promote a smooth and effective transition for young people.

Working with young people

Those involved in the care of young people often find themselves working within an organizationally led, arbitrarily set, chronological, restrictive definition set somewhere between adolescence and adulthood. Although adolescence is described as a recognizable phase of life and it has a wide range of definitions, some recognizing chronological descriptions, or phases, of adolescence, ranging from 10 to 24 years, most reflect an understanding that adolescence is essentially 'a stage, not an age' – a developmental stage described by the time period between the beginning of puberty and adulthood, which also enables a recognition that adolescence is a period of development unique to the individual rather than a specific age.

At the beginning of adolescence, the parents of young people are generally still mainly responsible for all aspects of the young person's care, but, by the end of adolescence, care issues will be mainly the responsibility of the young person, although there will probably still be involvement of parents/carers in that care. Other parents, for example those of young people with conditions such as severe cerebral palsy or severe developmental delay, will recognize that their child will never attain full independence, although the young person may choose to seek other care from paid carers to promote as much independence as possible and sometimes in recognition of the impact that caring for them has on their parents.

Work with this broadly defined age group requires an understanding of physical, emotional, social and cognitive development and a recognition that development continues in all or some of these areas for all young people, despite the impact of a life-threatening or life-limiting condition. During adolescence there are a number of developmental phases which lead to young people forming an understanding of their personal identity and value system and accepting a new body image, along with the development of skills and abilities and taking responsibility for their own behaviour. For young people with life-threatening or life-limiting conditions, adolescence may also bring concerns about physical appearance and mobility and a reliance on parents and others in relation to decision-making, which delays the development of independence, and there may also be limited opportunities for social interaction with peers or a sense of lack of acceptance or fear of rejection by peers. Young people may experience discrimination in employment or education opportunities and planning for the future has to begin much sooner to deal with the complexity of plans; at the same time, there is the threat of their condition changing or deteriorating and adversely affecting the plans, combined with the possibility of dying.

> ## Key point 🔑
>
> A life-limiting or life-threatening diagnosis adds complexity to a normal stage of development.

Young people's palliative care

Palliative care for young people with life-limiting conditions is described by ACT (the Association for Children's Palliative Care) as being an active and total approach to care, from the point of diagnosis or recognition, throughout the child's life, to death and beyond. It embraces physical, emotional, social and spiritual elements and focuses on the enhancement of quality of life for the child/young person and support for the family. It includes the management of distressing symptoms, provision of short breaks and care through death and bereavement (ACT 2009).

Care is provided for young people for whom curative treatment is no longer the main focus of care and, therefore, the care may extend over a relatively short period, for example for a young person who has a sudden traumatic episode for which no curative option is available, or may extend over many years, such as for those with Duchenne muscular dystrophy. The common factor to be reflected in their care is that they are expected to die prematurely, and plans have to be made to meet their individual and family needs.

Life-limiting or life-shortening conditions are those for which there is no reasonable hope of cure and from which children or young people will die. Some conditions cause progressive deterioration, rendering the child or young person increasingly dependent on parents and carers. Life-threatening conditions are those for which curative treatment may be feasible but that can fail, such as cancer (ACT 2009). In all cases, the degree of threat to life will be a significant factor.

Young people's palliative care has a number of similarities to children's palliative care and benefits from the core values of all services to children, including openness, honesty, respect and working in partnership with children, young people and families. It also has similarities to the palliative care of adults, such as self-help and support; user involvement; information giving; and social and spiritual support; as well as its own unique aspects of care with a focus on the impact of life-threatening or life-limiting conditions on young people's lives and how professionals deal with this.

Young people's palliative care is often provided by a variety of service providers from health, social care and education as well as from across the statutory, private and voluntary sectors (Price and McNeilly 2009).

Active palliative care approaches to support children, young people and families to lead as normal lives as possible include:

- symptom management
- partnership between the young person and family and professionals, to identify and meet the young person's needs in an individualized and flexible way
- listening to and responding to young people and their families
- services which are integrated and reflect the longer term continuing care pathway required by an increasing number of young people
- delivering care where the young person and family want it to be, e.g. in the home, hospital or hospice, school or education/employment setting
- psychological and social support, including formal counselling and therapy
- attention to cultural, spiritual and practical needs
- multiprofessional and multiagency teamwork and partnership
- supporting young people and their families and education professionals to enable children to continue to access education
- easy access to services and information; some minority groups may need extra assistance to enable this to happen, including translation services
- services appropriate to the age and development of the young person
- good communication
- provision or advice on childcare and travel assistance.

> **Principle for practice**
>
> Palliative care is an active, holistic approach to care, not simply a care process.

Defining transition

In 1993, Blum *et al.* provided a useful definition of the process of transition:

Transition is the purposeful, planned movement of adolescents and young adults with chronic physical and medical conditions from child-centred to adult-orientated health care systems.

(Blum et al. 1993, p. 573)

However, for the transition of young people with life-limiting or life-threatening conditions to adult services to be successful, the process needs to include a much wider range of services than just the healthcare services mentioned in the definition above. It needs to reflect the services required to meet the needs of the individual young person, from across the statutory and voluntary sector and a range of support which may include health, social, leisure, housing and education services.

McGrath and Yeowart (2009) describe a series of transitions that young people face; these are:

- from school to further or higher education
- from living at home or at school to living elsewhere
- from education to employment
- from children's services to adults' services.

Transition may describe the move from children's to adults' services or may represent the move from child to adult status within society, e.g. moving from school to work. Likewise, services may describe transition as occurring at a specific point, e.g. on a certain birthday or stage or on completion of education. Transition is unique to each individual and, in the context of this chapter, this term is used to describe the move from children's to adults' services. Effective transition must also allow for the fact that adolescents are undergoing changes far broader than just their clinical needs.

Although transition recognizes that young people strive to develop independence from their parents, many young people with life-limiting or life-threatening conditions remain dependent on their parents/carers for their everyday needs at the same time that they are striving to develop this level of independence.

Transition is recognized as a process rather than a single event; government documents recommend that transition should be a guided, educational, therapeutic process rather than an administrative one (Department of Health and Department for Education and Skills 2004a).

Principle for practice

- Transition should be an effective, efficient, timely process, working with young people and their families to transfer the young person's care from child-focused, family-centred children's services to patient-centred adult services.

Lost in Transition (Royal College of Nursing 2007) identified that services need to be flexible and based on the needs of the young person rather than focused on the needs of the service. This requires services to work in partnership and to examine what they provide – and do not provide – for young people and their families; this may lead to a service redesign or development. For palliative care services, this exploration will mean working across traditional boundaries and across statutory and voluntary sectors and will mean considering how to overcome barriers in service provision and how to develop the flexibility and accessibility required to meet the needs of young people and their families, friends and carers.

The criteria described in *You're Welcome Quality Criteria: Making Health Services Young People Friendly* (Department of Health 2007a) are based on examples of effective local practice working with young people aged under 20 and cover 10 topic areas:

- accessibility
- publicity
- confidentiality and consent
- the environment
- staff training, skills, attitudes and values
- joined-up working
- monitoring and evaluation, and involvement of young people
- health issues for adolescents
- sexual and reproductive health services
- child and adolescent mental health services.

The ACT recognized the specific needs of young people with life-limiting and life-threatening conditions and, in 2001, published its document *Palliative Care for Young People Aged 13–24 Years* (ACT 2001). This was followed in 2007 by the publication of *The ACT Transition Care Pathway: A Framework for the Development of Integrated Multi-Agency Care Pathways for Young People with Life-threatening and Life-limiting Conditions* (ACT 2007) in response to growing evidence of the:

- unmet needs and increasing numbers of young people living with a life-limiting condition into adult years (6–10 000 young people in the UK)
- poor outcomes for young people with complex and life-limiting conditions.

The ACT Care Pathway presents a framework that professionals can use to engage with the child's and family's needs and to make sure that everything is in place for families to access the appropriate support at the right time.

Case study

Jenny aged 20 and Jessica aged 21 years were sisters who both had a rare genetic condition; they remained in the Special School system until they were 18 and 19 years old, respectively. It appeared to their mother that, when the transport for Jessica ceased, the system seemed to 'lose sight' of Jenny too; their mother became reliant on the local children's hospice for short-break care as the only support she received. Her husband worked long hours and they had two younger sons. Following a review by the children's hospice, plans were put into place to discharge the two young women as they had reached the age limit set out in the hospice's registration documents. The hospice referred the sisters to adult social services. Social services tried to refer the sisters to the adult hospice service but the referrals were not accepted as the hospice focused on end-of-life care. With no equivalent service easily identified, the sisters were cared for wholly by their mother; when she injured her back lifting one of her daughters, the father gave up work to care for the family. A short time later, the family was referred to social services as the boys were truanting to work in local shops to help support the family financially. The lack of transition arrangements had led to a lack of any support for the family, including benefits advice, leading to severe financial difficulties, two other children missing education and two young women being totally reliant on their family for care.

Reflection point

When should transition planning have started for this family in this case study?

Key point

- There is growing evidence to show that transition is poorly managed.

Implementing an integrated care pathway to effectively manage transition

An ICP is a multidisciplinary outline of anticipated care, placed in an appropriate timeframe, to help a patient with a specific condition or set of symptoms to move progressively through a clinical experience to positive outcomes (Middleton *et al.* 2001).

In 2004, the ACT, the UK-wide organization for children's palliative care, produced the first ICP for children and young people with life-threatening and life-limiting conditions. The ACT Care Pathway (ACT 2004a) is designed to act as a tool to help professionals in planning appropriate care for children and young people with life-threatening or life-limiting conditions and their families and in coordinating the wide range of services and individuals that play a part in a child/young person's care. The ACT adopted recognized principles for the development of ICPs; namely, they:

- must be developed and 'owned' locally by a multidisciplinary team
- can cross organizational and inter-agency boundaries
- include a plan of anticipated care for an identified group
- make the patient the focus and allow for variation when appropriate
- incorporate evidence- or research-based standards or guidelines
- include systems for rigorous record-keeping
- include measurement of outcomes and promote continuous quality improvement.

This was followed in 2007 by the publication of *The ACT Transition Care Pathway: A Framework for the Development of Integrated MultiAgency Care Pathways for Young People with Life-threatening and Life-limiting Conditions* (ACT 2007). The aim of this transition care pathway was to complement the original ACT Care Pathway and engage with the emerging work from UK government departments that recognized the needs of young people.

The ACT Transition Care Pathway is guided by essential standards, based, where possible, on evidence, and provides information and guidance for those working with young people to improve the provision and consistency of care and support to young people, their families and their carers. The pathway provides a broad outline of the key events that happen, or should happen, on the journey made by young people and their families. It recognizes three phases of care:

1   the need to move on
2   moving on
3   the end of life.

It sets out six sentinel standards that should be developed as a minimum, with the aim of achieving equity for all young people and their families, wherever they live. Each of the six standards reflects a stage in the care journey and begins with a key event that is vitally significant to the family. These vital points on the care journey also identify the weakest points for many families. These are the points at which there are often difficulties with communication and integrated working by professionals and are, therefore, key actions that should be given the highest priority. The pathway follows the young person's care journey from recognition that the young person is approaching transition, through the process of moving on from children's to adults' services, to work on care at the end of life and into bereavement.

Each young person will take his or her own unique, individual care journey that reflects his or her own needs and circumstances. The pathway provides a template to enable local services to develop essential components to underpin more detailed local and individual pathways. There is a focus on ensuring that the young person's needs are central to the planning process, and the pathway aims to ensure that the young person receives integrated, personalized services to meet his or her individual needs.

The number of young people in need of palliative care and effective transition

The *Palliative Care for Young People Aged 13–24 Years* report (ACT 2001) described the annual mortality rate for this group as 1.7 per 10 000 young people, with a much higher prevalence of young people living under the threat of death who require symptom management and daily care, which is estimated to be between 6000 and 10 000. In 2007, the resident population of the UK was described by the Office for National Statistics (2008) in *Social Trends* as just under 61 million; young adults aged 16–24 years accounted for 12% of that number (7.4 million), with an estimate that 700 000 young adults, aged 16–24 years, have a disability, and further studies identifying that some 10–15% of children under the age of 16 are affected by chronic, long-term health conditions (Weiland *et al.* 2007).

It is widely recognized that, as new technologies emerge, an increasing number of children with life-limiting and/or life-threatening conditions are surviving into adulthood (Botting 1995; While *et al.* 1996; ACT 2001). There are children with a number of different impairments or conditions who need long-term care and support (Morris 1999), with over 85% of children with chronic illnesses (Betz 1999) and 90% of those with disabilities (Bloomquist *et al.* 1998) surviving into adulthood. It is expected that these numbers will increase as earlier diagnosis and improved care and management lead to higher rates of survival. New developments in the care of young people with Duchenne muscular dystrophy including non-invasive assisted ventilation means that the life expectancy for this group of service users has risen to 25 years, compared with 14 years during the 1960s, with further predictions that this will rise further to 40 years. Children and young people with cystic fibrosis (CF) are currently not typical users of children's palliative care services, although a study by Jaffe and Bush (2001) reported that the median estimated life expectancy of children with CF born in 1990 is now predicted as 40 years, which represents a doubling in the last 20 years. There is also evidence that use of anthracyclines can cause congestive cardiac failure in later life, with adverse effects increasing over time (Scottish Intercollegiate Guidelines Network 2004).

Currently, many adult palliative care services are considering how to widen access to their services, including developing services for people with cardiac and neurological conditions, with patterns of service changing to care for patients who deteriorate over a long period of time and then death coming quite unexpectedly and suddenly when compared with patients with cancer who require terminal and end-of-life care.

In addition to the more typical 'graduates' from children's palliative care services, there are also those who develop a life-threatening or life-limiting condition in early adulthood. 'Second cancers' are the leading cause of death in long-term survivors of Hodgkin's disease, with exceptionally high risks of breast cancer among women treated at a young age. One in three people will be diagnosed with cancer during their lifetime. Although cancer is a disease that affects mainly older people, with 64% of cases occurring in those aged 65 and over, in young men aged 20–39 years testicular cancer is the most frequently occurring cancer. However, current usage of palliative care services is low for children with malignant conditions, and it is unknown whether this would be different in the young person's group; anecdotal evidence suggests an increasing use from within this care group.

Such predictions include young people who will die prematurely as a result of the life-limiting nature of their illness or disorder. Most will fall into one of the groups shown in Table 12.1 (ACT 2009). These four categories are described as a guide to the young people who are likely to have palliative care needs; many young people with chronic progressive conditions reach a crisis in terms of physical deterioration in adolescence or early adulthood, with a number dying in their late teens or twenties. It should be noted that this age group has a higher proportion of those needing

Key point 🔑

The lack of real-time data, as more young people survive into adulthood, leads to an inability to plan services to meet needs and a subsequent gap in care.

Table 12.1 ACT categories of life-threatening conditions

Category	Description of conditions
1	Life-threatening conditions for which curative treatment may be feasible but can fail. Where access to palliative care services may be necessary when treatment fails or during an acute crisis, irrespective of the duration of that threat to life. On reaching long-term remission or following successful curative treatment, there is no longer a need for palliative care services *Examples: cancer, irreversible organ failures of heart, liver, kidney*
2	Conditions in which premature death is inevitable, where there may be long periods of intensive treatment aimed at prolonging life and allowing participation in normal activities *Examples: cystic fibrosis, Duchenne muscular dystrophy*
3	Progressive conditions without curative treatment options, in which treatment is exclusively palliative and may commonly extend over many years *Examples: Batten disease, mucopolysaccharidoses*
4	Irreversible but non-progressive conditions causing severe disability leading to susceptibility to health complications and likelihood of premature death. *Examples: severe cerebral palsy, multiple disabilities such as following brain or spinal cord injury, complex healthcare needs and a high risk of an unpredictable life-threatening event or episode*

palliative care than do younger children or 'young adults' – a term used by the Office for National Statistics (2008) for those under the age of 65.

For professionals working with young people, there is also a potential challenge of working with individuals across a wide spectrum of cognitive ability: some will have severe cognitive impairment related to their underlying disease, whereas others will have no cognitive delay. Identifying the actual number of young people with palliative care needs is problematic because of a lack of statistical information. The prevalence of young people who are ill and who have palliative care needs is much higher than the mortality rate, although accurate data are not available. In 2001, ACT estimated that the number is between 6000 and 10 000, based on evidence from children's service providers. It is also clear that the patient population is inevitably growing since earlier diagnosis, improved feeding techniques (especially gastrostomies), clinical intervention and medication lead to greater survival into adulthood. There are also data for young people with congenital heart disease, 70% of whom now reach adolescence and adulthood. Many have complicated conditions and need expert cardiological support (Somerville 1997).

In recognition of the difficulty in identifying the data, the Department of Health (2007b) report *Palliative Care Statistics for Children and Young Adults* included information on young adults aged 20–39 years, confirming that there were 42 400 deaths in England of children and young people aged 0–39 years from causes likely to have required palliative care during 2001–5, i.e. an annual mortality of 8480. Importantly, this analysis also highlighted that these account for 50% of deaths from all causes in this age group and reflects previous estimates compiled by the ACT in 2001.

Improving transition: policy and practice

Over recent years, a number of levers for change in children's services have emerged, building from the *Learning from Bristol* report (Department of Health 2001), which recognizes the need for children and young people's needs to be appropriately addressed and touches on staffing issues. This was followed by the White Paper *Every Child Matters: Change for Children* (Department for Education and Skills 2004a), the *National Service Framework for Children, Young People and Maternity Services* (Department of Health and Department for Education and Skills 2004a), the *National Service Framework for Long Term Conditions* (Department of Health 2005) and *Transition: Getting it Right for Young People* (Department of Health and Department for Education and Skills 2006).

An increasing number of children with life-limiting or life-threatening conditions are surviving into adulthood and smooth transition to adult services requires cooperative planning across services well ahead of the time when transfer to other services is anticipated. The Health Select Committee (House of Commons 2004) inquiry into palliative care acknowledged the particular difficulties of the transition from adolescent to adult services and recognized the gap in provision between children and young adults. A number of reports identify common themes to be considered in the transition to adulthood, including:

- the apprehension of young disabled people
- the changing roles of families
- the failure of different agencies to work together

- recognition that children's services for rare conditions are usually more highly developed than adult services
- insufficient time for transition planning.

Involving young people and their parents/carers in the transition process

In the UK, growing importance is given to the involvement of young people in decision-making about their care and service developments within local government and the NHS.

Growing evidence regarding poor transition planning processes and poor outcomes of transitions for disabled young people (Beresford 2004) has meant that improving the transitions to adult services and adulthood for disabled young people is an increasing priority within government (e.g. Department for Education and Skills 2004b; Department of Health and Department for Education and Skills 2004b). The cross-government report in England *Aiming High for Disabled Children: Better Support for Families* (HM Treasury & Department for Education and Skills 2007) concluded that more needed to be done to coordinate services for disabled young people in transition to adult life, and to ensure that young people and families can access high-quality information at key transition points. Also, cross-government guidance with regard to transitions, and specifically health transitions, has recently been published (Department for Children, Schools and Families and Department of Health 2008; Department of Health 2008).

Young people identified that they want (ACT 2007):

- to be viewed as a young person first and as being unwell as a secondary consideration
- to receive emotional and psychological support
- to live independently
- to go to school or college and have a career
- to be involved in the process of transition and make decisions about their care
- to have leisure opportunities and develop a social life, e.g. seeing friends
- to have opportunities to do things that other young people do, including developing personal relationships and having sexual experiences
- not to have to wait for services
- to have an efficient wheelchair service
- to have an advocate or key worker to coordinate services
- to have access to short breaks that are appropriate for young people.

Beresford (2004) identified that services which successfully manage the challenge of moving from children's to adults' services include:

- for young people:
  - specific service provision
  - development of skills of self-management and self-determination
  - supported psychosocial development
  - involvement of young people
  - peer involvement
  - support for changed relationships with parents/carers
  - provision of choice

- provision of information
- focus upon the young person's strengths for future development
- for parents:
  - support for adjustment to changed relationships with young people
  - parental involvement in service planning
  - a family-centred approach
  - provision of information.

McGrath and Yeowart (2009) identified the following problems if transition is managed badly:

- a lasting negative impact on young people's well-being and chances in life
- increased costs of care
- the benefits of early work with disabled children will be lost
- disabled young people can become socially and economically excluded
- the development of psychological and physical problems
- lack of help led to greater support needs later on in life
- distress and disruption to families
- possible increased reliance on health and social services
- significant financial repercussions.

Principle for practice

- Young people, wherever possible, and their parents/carers must be involved in the transition process as partners with professionals.

Models of care

A number of different models of care have evolved over recent years to provide young people's palliative care, often reflecting the services available in the local setting, as very little additional, directed funding has been made available for service development. Most service developments have emerged from children's services; however, with the establishment of the widening access agenda in adult palliative care and with hospice services considering how to provide better equity of services for people with palliative care needs, services are being developed which provide more appropriate services for younger people. In children's services and at the beginning of the transition process, young people with life-limiting conditions usually remain under the care of a paediatrician, often a community paediatrician or a disease-focused specialist such as a paediatric oncologist, neurologist or metabolic specialist, with input from a multiprofessional team, including therapists and psychology services and social care (McNeilly and Gilmore 2009).

Community teams, often nurse-led, provide ongoing care; such services continue to gradually grow in number and provide a key focus for care delivery. Within adult services, the young person's care is overseen by a specialist, with coordination from generalists such as GPs and district nurses. Children's community nursing teams are regarded as the bedrock for children's palliative care, but, in adult services, district nursing services are seen as a more generic support to specialist palliative care services.

The care of young people is delivered in many settings such as home, school or educational placements and short-break settings, of which hospice services and other voluntary services provide an important component or residential care.

The ideal service model for young people is one which brings together all players to deliver individualized packages of care to meet assessed needs and formalizes standards and quality assurance. If such models are going to be developed, commissioning and delivering palliative care to young people needs to be planned in partnership within the NHS, and with social services, education and the voluntary sector, to take account of the life-long and changing developmental needs of young people, based on accurate, real-time data to recognize the needs of service users.

The following models of care illustrate how a whole system of support to the young people and family can be based on choice and access.

- Local multidisciplinary palliative care teams which often include community nurses, hospital specialists, hospices, social workers, psychologists and therapists to deliver community-based care.
- Outreach nurse specialists working from a tertiary or shared care centre.
- Cardiac centres often provide good transition services which enable the young person to be supported by familiar carers (in a key worker role) as they bridge the gap between children's and adults' services.
- Medical back-up from a variety of services, including oncologists, general paediatricians, GPs and, sometimes, adult or paediatric palliative care consultants. It is essential to ensure that GPs and their teams are kept informed about the care of their patients to facilitate the provision of seamless care and services.
- Paediatricians with an interest in disability and long-term conditions are increasingly involved in the local clinical management of young people with life-limiting conditions, supporting the primary care team for whom the young person's condition may be rare and unfamiliar; this support can also be provided to adult palliative care services to ensure that their expertise can be adapted to meet the needs of the young person.
- Clinical nurse specialists based in specialized service centres, supporting a particular life-limiting condition, can work effectively with families through close liaison and coordinated working with local community nursing teams and work across children's and adults' services.
- Services to support the siblings of young people who are dying are an important part of supporting the whole family.
- Bereavement support for parents, family, siblings and other carers involved with the young people is also a part of palliative care.

Key point

There are a number of models of care which can be combined to provide the care needed by young people.

Using a care pathway approach to effect successful transition

There are a variety of different models of care that can provide support to meet the needs of young people with life-limiting or life-threatening conditions. The key challenge is to find a coordinated process which can be adapted to differing circumstances to ensure that the needs of the young person are systematically considered to ensure their care needs are met throughout their transition to adult services, focusing on the needs of the young person regardless of the name of the condition.

The challenge of ensuring that transition planning focuses on the fulfilment of the hopes, dreams and potential of the life-limited or life-threatened young person, enabling them to maximize education, training and employment opportunities, to enjoy social relationships and to live independently, calls for innovative, flexible and collaborative care solutions. For nurses, the professional challenge is to work alongside young people and their families and carers, within health and other settings, to support and provide appropriate young person's services with a view to enabling smooth transition to comprehensive adult multidisciplinary care.

In Doug *et al.* (2009) there is recognition that there are differing condition-dependent viewpoints on when transition should occur, but agreement on major principles guiding transition planning and probable barriers. In 2003, the Royal College of Paediatrics and Child Health recognized that transition is a lengthy process and should continue on into adult care (Royal College of Paediatrics and Child Health 2003). The responsibility for ensuring effective transition does not stop at the point of transfer of the young person to a different consultant.

Improving the Life Chances of Disabled People, published by the UK government's Strategy Unit (Cabinet Office 2005), identifies that future strategy should facilitate a smooth transition into adulthood. The three key ingredients to ensure effective support of disabled young people were described in the report as:

1   planning for transition focused on individual need
2   continuous service provision
3   access to a more transparent and appropriate menu of opportunities and choices.

It expects that this will be achieved by:

- putting in place improved mechanisms for effective planning for the transition to adulthood and the support that goes with this
- removing 'cliff edges' in service provision
- giving disabled young people access to more information for young people; this information should be in a suitable format and should include accessible local and national information on transition processes, services and opportunities.

The ACT Transition Care Pathway

The case for using a systematic, but individualized, person-centred approach to care planning has been put forward as the most effective way of ensuring that care and services are in place to assist with the successful transition from children's to adults' services. In this respect, the ACT Transition Care Pathway (Fig. 12.1) has been developed specifically to meet these needs. As will be shown by a series of sentinel standards throughout the pathway that mark important milestones in the care journey, each standard is then supported by care goals that suggest ways to help the practitioner work towards achieving the standard for each young person.

The following sections demonstrate how the ACT Transition Care Pathway may be used effectively through each phase and how this is underpinned by the six sentinel standards.

Entry to the Pathway

Many young people enter the ACT Transition Care Pathway following attendance at, or admission to, hospital for medical assessment and investigations, and the young person and his or her family will probably have already had contact with a number of different professionals before any diagnosis is made. Usually, the pathway begins with the devastating news that the young person has been diagnosed with a life-threatening or life-limiting condition. Breaking this news to the young person and the family requires skill and sensitivity (Davies *et al.* 2003). For many young people approaching adolescence, this diagnosis and news sharing will have happened during childhood, and they will have grown up with the knowledge that they have a life-threatening or life-limiting condition. However, for some young people, this will be the first recognition of the likelihood of their early death. This is the first milestone on the pathway. Some families may then proceed immediately to the final stage in the pathway (end-of-life care) whereas others may need to be supported for varying periods of time through multiagency needs assessment and long-term care plans.

Standard 1: Sharing significant news

In cases of new diagnoses, or when revisiting a prognosis made earlier in childhood, every family should receive the disclosure of their child's prognosis in a face-to-face discussion in privacy and should be treated with respect, honesty and sensitivity. Information should be provided both for the young person and family in language that they can understand.

(ACT 2007, p. 16)

Diagnosis/recognizing the need to move on

In cases of new diagnoses or when revisiting a prognosis made earlier in childhood every family should receive the disclosure of their child's prognosis in a face-to-face discussion in privacy and should be treated with respect, honesty and sensitivity. Information should be provided both for the young person and family in language that they can understand

There is no one 'right' time or age for completion of transition. It should happen at the appropriate developmental stage for each young person. However it is vital that transition does not come as a surprise to young people, and that they are prepared long before they reach it. Every young person should be supported by an identified key worker to prepare for the move onto adults' services *from* their 14th birthday

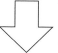

Moving on

Every young person with a life-limiting or life-threatening condition has a right to plan proactively for their future

Every young person has a timely multiagency plan for an active transition process to take place within an agreed time frame. A coordinated care plan is developed to meet the young person's individual needs. A key worker and adult key worker designate are identified to work alongside the young person/family to facilitate this process

The young person is appropriately supported in adult services, with a multiagency team fully engaged in facilitating care and support. There is confidence from the young person, family and professional perspective in the future plan and provision of care

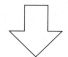

End-of-life care

When end of life is recognized there should be a review of the young person and family's needs and goals and an end-of-life plan drawn up. This should be a multidisciplinary/multiagency meeting with the active involvement of the young person and family. The meeting should take place within 2 weeks of recognition of end of life approaching or sooner if the young person's death appears imminent

Figure 12.1 The ACT Transition Care Pathway stages and standards of care.

This standard recognizes the need for sensitivity and confident, but caring, communication with the young person and his or her family. Information should also be provided in a format and language that the young person and family can understand; examples of good practice include the recording of conversations with clinicians, so that families can revisit the information when they want to.

Professionals should be aware of the impact that communication styles may have on the well-being of the young person and family. Sharing significant news is one of the more difficult tasks that professionals have to undertake. When news is broken well, it can form the basis for a helpful and constructive partnership between the young person, the family and the staff involved in their care. If it is done badly, this may affect future contact with the professionals involved in their treatment and may impair their quality of life and well-being. Professionals involved in sharing significant news should have access to appropriate training to enable them to develop the necessary skills, knowledge and understanding to undertake their role.

Young people and their parents or carers will usually be seen together, often with the parents and carers taking a key role in leading care discussions and acting, or seen by professionals as key advocates, for the young person. The process of transition should assist young people in taking increasing responsibility for their care decisions and at the same time support parents in their changing role, as decisions are increasingly made by the young person. In families in which the first language is not English, one or two family members, sometimes the young person themselves, act as interpreters, which may not be appropriate when considering difficult discussions about diagnosis or prognosis. The Disability Discrimination Act 2005 (Her Majesty's Government 2005) expects that service information should be available in appropriate formats for people with physical disabilities or sensory impairments in an appropriate format.

There is no right age for the completion of transition, but the process should be started by the young person's 14th birthday, as this also links into education review processes.

Reflection point

Consider the skills that nurses working with young people need to be able to facilitate discussions between young people and their family members.

Case study

Alfie was a 14 year old boy with Duchenne muscular dystrophy. He attended a local school that had a special support unit attached for children with a range of disabilities. He was offered a referral to the local children's hospice, which his mother accepted, feeling it would help to open discussions with Alfie about his prognosis as she did not know how to explain that he had a life-limiting condition. Alfie told his teaching assistant that he was pleased he had been referred to the children's hospice. He thought that it might help him to explain his condition to his mother as she did not seem to know that Duchenne muscular dystrophy was likely to cause his early death, as it had to some of the other boys who had attended the school, and he might get someone to help tell her about this.

Standard 2: Approaching adolescence

There is no one 'right' time or age for completion of transition. It should happen at the appropriate developmental stage for each young person. However it is vital that transition doesn't come as a surprise to young people, and that they are prepared long before they reach it. Every young person should be supported by an identified key worker to prepare for the move onto adult services from their 14th birthday.

(ACT 2007, p. 18)

Transition should be an actively managed process and the appointment of a key worker can help to support the young person and their family through the process. Care Coordination UK (CCN UK), a networking organization promoting and supporting key working for disabled children/young people and their families in England, Northern Ireland, Scotland and Wales, has developed standards for key workers (Care Coordination UK 2009). Once the transition process has commenced, there is a need to empower the young person, wherever possible, to plan proactively for the future.

Case study

Samir, aged 15, approached her school nurse to ask how she would be able to arrange her care so that she could attend the local college following her GCSEs rather than continuing at school. This care included personal care, assistance with mobility, toileting, feeding as well as assistance with educational activities and using a personal computer. Samir wanted to be involved in the discussions about the plans for her future. A planning meeting was arranged with the Connexions adviser, as the adviser took a lead in transition planning with the school and health staff, Samir and her parents. At the beginning of the meeting, Samir was asked to outline her hopes for the future and the support she needed to be able to achieve these plans. Samir asked that her teaching assistant could act as her key worker as she had a good relationship with the assistant and trusted her; also, the teaching assistant understood her day-to-day needs and was in regular contact with her and her family. The teaching assistant was willing to act as the key worker, but had no experience in arranging transition; therefore, the Connexions adviser mentored the teaching assistant in the key worker role and a successful transition took place. Samir achieved her plan to move to college, with an appropriate, personalized plan and transition occurring smoothly.

Reflection point

★ What skills does a key worker need to have?

The process will also provide an opportunity to develop a young person's decision-making skills and to support the family as the young person develops a more independent lifestyle. The process should also take into account how cultural attitudes may affect the development of independent lifestyles and ensure that the transition process considers this in individual cases; throughout the process the support needs of young people and families from diverse backgrounds should be considered. Gandhi-Rhodes and Odogwu (2009) identified that language barriers can be one reason people stay away from using services, but there is also a need to be aware of religious and cultural norms to try to overcome potential problems. For example, religious and cultural norms can mean that an inappropriate pairing of client/translator in some communities inhibits full discussion, e.g. men translating for women.

At the beginning of the process, and throughout transition, professionals must work with the young person and his or her family to identify their views and consent to how information will be shared and who that information will be shared with. It is also useful for key workers to promote an understanding of the roles of other professionals and agencies who will be involved in the transition process.

Standard 3: Proactive planning

Every young person with a life-limiting or life-threatening condition has a right to plan proactively for their future.

(ACT 2007, p. 19)

The concept of proactive planning encourages planning to continue during times of uncertainty. This will help to ensure crises do not stop the planning and lose the momentum to find the services to meet the young person's assessed care and education needs. This planning may need to be a parallel process of planning for care at the end of life if the young person's physical condition deteriorates. Advanced care planning is considered further within Standard 6.

Young people often question the meaning of their life and look for reasons for pain and suffering. For young people with life-limiting or life-threatening conditions who are facing the probability of a premature death, the meaning of life may gain extra significance and the young person may want to explore their own beliefs system; workers should consider when it is best to offer spiritual support.

While engaging with services and planning for the future, it is important that professionals involved with young people recognize the need for the transition process to remain a part of the young person's life, rather than taking over the whole life of the young person. Often, specialist advisers such as Connexions advisers, do not have specialist knowledge of life-limiting or life-threatening conditions and how this can affect the young person's transition process.

Some young people's plans for the future may include plans to attend university or college, or to take up employment, in a new location. The transition process should take this into consideration and ensure that the young person is able to find out about services in the new area, make links to move to these services or consider whether this will involve a move to services away from the existing area. This may also include considering the roles of services such as University Health Services or Occupational Health Services in the later stages of the transition plan.

Case study

Hanna, a 16 year old newly diagnosed with Wolfram (diabetes insipidus, diabetes mellitus, optic atrophy and deafness; DIDMOAD) syndrome, has completed her school examinations and wants to plan for a university application. Her parents are reluctant for her to move away from home in the light of her life-limiting diagnosis. A family conference is arranged by the diabetic nurse specialist and includes the family GP and Hanna's head of year at school. During discussions, it is apparent that Hanna is aware of her prognosis, but desperately wants to attain a degree and gain some independence and move away from home. The head of year believes that it is highly likely that Hanna can achieve the educational requirements to go to university. The diabetic nurse specialist is able to confirm that the local hospital in the university town has a good diabetic service. Plans are made for Hanna to progress with university applications, with support from the head of year, and for the diabetic nurse specialist to liaise with Hanna's GP and the family to arrange for healthcare support from the University Health Service when university placements are being planned.

Reflection point

★ How can home and university health services work together to ensure optimal care?

Standard 4: Multiagency care plan

Every young person has a timely multi-agency plan for an active transition process to take place within an agreed time frame. A co-ordinated care plan is developed to meet the young person's individual needs. A key worker and adult key worker designate are identified to work alongside the young person/family to facilitate this process.

(ACT 2007, p. 28)

This standard introduces the concept of a key worker designate, described as an identified worker to act as a link person working in an adult service who works closely with the children's services key worker and through whom adult services can be effectively accessed. The key worker designate is also ideally placed to be able to take forward the coordinated planning of care within adult services and implement the multiagency care plan required. It is essential that there is clarity over the lines of responsibility and communication within and between the young person and their family/carers and agencies and professionals during this period, and that this is reviewed as transition occurs and roles change.

The development of a person-centred plan is an important aspect of successfully achieving this standard; the plan should be developed by the multidisciplinary team and reflect the holistic needs of the young person.

During the assessment process, the identification of the young person's current and predicted needs should enable care planning to take place. Consideration should be given to their needs and identification of the service provider(s) who can meet these. Often, at the start of transition, children's services provide for the majority of needs; from the point of view of familiarity, this may be seen as the model of care, i.e. from a single provider, that is desirable for the future. However, it is advisable that broader consideration is given to identify the most appropriate provider and that a care plan is drawn up to coordinate service provision and provide a seamless approach to the young person's care.

Holistic assessments should also address the sexual health needs of the young person. All young people with life-limiting or life-threatening conditions have the right to receive information and support to develop their self-esteem, a positive body image and self-confidence in relation to their sexuality and relationships.

Support should be provided to help them develop skills such as decision-making, communication, assertiveness and understanding personal safety to underpin their ability to develop relationships. They should be assisted to understand their sexual feelings and learn about acceptable and appropriate behaviour and respect for others. Information, advice and support should be given to parents and carers to enable them to deal with their child's emerging sexuality.

Case study

Ben, who is 15, is invited to join a transition programme being run by the local children's hospice service. The programme involves a small group of young people arranging a programme of activities for themselves over the year ahead. The programme has a budget for the young people to use. The process is facilitated by one of the hospice staff, who encourages group discussion in the initial stages. During the year, the young people learn and develop negotiating skills, working together to plan budgets and arrange events, including transport; this is a range of skills which can be utilized in other settings. Also during the year, a group for parents of teenagers considers the challenges of parenting teenagers and encourages parents to explore how to support their child as he or she moves towards a more independent lifestyle as a young adult.

Reflection point

★ What barriers can there be for young people using hospice services?

Standard 5: Multiagency support

The young person is appropriately supported in adult services, with the multiagency team fully engaged in facilitating care and support. There is confidence from the young person, family and professional perspective in the future plan and provision of care.

(ACT 2007, p. 33)

Workers within children's and adults' services have a role to play in ensuring that the young person and his or her family have been recognized as equal partners in the care-planning process and that their views have been considered fully. Young people should also be provided with the same information relating to health promotion as other young people of the same age, and they should be aware that they have the same rights to confidentiality as their peers.

The key worker should work with the young person to consider how the young person wants to share information with professionals and agencies, from across the children's and adults' sectors. The key worker should consider how the young person will hold that information, whether they want to receive copies of all letters and reports or whether they want their parents/carers to hold the information for sharing, and how their views are included and shared at statutory reviews, e.g. special education needs (SEN) reviews or transition plan reviews. This should be kept under review as the young person may change his or her mind as transition progresses and the young person develops more confidence in becoming self-advocating.

Decision-making with young people is often a matter of negotiation between the young person and those with parental responsibility and clinicians. Young people should never feel that decisions are being made over their heads. Even when young people are not able to give valid consent for themselves, it is very important to involve them as much as possible in decisions about their own health. The key issue is to consider whether the young person has sufficient comprehension and intelligence to understand fully what is proposed. A young person of any age can give valid consent to treatment or examination provided he or she is considered to be competent to make the decision. Negotiation and explanation of the issues is essential to help the young person make decisions. Professionals' decision-making should be transparent, justifiable and well recorded.

Care planning is an important process for both the young person and parents/carers as it offers an opportunity for the young person to make choices about their future care wishes, while still supported by their parents. The desire to gain independence from parents is a normal phase of adolescence, but many young people with life-limiting or life-threatening conditions remain dependent on their family for considerable care. Nevertheless, professionals should consider how they can enable more independence for the young person, e.g. the provision of self-operated hoists or turning beds, which also relieves the family of some of the physical demands of care. The care-planning process also provides an opportunity for discussions about how to use benefits to employ carers.

Case study

Mo is 19 years old and is studying information technology at university; he has a 24 hour package of care arranged by the local social services team. He is dissatisfied with the package as carers often change at the last moment and are unwilling to support him socially, leaving him isolated. He decides to arrange his own package of care, supported by his social worker. He creates this using a range of benefits, including Direct Payments, Independent Living Fund, Disability Living Allowance and Local Education Authority allowances, and employs his own team of carers. He reports that this brings more continuity of care and enables him to employ carers who are willing to support his university lifestyle and meet both the academic aspects and social aspects of his life.

The Care Pathway also commends the use of a person-centred planning approach, described as a process for continual listening and learning, focused on what is important to someone now and for the future, and acting upon this in alliance with family and friends.

Reflection point

★ How can young people access training to develop skills to be able to coordinate their care?

Predicting the time when a young person is likely to move into their end-of-life phase is not easy. For some young people, there may have been a series of peaks and troughs in their condition where they have returned to periods of stability following a period of serious decline; for this reason, parallel planning may have considered the need for care at end-of-life planning for some time. For other young people, the recognition that death is imminent may be quite sudden, possibly only hours or days before death.

This unpredictability is difficult for professionals to manage, but for family members it may mean that they have had little time to acknowledge this reality or plan for the death. Professionals working with these young people, their families and their carers should be honest and open about the probability that the young person's life is nearing an end. Families and young people, when appropriate, should be supported to plan for death. The young person, family and carers should be empowered to exercise informed choice and receive full care and support in that choice. It is essential that they are provided with information about the choices available to them and for a care plan to be developed, based on the young person's and family's needs and wishes.

The specific needs of siblings should be considered as they may be young carers (described as a child or young person under the age of 18 who looks after someone in their family who has an illness, disability, mental health problem or drug and alcohol abuse/misuse problems) who share the practical and/or emotional caring responsibilities for their brother or sister with parents and other family carers. Explain to parents and children that they may both be entitled to an assessment of their needs from social services. Parents and other young carers who are 16 or over are entitled to a carer's assessment, and professionals should offer them the opportunity to be referred for an assessment and support (Her Majesty's Government 2000). Younger carers can also access support through social care and voluntary organizations.

Professionals should also be aware that the life-limited or life-threatened young person may have caring responsibilities for other children within the family, which may further restrict their choices in developing independence. It should also be recognized that young people may want to formally say goodbye to children's services as they move on to adult care.

Standard 6: End-of-life care

When end of life is recognised there should be a review of the young person and family's needs and goals and an end-of-life plan drawn up. This should be a multi-disciplinary/multi-agency meeting with the active involvement of the young person and family. The meeting should take place within two weeks of recognition of end-of-life approaching or sooner if the young person's death appears imminent.

(ACT 2007, p. 37)

Supporting individuals and families when the death of a young person is anticipated is challenging. One of the challenges faced by young people, and their families, who have life-limiting conditions is making a plan for death. Families may wish for their child to die at home, in a hospice or in hospital; they want to know that they will have access to the support they require and that their wishes will be treated with respect. Professionals should aim to offer all families an opportunity to talk about end-of-life issues (concerns or wishes), but with the awareness that, in some cases, families will not want to take this up, or may need more time before they are ready to do so.

Professionals often find it hard to decide when to start conversations about care at end of life and may find it useful to consider and then reflect on the following questions.

Reflection points

★ Would you be surprised if a young person you were caring for died prematurely as a result of a life-limiting or life-threatening illness?

★ Would you be surprised if this young person died within a year?

★ Would you be surprised if this young person died during this episode of care?

★ Do you know what the young person's and family's wishes are for the end of life?

★ Answering 'No' to any of the questions should encourage the professional to consider discussing Advance Care Planning with the young person and family. Making an Advance Care Plan can help to mitigate some of the young person's and family's anxieties and ensure that events happen as they want.

An Advance Care Plan is a document that sets out an agreed plan of care to be followed as the young person's condition deteriorates. It can be difficult to make rational and informed decisions during a crisis, so the benefit of an Advance Care Plan is that a plan of action can be made before the situation occurs (ACT 2004b).

Every young person with a life-limiting condition and their family should be helped to decide on an end-of-life plan, and should be provided with care and support to achieve this as closely as possible. The end-of-life plan should consider the young person's wishes and holistic needs, and those of their family, in the terminal phase of their illness, at the time of death, and after death. In many circumstances, it should include discussion and decision-making about withdrawing or withholding life-sustaining treatment, and allowing a natural death. The outcome of this discussion should result in the development of a personal Emergency/Advance Care Plan. Sometimes, young people will want friends to be present during discussions because they play an important role in the young person's life as emotional separation from their parents continues and adolescence moves on and, at the same time, identification with peers increases.

Young people and families should expect to be able to access good palliative care in all environments and to discuss care options with the care team from early in the young person's care, and for these discussions to be ongoing throughout that care.

The Gold Standards Framework (GSF) and Liverpool Care Pathway (LCP) are tools which support the delivery of palliative care to adults approaching their end of life.

The GSF is described as a systematic evidence-based approach to optimizing the care for patients nearing the end of life delivered by generalist providers. It is concerned with helping people to live well until the end of life and includes care in the final years of life for people with any end-stage illness in any setting. The GSF is extensively used in the UK as an approach to palliative care for adults. The LCP is an ICP that is used at the bedside to drive up sustained quality of care of the dying in the last hours and days of life. It is a means to transfer the best quality for care of the dying from the hospice movement into other clinical areas, so that wherever the person is dying there can be an equitable model of care. Both tools have been designed as generic tools to promote the care of adults and do not consider the specific needs of young people.

General practitioners and the primary care team should be included in the plans for care, but they may lack experience and specialist support may be difficult to acquire. Children's nurses also sometimes lack confidence in the symptom management of young people, and adult community and Macmillan nurses may share these or similar concerns when caring for a young adult at end of life, especially in cases when the patient is dying from a non-malignant disorder.

The young person's quality of life up to the point of death must be a major consideration, and there may be associated difficult decisions surrounding the withdrawal of non-essential drugs or other invasive interventions. The Royal College of Paediatrics and Child Health has published guidance on withdrawing treatment in children (Royal College of Paediatrics and Child Health 2007) and the British Medical Association has also published a series of guidance documents which provide extensive discussion of the ethics around end-of-life care (British Medical Association 2007a,b).

It is desirable to develop a written Advance Care Plan with the consultant and other people looking after the child, to assist in communication between different professionals. The family may also wish to discuss the options with regard to organ donation and the subject of post-mortem; in cases in which the young person is under 18, Child Death Review Processes may need to be explained. Workers should ensure that the advice and support takes into account cultural views as organ/tissue donation may be considered taboo. Parents should be fully informed about these issues and should feel that their decisions are understood and respected by all concerned. Young people with the capacity to decide independently should be involved in making decisions about end-of-life choices.

Care at end of life

The time of death will be an extremely painful time for the family and friends of the young person. The young person will need to have loved ones close by, with the necessary privacy and space. Sometimes, the young person or the family may decide they wish to transfer to another setting, such as a hospice or hospital, and this should be supported wherever possible (Davies 2009).

The family will also need to consider what they want after the young person's death: where would they prefer the young person's body to be cared for; who will need to be contacted; who will deal with the death certificate; is there to be a post-mortem; has organ donation been discussed? If the family wishes to take the young person home after death in a hospice or hospital this should be recorded in the young person's notes and the process for this to happen should be commenced.

Principles for practice

- The young person's needs are assessed and a plan of care is discussed and developed with the young person, family and carers, including choice of place of care. Within this assessment, the ability of the young person, family and carers to communicate must be considered and appropriate interpreting services ensured.
- The religious and spiritual needs of the young person, family and carers are assessed.
- The insights of the young person, family and carers into the young person's condition are identified and their wishes and views are incorporated into the care plan.
- Emergency contact details for the staff to be contacted are confirmed for the family and carers of the young person.
- Current medications are assessed and non-essentials discontinued.
- 'As required' subcutaneous and other medication is prescribed according to an agreed protocol to manage symptoms including pain, agitation, nausea and vomiting, and respiratory tract secretions.
- Decisions are taken as to whether to discontinue inappropriate interventions, including blood tests, intravenous fluids and observation of vital signs.
- The family and carers are given appropriate written information.
- The GP's practice, care team (e.g. community nursing services, consultants) and others (e.g. ambulance trust), including out-of-hours services, are made aware of the young person's condition.
- The family are given an opportunity to discuss their plans for after-death care, including who to call, what to do immediately and what can wait.

After the young person's death it is vital that parents retain control and choice in the care of their child's body (Davies 2005). Families need to have time and privacy with their child in the hours and days following the death. Families will also appreciate advice from the care team or funeral director about care of the body at home (Dominica 1997). For example, it may also be possible to arrange for a mobile cooling device in the family home so that the young person's body can remain at home for a period.

Professionals should also ensure that the family's religious or cultural beliefs and rituals are respected. Families should be consulted about whether they want to be involved in laying out the young person and choosing the clothes to be worn. They will need reassurance that their child will be treated with dignity and respect by any professional handling the body.

Siblings should be given opportunities to express their emotions openly and ask questions. They should be asked whether they wish to see their brother's or sister's body and should not be excluded from decisions about funeral arrangements. Grandparents also need sensitive consideration.

There will be an immediate need to inform all those in contact with the family that the young person has died. The family's key worker or another member of the team can assist in this if the family wishes. People to contact may include the GP, community or specialist nurses, health visitor, social worker, school/education placement, short break service, and transport and ambulance service. It is also important to ensure that any department or service expecting the young person at an appointment is informed to ensure that 'did not attend' letters are not sent out. Where appropriate, benefit agencies should be informed as soon as possible.

The environment in which the family feels most comfortable will also be a consideration. Many wish to be at home, but others may choose a children's hospice or a hospital where they feel more confident to deal with emergencies. A combination of these places is also possible, and this will require efficient collaborative working. Whatever the choice, the family will need 24 hour access to care in the terminal stage. Clarification will be needed about who will be prescribing and that they have the appropriate skills and knowledge or, if not, will be supported by a physician who has. Planning will be required for supplies of medication and provision of out-of-hours pharmacy needs.

Plan for providing terminal care

The child or young person must receive effective pain and symptom control. The key will be ensuring that regular symptom reviews are undertaken and the right treatment administered. The appropriate analgesia should be administered at regular dosing intervals with adjunctive drug therapy for symptom and side-effect control. There is a range of pain assessment tools appropriate to the age and understanding of individual infants, children and adolescents, in particular those produced by the Royal College of Nursing. It may sometimes be necessary to request advice and this is far preferable to getting something wrong and jeopardizing the family's trust. The family's decision to provide terminal care at home may be thwarted if there is a breakdown in symptom control resulting in admission to hospital. There will also be the possibility of other distressing symptoms, and the child and family will need reassurance that these can be managed effectively. It is important that the family and the team have 24 hour access to a paediatric palliative care specialist, paediatrician or specially trained GP so that symptoms and pain can be controlled outside normal working hours and unnecessary emergency admissions to hospital can be avoided.

Complementary therapies such as music therapy, play therapy, story-telling, visualization or relaxation techniques and even hypnosis may have a role to play and should be considered as part of the care if the family wish. The agreed end-of-life care plan will need to be documented, including the personalized resuscitation plan setting out what emergency treatment is to be used and what is not to be used by ambulance crews and local accident and emergency departments. It may be helpful to discuss this with the local emergency services and provide them with a copy of the document. The plan should allow for ongoing review of care and changing goals to comply with the wishes of the family. It is essential that all in the team are informed of changes and kept up to date with the child's care.

Supporting the child's and family's choices for quality of life

Parents and other significant family members should be encouraged and supported to continue their caring role with the child or young person. Depending on the age of the child, the school community may continue to be involved and informed. The child may wish to continue with school work and this should be facilitated. He or she may want to continue seeing friends, and carry on with other pleasurable activities for as long as possible. Siblings and grandparents, where appropriate, should be included in discussions about choices on quality of life.

Written information should be provided for the family about procedures and entitlements following the death, to include:

- registering the death
- the procedure required for cremation
- the contact details of the funeral director
- advice on benefits or entitlements.

Case study

Sophie, 16 years old, is admitted to hospital with a chest infection, following a relapse of leukaemia; she is recognized to be approaching the end of her life. Discussions between Sophie's parents and the clinicians caring for her identify that Sophie had not wanted to be admitted to hospital and had expressed her wish to die at home. Her parents are concerned that they may not be able to cope with caring for her at home. A multiagency case conference is arranged and includes the local CCN team, local district nursing team, oncology nurse specialists, oncologists and GP. A care plan is developed and Sophie's opinions are sought about where she wants to be cared for. The local CCN team works Monday to Friday, 9 a.m. to 5 p.m., with cover for end-of-life care; the care plan ensures that Sophie's parents have 24 hour access to advice from the CCN team and the oncology nurse specialists who have been involved in Sophie's long-term care. The district nursing team offers back-up to the CCN team, to ensure equipment availability and support. Sophie's parents do not feel able to work; the oncology unit social worker helps them identify the best way of dealing with their absence from work, which includes Sophie's father taking special leave and her mother getting a medical certificate from the GP. A symptom management plan is developed, with Sophie's parents aware that 24 hour support is available from the oncology team and that their GP is also aware of the plan. A pharmacy box is arranged so that all the drugs Sophie is likely to need are readily available. Sophie is taken home by ambulance and is cared for by her family, supported by the CCN team and nurse specialists from the hospital, until her death 72 hours later. Following death, she is transferred to the local children's hospice for care in their 'special bedroom', which is chilled and which enables Sophie's family to say their goodbyes to her in their own time, until her funeral.

Reflection point

★ Where can the care team access specialist support for symptom management out of hours?

It has been shown that the ACT Transition Care Pathway can be used effectively to plan, implement and deliver effective evidence-based care. The role of the children's nurse in ensuring that this does happen is discussed in the following section.

The role of the children's nurse in promoting effective transition

The Nursing and Midwifery Council (2008) confirmed a series of principles to underpin work with children and young people, namely:

- making the care of children, young people and their parents the first concern, treating them as individuals and respecting their dignity
- working with others to protect and promote the health and well-being of those in their care, their families and carers, and the wider community
- providing a high standard of practice and care at all times
- being open and honest, acting with integrity and upholding the reputation of the profession.

When working with young people, this means getting to know the young person as an individual and accepting that all families are different, promoting a need for individualized and collaborative approaches to care. Young *et al.* (2003) identified the difficulties in managing communication with young people who have a chronic, life-threatening illness and in the role parents take in relation to facilitating and constraining communication between the professional and the young person. They also identified the potential for the parental role to hamper the development of successful relationships between professionals and young patients.

Nurses who work with young people should be aware of the barriers that the young people may face, such as social isolation, lack of employment/education and leisure opportunities, and work to support them and their families to try to overcome the barriers and the impact they have on the young people's lives and care needs.

Nurses working with young people will need to balance the rights of the young person with those involved in their care. They will need to apply professional codes of practice and legal requirements relating to the care of young people, such as confidentiality, information sharing, consent, service provision, young people's rights, antidiscriminatory practice and safeguarding issues, to the practical provision of care and support of individual young people and their families. Nurses have a duty of care to act with appropriate skill and judgement and to take all reasonable steps to ensure that the young person does not suffer harm as a result of their actions or failure to act; nurses should also work within the professional code of ethics regarding working with young people. The care of life-limited or life-threatened young people will require the nurse to apply a practical consideration and implementation of ethics in relation to consent and confidentiality, including capacity issues, combined with an ability to communicate effectively with young people and those involved in their care.

Nurses working with young people with life-limiting or life-threatening conditions and their families are ideally placed to act as a care/service navigator to guide and support young people and their families, friends and carers through the transition maze. They can promote an understanding of palliative care approaches and attitudes, within specialist and generalist services. Nurses can help the young person to develop skills in communication, decision-making, assertiveness, self-care and self-advocacy to assist with the transition process. They are also ideally placed to recognize any gaps in the young person's readiness to move between children's and adults' services and to help address any such gaps, by working with the young person, their family and other supporters, including other professionals, and by making appropriate referrals to other services, when needed. They can also help to manage expectations that young people and their families have about the move to adult services and give the young person time to adjust to the new services. Finally, they have a crucial role in ensuring that the young person has a 'good death', i.e. one which is pain free and dignified, in the environment of their choice and with those they love around them (Davies 2009).

Nurses can also play a key role in helping services establish and develop processes, systems and attitudes to support young people and their families/carers to adjust to, prepare for, and move on to adult services, as well as contributing to the commissioning of services for young people.

Conclusion

Young people with life-limiting or life-threatening conditions have specific palliative care needs and physical, psychological and developmental needs that are significantly different from those experienced by children and adults. However, although the number of young people who meet the criteria for palliative care has increased significantly, transition for many is poorly managed and this has a detrimental effect not only on the individual but also on their family/carers.

It is clear that young people and their families/carers require an integrated, person-centred approach to guide and support them through what may be described as the transition maze. Such an approach can help ensure that they receive a coordinated and person-centred approach to care and support throughout their care journey. As this chapter has shown, the ACT Transition Care Pathway may be used to plan, implement and deliver effective evidence-based care throughout. In doing so, the role of the children's nurse in ensuring this has been highlighted. Finally, using case studies, it has been shown how the pathway may be applied in practice so that the young person and their family/carers are not lost in the process of transition but have ongoing support from within primary, secondary and tertiary care for long as is needed.

From this discussion several key principles for practice can be clearly articulated.

Summary of principles for practice

- Children and young people's nurses must be informed that coordinated approaches to care require clear communication and partnership working; this takes time and nurses need to allocate time to the process of transition and to partnership working.
- Children and young people's nurses must understand that continuity of care is essential for young people and their families and requires parallel planning, with the young people and families recognized as equal partners in the planning process; nurses need to develop communication skills to be able to work effectively with young people, families and co-workers.
- Children and young people's nurses must understand that communication provides a firm foundation for a smooth transition and should continue during times of uncertainty.
- Children and young people's nurses must be aware that it is difficult to predict when a young person may enter the end-of-life phase, but professionals should be honest and open about the probability that the young person's life is nearing an end.

References

Association for Children with Life-Threatening or Terminal Conditions and their Families (2001) *Palliative care for young people aged 13–24 years*. A joint report by the ACT, National Council for Hospice and Specialist Palliative Care and Scottish Partnership Agency for Palliative and Cancer Care. Bristol: ACT.

Association for Children with Life-Threatening or Terminal Conditions and their Families (2004a) *A framework for the development of integrated multi-agency care pathways for children with life-threatening and life-limiting conditions*. Bristol: ACT.

Association for Children with Life-Threatening or Terminal Conditions and their Families (2004b) *The ACT charter for children with life-threatening or terminal conditions and their families*. Bristol: ACT.

Association for Children with Life-Threatening or Terminal Conditions and their Families (2007) *The ACT Transition Care Pathway: A framework for the development of integrated multi-agency care pathways for young people with life-threatening and life-limiting conditions*. Bristol: ACT

ACT (2009) *A guide to the development of children's palliative care services*, 3rd edn. Bristol: ACT.

Beresford B (2004) On the road to nowhere? Young disabled people and transition. *Child: Care, Health and Development* **60**: 581–7.

Betz CL (1999) Adolescents with chronic conditions: linkages to adult service systems. *Pediatric Nursing* **25**: 473–6.

Bloomquist KB, Brown G, Peerson A, Presler EP (1998) Transitioning to independence: challenges for young people with disabilities and their caregivers. *Orthopaedic Nursing* **17**(3): 27–35.

Blum R, Garell D, Hodgman C, *et al.* (1993) Transition from child-centered to adult health-care systems for adolescents with chronic conditions. A position paper of the Society for Adolescent Medicine. *Journal of Adolescent Health* **14**: 570–6.

Botting B (ed.) (1995) *The health of our children decennial supplement*. OPCS Series DS No. 11. London: HMSO.

Bristol Royal Infirmary Inquiry (2001) *The inquiry into the management of care of children receiving complex heart surgery at the Bristol Royal Infirmary: learning from Bristol*. London: The Stationery Office.

British Medical Association (2007a) *Advance decisions and proxy decision-making in medical treatment and research*. London: BMA.

British Medical Association (2007b) *Withholding and withdrawing life-prolonging medical treatment: guidance for decision making*. London: BMA.

Cabinet Office (2005) *Improving the life chances of disabled people*. London: Cabinet Office.

Care Coordination UK (2009) *Key worker standards*. York: Care Coordination UK.

Davies R (2005) Mothers' stories of loss: their need to be with their dying child and their child's body after death. *Journal of Child Health Care* **9**(4): 288–300.

Davies R (2009) Care of the child at the end of life. In: Price J, McNeilly P (eds) *Palliative care for children and families: an interdisciplinary approach*. Basingstoke: Palgrave Macmillan.

Davies R, Davis B, Sibert J (2003) Parents' stories of sensitive and insensitive care by paediatricians in the time leading up to and including diagnostic disclosure of a life-limiting condition in their child. *Child: Care, Health and Development* **29**(1): 77–82.

Department for Children, Schools and Families and Department of Health (2008) *Transition: moving on well. A good practice guide for health professionals and their partners on transition planning for young people with complex health needs or a disability*. London: Department of Health and Department for Children, Schools and Families.

Department for Education and Skills (2004a) *Every child matters: change for children*. Nottingham: Department for Education and Skills Publications.

Department for Education and Skills (2004b) *Every child matters: next steps*. Nottingham: Department for Education and Skills Publications.

Department of Health (2001) *Learning from Bristol: the Department of Health's response to the Report of the Public Inquiry into children's heart surgery at the Bristol Royal Infirmary 1984–1995*. London: Department of Health.

Department of Health (2005) *The National Service Framework for long term conditions*. London: Department of Health.

Department of Health (2007a) *You're welcome quality criteria: making health services young people friendly*. London: The Stationery Office.

Department of Health (2007b) *Palliative care statistics for children and young adults*. London: Department of Health.

Department of Health and Department for Education and Skills (2004a) *National Service Framework for Children, Young People and Maternity Services: the mental health and psychological wellbeing of children and young people.* London: Department of Health.

Department of Health and Department for Education and Skills (2004b) *National Service Framework for Children, Young People and Maternity Services: disabled children and those with complex health needs.* London: Department of Health.

Department of Health and Department for Education and Skills (2006) *Transition: getting it right for young people.* London: DH/DfES.

Dominica F (1997) *Just my reflection: helping parents to do the things their way when their child dies.* London: Darton, Longman and Todd.

Doug M, Adi Y, William J, *et al.* (2009) Transition to adult services for children and young people with palliative care needs: a systematic review. *Archives of Disease in Childhood* [Epub ahead of print]

Gandhi-Rhodes K, Odogwu CR (2009) *The diversity toolkit.* Bristol: Children's Hospices UK.

Her Majesty's Government (2000) Carers and Disabled Children Act. London: The Stationery Office.

Her Majesty's Government (2005) Disability Discrimination Act. London: The Stationery Office.

HM Treasury and Department for Education and Skills (2007) *Aiming high for disabled children: better support for families.* London: HM Treasury.

House of Commons (2004) *Report on palliative care: fourth report of Session 2003–4.* London: The Stationery Office.

Jaffe A, Bush A (2001) Cystic fibrosis: review of the decade. *Monaldi Archives for Chest Disease* **56**: 240–7.

McGrath A, Yeowart C (2009) *Rights of passage: supporting disabled young people through the transition to adulthood.* London: New Philanthropy Capital.

McNeilly P, Gilmore F (2009) Interdisciplinary working. In: Price J, McNeilly P (eds) *Palliative care for children and families: an interdisciplinary approach.* Basingstoke: Palgrave Macmillan.

Middleton S, Barnett J, Reeves D (2001) What is an integrated care pathway? *Evidence-based Medicine* **3**(3): 1–8.

Morris J (1999) *Hurtling into a void: transition to adulthood for young people with complex health and support needs.* York: Joseph Rowntree Foundation.

Nursing and Midwifery Council (2008) *Advice for nurses working with children and young people.* See http://www.nmc-uk.org/Nurses-and-midwives/Advice-by-topic/A/Advice/Advice-on-working-with-children-and-young-people/

Office for National Statistics (2008) *Social trends.* Report No. 38. Basingstoke: Palgrave Macmillan.

Price J, McNeilly P (eds) (2009) *Palliative care for children and families: an interdisciplinary approach.* Basingstoke: Palgrave Macmillan.

Royal College of Nursing (2007) *Lost in transition.* London: RCN.

Royal College of Paediatrics and Child Health (2003) *Specialist health services for children and young people: a guide for primary care organisations.* London: RCPCH.

Royal College of Paediatrics and Child Health (2004) *Withholding or withdrawing life sustaining treatment in children: a framework for practice,* 2nd edn. London: RCPCH.

Royal College of Paediatrics and Child Health (2007) *Withholding or withdrawing life saving treatment in children: a framework for practice.* London: RCPCH.

Scottish Intercollegiate Guidelines Network (2004) *Long term follow up of survivors of childhood cancer: a national clinical guideline.* Edinburgh: SIGN.

Somerville J (1997) Management of adults with congenital heart disease: an increasing problem. *Annual Review of Medicine* **48**: 283–93.

Weiland SK, Pless IB, Roughman KJ (2007) Chronic illness and mental health problems in paediatric practice. *Pediatrics* **89**: 445–59.

While A, Citrone C, Cornish J (1996) *A study of the needs and provisions for families caring for children with life-limiting incurable disorders.* London: Department of Nursing Studies, King's College.

Young B, Dixon-Woods M, Windridge KC, Heney D (2003) Managing communication with young people who have a potentially life threatening chronic illness: qualitative study of patients and parents. *British Medical Journal* **326**(7384): 305.

PART 4

Advancing practice and developing a career in children and young people's nursing

Chapter 13

Developing a professional portfolio

Alyson Davies and Gary Rolfe

Overview

This chapter will examine the use of portfolios as part of professional development and progression within nursing careers. This will include discussion of the issues and debates surrounding the use of portfolios and how these tensions may be resolved for post-registration children and young people's nurses during their professional development and lifelong learning.

Introduction

Portfolios have been used widely for many years in a variety of disciplines to demonstrate individual progression and development. Portfolios have become increasingly popular in nursing as a means of recording and enhancing learning, the integration of theory with practice, critical thinking and personal professional development (Jasper 2006; Nairn *et al.* 2006; Byrne *et al.* 2007; Nursing and Midwifery Council 2008a; Timmins and Dunne 2009). Nurses are under a professional obligation to ensure that their knowledge and skills are safe, current and effective (Welsh Assembly Government 2004, 2009; Nursing and Midwifery Council 2008b), and this requires them to engage in appropriate learning and practice-oriented activities that develop and maintain competence and performance (Nursing and Midwifery Council 2008b,c; Timmins and Dunne 2009). Thus, as educational courses move towards more competency-based assessments, so the portfolio has come to play a vital role in making the process and development of learning transparent through its components, including reflective writing (Endacott *et al.* 2004; Jasper 2006; Nursing and Midwifery Council 2008a). Such an approach is based upon andragogical principles whereby the learner takes responsibility for the scope and shape of their learning. The learner is recognized as being in control of his or her learning, contributing personal knowledge and experience to the process (Knowles 1990). Thus, nurses are responsible for directing their own learning experiences and providing evidence of their competence. This demands a degree of self-directed learning, with the portfolio being used as a dynamic, flexible, highly individualized document of the learner's development (Endacott *et al.* 2004; Jasper 2006; Timmins and Dunne 2009).

A number of debates surrounding the use of portfolios have emerged during the past decade, and they have been adopted enthusiastically but with little evidence to support their use and the claims made for them (Timmins and Dunne 2009). Indeed, their use is contentious at a time when there is still considerable debate about the value of competence and competence-based assessments (McMullan *et al.* 2003; Timmins and Dunne 2009). Assessment of the portfolio has proved to be a challenging aspect, with discussion focusing on frameworks, language used to assess the portfolio, standardization of assessment and formalization of the process (Endacott *et al.* 2004; Scholes *et al.* 2004; Byrne *et al.* 2007). Critics have questioned the rigour of the portfolio as well as the reliability and validity of the assessment process. Supporters of their use claim that they enable students to develop reflective skills and take ownership of their lifelong learning following the social, political and professional imperatives placed upon them; that they facilitate the acquisition of skills and knowledge; that they give insight into competence; and that they provide a means of integrating theory with clinical practice, thus developing a practitioner who is insightful and critically aware and who matures professionally with each experience (Jasper and Fulton 2005; Joyce 2005; Byrne *et al.* 2007; Kicken *et al.* 2009). What emerges from the literature is that there is little empirical evidence to support such claims, yet educational and clinical assessment is now based on such a method of assessment (McColgan 2008; Timmins and Dunne 2009).

The origins and purpose of portfolios in nursing

Historical development

The term 'portfolio' is derived from the Italian words *portare* 'to carry' and *foglio* 'leaf' or 'sheet', and has come to mean both the folder in which sheets of paper are carried and also the papers themselves. The concept of a portfolio was formally introduced into nurse education in the early 1990s, first by the Welsh National Board for Nursing (WNB) as part of its continuing educational framework, and shortly after by the English National Board (ENB) as part of its 'Higher Award'. The purpose of the portfolio in relation to these initiatives was predominantly a way of demonstrating prior formal and experiential learning within the Credit Accumulation and Transfer Scheme (CATS), and was generally defined in terms of previous learning. For example, Snadden and Thomas (1998) defined a portfolio as 'the collection of evidence that learning has taken place'. This retrospective function of recording prior learning was also emphasized by the United Kingdom Central Council (UKCC) governing body for nursing and midwifery in 1995, when it introduced the portfolio as a means for registered nurses and midwives to demonstrate that they had met the UKCC's requirement for a minimum of 5 days of updating.

Portfolios were initially introduced as a statutory requirement and the UKCC could demand to see them at the point of re-registration. Writing at the time, Hull and Redfern (1996) predicted that portfolios were therefore set to 'become an integral part of professional behaviour', and noted the rapidly increasing market in professionally produced portfolios, many of which were little more than binders (hence emphasizing the definition of a portfolio as the folder in which the documents were kept rather than the documents themselves). However, the statutory requirement for nurses and midwives to keep and submit a portfolio ended when the UKCC was replaced in 2002 by the Nursing and Midwifery Council (NMC), and the requirement to submit a portfolio was replaced with a requirement to fill in a form asking for 'a brief description of the CPD [continuing professional development] they have undertaken and its relevance to their work' (Hull *et al.* 2005). However, Hull *et al.* remained hopeful that the portfolio would continue to be an integral part of professional behaviour and pointed out that 'without a Personal Professional Portfolio with clear records of CPD activities to refer back to, the task would be far more difficult!' (Hull *et al.* 2005, p. 3). Despite the positive gloss given to portfolios, it is difficult to escape the implication here that their primary function is as a retrospective record of educational and professional activity kept primarily for the purpose of remaining on the active register of nurses and midwives. In fact, this retrospective documentary nature of portfolios was being emphasized even before they ceased to be a statutory requirement for re-registration, and features in many definitions from the time. So, for example, Brown (1995), Redfern (1998) and Snadden and Thomas (1998) each describe a portfolio in more or less identical words as the collection of evidence that learning has taken place.

Jasper (2006) appears at first to agree with this definition of a portfolio when she writes that 'A portfolio, when used in a professional context, is simply a collection of documents that present a picture of the practitioner. It is like a photo album, but in word, not visual, pictures'. If this were indeed the case, then the purpose and motivation for keeping a portfolio would be extremely limited and would hardly merit a chapter in a textbook. However, Jasper (2006) swiftly corrects herself and 'moves the concept of a portfolio on from being a recording device, to one of activity and interaction used on a continuous basis throughout a practitioner's life'. This view is in keeping with her earlier work undertaken for the ENB shortly before it was disbanded (Webb *et al.* 2003). That paper took as its starting point the definition of portfolios offered by McMullan *et al.* (2003) as:

> *A collection of evidence, usually in written form, of both the products and processes of learning. It attests to achievement and personal and professional development, by providing critical analysis of its content.*

> *(McMullan* et al. *2003, p. 288)*

That definition develops from being merely a collection of evidence for prior learning to including a critical analysis of that content. In other words, it provides the opportunity for *ongoing* learning through critical reflective writing – the concept of a portfolio.

Principles for practice

- Portfolios are now recognized as a tool for professional and personal development.
- Portfolios provide opportunities to reflect analytically and write critically.

The purpose of the portfolio

Although Webb and colleagues had been commissioned by the ENB to examine certain educational aspects of portfolios, most writers acknowledge that many of the issues relating to formal post-qualifying education apply equally to the sphere of informal professional development. For example, Neades (2003) suggests that portfolios have three major roles to play in post-qualifying education. First, they resonate with the aims of adult education insofar as they promote self-directed learning from previous experience of real-life problems. Second, Neades regards portfolios as a means of bringing theory and practice closer together and of facilitating practice development. And, third, she claims that 'the production of a portfolio can facilitate the development of reflective learning skills allowing the practitioner to learn from experience and clinical practice' (Neades 2003). Now clearly, these educational issues which portfolios are seen to address are also issues of concern to *all* qualified nurses, regardless of whether they are formally enrolled on an educational course. Thus, although portfolios have a role to play at all stages of a student's progression through a course of study and can be used variously as a means of gaining access to a course, of being exempted from some elements of it, as a tool for learning and as a means of assessment, they are also arguably of benefit to all registered nurses, not only as a record of their continuing professional development (CPD), but more importantly as an ongoing part of it. As Webb *et al.* (2003) point out, 'the value of the portfolio lies in the nature of the process, rather than the end product per se'.

This shift in the focus and purpose of portfolios has not been without difficulties. Assessment of post-registration nursing courses has traditionally been undertaken through prescriptive and highly structured written assignments, and the shift to a portfolio-based system has demanded far greater autonomy and accountability from the students, who are expected to play a leading role in identifying their own learning needs, outcomes and development in relation to the objectives or competencies set by the course or regulatory body (Knowles 1990; Endacott *et al.* 2004; Scholes *et al.* 2004; Joyce 2005). This in turn should provide the foundations for lifelong learning and continued use of the portfolio to demonstrate development in a number of personal and professional areas (Endacott *et al.* 2004; Jasper 2006; Nursing and Midwifery Council 2008c).

However, the guidance offered by the NMC for post-registration children's nurses fails to emphasize these active developmental aspects of the portfolio, and following the NMC (2008c) guidelines would potentially result in a portfolio which is little more than a collection of incidents, descriptions of events and the learning which occurred. It would appear that the vital reflective component highlighted by many writers is not emphasized strongly enough, and the requirement to demonstrate the use of underpinning knowledge through reflective writing is not apparent. A portfolio that adheres to the NMC guidelines may not develop in such a way as to demonstrate a progression and maturation of learning and an appreciation of the nuances of practice which is its primary aim (Bowers and Jinks 2004; Joyce 2005; Jasper 2006). Thus, it is anticipated that portfolios will vary significantly and substantially in quality between practitioners, where some will demonstrate reflective practice and others merely describe incidents, resulting in discrepancies and variations in the standard of knowledge acquisition and utilization by registered nurses. It can be argued that the current regulatory requirements encourage the production of a portfolio which is a collection of artefacts with little guidance on how the practitioner might develop it further.

Principles for practice

- Portfolios allow the practitioner to learn from experience.
- Portfolios 'recognize' the individual nature of the learner/practitioner's experience and have the flexibility to reflect this in their construction.

Portfolio construction

Reflection points

★ Do you keep a portfolio?

★ What is in the portfolio?

★ How is it arranged?

★ What criteria did you use to organize your portfolio?

Clearly, the purpose for which the portfolio is kept will have an influence on the way that it is structured. If the portfolio is seen merely as a way of recording prior learning, and if there is no requirement to reflect on or integrate that learning, then there is a danger of producing a 'shopping trolley' or 'toast rack' portfolio rather than a 'spinal column' or 'cake mix' (Endacott *et al.* 2004), as set out in Box 13.1. This can give rise to tension and confusion in relation to structure. At post-registration level the portfolio is designed to be flexible, individual and creative, and thus no particular structure is prescribed. The student is free to design the portfolio to meet his or her own professional needs and experiences (Jasper 2006), but with this freedom comes a number of problems.

First, many nurses may have previously been assessed traditionally through structured essays and may be novices in portfolio construction. Although being capable of studying, thinking and practising at post-registration or Masters level, they may struggle to produce the requisite 'cake mix' portfolio which demands well-developed self-directed learning skills, including the ability to diagnose their learning needs in light of performance standards, formulate meaningful goals, diagnose and monitor their own performance, and identify resources and learning strategies appropriate to the competency and knowledge required (Kicken *et al.* 2009).

Second, some students have great difficulty in fulfilling the requirement to determine the structure and the content of their portfolios. The lack of structure becomes frustrating and disorienting as students struggle to find direction (Bowers and Jinks 2004). The portfolio must have some 'structure' or framework in order to

Box 13.1	Portfolio models

- Shopping trolley
  — Collection of items
  — Repository of artefacts
  — Chosen by student
  — Little attempt to link evidence to outcomes/competencies
  — Reflective accounts stand alone

- Toast rack
  — Discrete elements assessing theory and practice
  — Placed into separate sections of a binder, e.g. skills log, competencies, reflective accounts
  — Reflective accounts stand alone, not integrated with other elements
  — Different people participate in the assessment

- Spinal column
  — Structured around practice competencies/learning outcomes

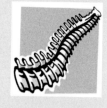

  — Evidence slotted in to demonstrate each competency
  — Reflective accounts consider more than one competency
  — Explicit evidence of learning and competence
  — Multiple pieces of evidence for overarching competencies
  — Emphasis on original work

- Cake mix
  — Evidence from theory and practice integrated into portfolio

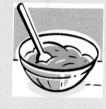

  — Overarching narrative
  — Reflective commentary
  — Demonstrates critical and analytical skills
  — Reflectivity, practice and professional development are features

(Endacott et al. *2004)*

understand what is to be assessed, and Kicken *et al.* (2009) point out that if the student does not know what knowledge they lack then it is difficult to identify what needs to be known. Conversely, if the structure of the portfolio is too prescriptive it may cause negativity in the nurse, who may feel it to be restrictive and stifling of creativity (Nairn *et al.* 2006). In addition, there is a danger that the portfolio could be assessment driven and focus on the submission of work by specified deadlines, i.e. it could become product rather than process led (Scholes *et al.* 2004; Joyce 2005), in which case the richness and potency of the portfolio as a developmental learning tool may be lost. As Scholes *et al.* (2004) argue, the portfolio then becomes an intellectual exercise geared more towards prescribed activities rather than facilitating a critical analysis of practice. This may result in a loss of identity and ownership of the portfolio as it is tailored to suit the needs of the course and practice assessor rather than those of the writer (Endacott *et al.* 2004; Scholes *et al.* 2004).

Research evidence tends to support these concerns. Nairn *et al.* (2006) found final-year student nurses in their study were unsure about the structure and the purpose of the portfolio and were less optimistic about its use than first-year students. They were also sceptical about its importance as an aid to communicate learning, but felt that it did provide a cathartic function by enabling feelings and difficult experiences to be explored. Likewise, McMullan (2006) found that ongoing support and guidance is required to facilitate the development of the portfolio and reflective and critical-thinking skills. However, such support and guidance should not be at the cost of relevance, creativity, personal identity and ownership (Bowers and Jinks 2004; Endacott *et al.* 2004; Jasper 2006; Nairn *et al.* 2006). While these studies focus on pre-registration students, the arguments can be extrapolated to post-registration children's nurses who are compiling portfolios either as part of a formal course or informally to provide evidence to ensure re-registration occurs (Nursing and Midwifery Council 2008b,c).

Principles for practice

- Portfolios do not have a prescribed structure, thus support may be needed to construct one.
- Portfolios follow one of four models; the 'cake mix' portfolio is the hallmark of an analytical, critical learner/practitioner.

Controversies in portfolio development

It can be seen that, although portfolio writing can be a powerful method of facilitating and recording learning, it is not without its critics. Several writers have raised concerns about the usefulness of portfolios in both educational and CPD settings as the means both to develop practice and to assess and evaluate educational or practice developments. Gannon *et al.* (2001) point out that portfolios are used not only to identify and record *theoretical* learning, but also as a means of critically evaluating and assessing *clinical* competence. They identify a number of reasons why the educational assessment of clinical competence in pre- and post-qualifying students is 'inherently problematic', and many of their concerns apply equally to situations in which the portfolio is being used primarily as a 'reflective diary' for personal CPD reasons.

Gannon *et al.* (2001) point out that there is a great deal of confusion and leeway over terminology, particularly concerning the terms 'portfolio' and 'profile', leading to problems of standardization if portfolios are to be used as assessment instruments. However, although it is true that the terms were used more or less interchangeably during the 1990s, 'portfolio' is now the standard term used in nurse education to describe an assignment which involves a critical reflection on a collection of documents. Nevertheless, Gannon *et al.* (2001) are correct insofar as a lack of standardization with regard to portfolios remains an issue, and a number of disagreements about the structure, content and purpose of portfolios have already been discussed. However, as Snadden and Thomas (1998) point out, the question of whether the portfolio is primarily a developmental tool (formative), an assessment tool (summative) or both is particularly problematic, and lies at the root of a number of fundamental concerns about the use of portfolios, particularly in relation to honesty and confidentiality (Gerrish 1993; Gannon *et al.* 2001).

Honesty

Reflection points

★ Are you truly honest in your reflective writing?

★ Do you write for yourself (privately) or with an audience in mind (publicly)?

★ Think about your answers and the impact on your learning and clinical practice.

It can be argued that if nurses do not write about practice in an insightful, incisive manner then children and young people's nursing practice specifically and nursing practice generally will not develop in an innovative, dynamic way. Children and young people's nurses need to scrutinize what they do in order to identify innovative practice personally and on a wider professional level to ensure their own CPD, career progression and the development of services and care delivery to the most vulnerable members of society – children and young people (Storey and Haigh 2002; Department of Health 2004a; Welsh Assembly Government 2004, 2005, 2009).

This requires honesty and the confidence to confront those elements of practice and knowledge deficits which make practitioners feel uncomfortable. While positive incidents do facilitate learning, it is often the 'negative' events which provide the richest learning experience and the opportunity to reflect at a deeper level (Harris *et al.* 2001; McMullan 2006). Children's nursing practitioners may begin to question their values and beliefs concerning children's nursing when events or actions appear to conflict with those values. Thus, such scrutiny may result in a changed perspective and the development of new practice and new ways of using knowledge.

If the purpose of the portfolio is primarily as a personal means for the writer to explore her/his own practice through a process of critical reflection, then an honest examination of practice is relatively unproblematic. In other words, if the practitioner is writing solely for his or her own benefit and no other eyes are likely to see the contents of the portfolio, then the writer will have no cause to elaborate or fabricate what is being recorded and reflected on. However, in cases in which the portfolio is used for assessment purposes, students often feel threatened about expressing their innermost thoughts and feelings and are reluctant and uncertain about engaging in self-reflection (McMullan 2006; Byrne *et al.* 2007), in some cases feeling that the portfolio was an 'invasion of privacy'. Thus, they write for a perceived audience, the assessor, according to their perception of what they think the assessor should read (Scholes *et al.* 2004; McMullan 2006; Byrne *et al.* 2007). As Gannon *et al.* (2001) point out:

> *there may be an inverse relationship between the use of portfolios in the assessment process and the honesty of the records which the keeper of the portfolio may maintain.*
>
> *(Gannon et al. 2001, p. 536)*

In other words, the pressure on a student to pass a portfolio-based assignment might well compromise the honesty of the account.

McMullan (2006) found that students expressed this concern that they could not be truly honest and critical in their writing if anyone in authority or power was likely to see the portfolio. This creates a paradox. The portfolio is a means to develop knowledge and practice that requires honesty with oneself, but as an assessment and learning tool it also requires facilitation by a mentor. However, the very fact that the mentor is also a tutor and assessor places them in a position of covert or explicit authority and power, which in turn leads the student to censor their own writing in order to avoid criticism and the exposure of practices and private thoughts (Gannon *et al.* 2001; Dolan *et al.* 2004; McMullan 2006; Timmins and Dunne 2009).

Principles for practice

- Portfolios enable the practitioner to illuminate practice and should be honest in their analysis.
- Avoid writing for an audience – write for yourself.

Confidentiality

Reflection points

★ Who has access to your portfolio?

★ Where is the information stored?

★ How do you ensure the confidentiality of your portfolio?

One possible solution to this problem is to offer the writer a promise of confidentiality by restricting the readership of the portfolio to a few selected internal markers. If writers are not assured of confidentiality regarding the portfolio's contents, then it becomes flawed as an assessment tool (McMullan 2006; Dolan *et al.* 2004). Summative assessment could lead to a reduced sense of ownership and compromise its use as a developmental tool. We have seen that the knowledge that the work will be seen by a number of assessors can stifle thinking and writing as the author begins to analyse which information should be disclosed to specific people and which remains hidden from scrutiny. The spectre of censorship is apparent at this juncture. Censorship leads to impoverished reflective writing as key elements are omitted for fear of exposing poor practice and other ethical concerns. However, although a confidential approach might perhaps increase the likelihood of an honest account,

Johns (1999) pointed out that, even when writing for no one's eyes except our own, there is a still a (sometimes subconscious) tendency to elaborate on or refrain from the truth in order to protect our own self-esteem.

However, the issue of confidentiality has to be considered not only from the writer's perspective but also from that of the people being written about. The NMC Code of Conduct (2008b) states:

> *You must respect people's right to confidentiality; you must ensure people are informed about how and why information is shared by those who will be providing their care; you must disclose information if you believe someone may be at risk of harm, in line with the law of the country in which you are practising.*

(*Nursing and Midwifery Council 2008b*)

It can be argued that the use of reflective writing and its presentation within the portfolio compromises this standard as soon as the portfolio is submitted for examination or scrutiny by a third party. Despite making material anonymous, patient information and that of working colleagues is presented for assessment without their knowledge or consent. Such issues need to be addressed in order to maintain the integrity of working relationships with colleagues and patients, who should retain consent over the disclosure of information involving their practice, particularly where poor practice is highlighted (Timmins and Dunne 2009). The evidence shows that practitioners are reluctant to disclose or write about poor practice, preferring to reflect on positive incidents of care. Thus, practitioners have to consider carefully what they are prepared to make public and what they wish to keep private (Bowers and Jinks 2004; Endacott *et al.* 2004; Joyce 2005).

The children's nursing world is small and confined, and therefore incidents, locations and patients themselves may be easily recognizable despite the best attempts to conceal identities. As a result, the practitioner is presented with a conundrum: they need to reflect to learn from the incident, a private activity; yet they are also expected to produce written reflections to demonstrate learning and the development of practice, a public activity. This could lead to the development of parallel portfolios to avoid compromising confidentiality, and in turn result in two separate arenas of learning. 'Real' learning could be restricted to the private portfolio, whereas the public portfolio might result in 'public learning' led by the assessment process, which then becomes an intellectual activity rather than a scrutiny of the key personal and practice-led issues (Scholes *et al.* 2004; Nairn *et al.* 2006).

Principles for practice

- Confidentiality must be maintained and must not be compromised in the reflective writing.
- Access to the portfolio must be controlled by the learner.

PART 4

Stakeholder interest/control of learning through portfolio use

Reflection points

★ Who/what shapes your learning – your needs, the patient's needs, the organization's needs?

★ Is this reflected in your portfolio?

We have seen that portfolios should be personal and concerned with the personal learning which the children's nurse needs to undertake. However, there is an issue of social control and monitoring of learning by the stakeholder who funds the CPD. Nurses are under an obligation to constantly refine their developmental learning, critical thinking and delivery of care commensurate with their experience and level of expertise (Nursing and Midwifery Council 2008a–c). However, as the NHS evolves, nurses may find themselves undertaking education and training which is shaped by the organization rather than their own professional needs and the needs of the children and families in their care. The learning may be shaped by local organizational policy and the need to standardize roles, particularly at advanced levels (Bowers and Jinks 2004; Department of Health 2008a; Welsh Assembly Government 2009). The document *A High Quality Workforce* (Department of Health 2008b) sets out to improve access to funding for education to support diverse educational experiences designed to promote CPD. It has been suggested that nurses now have the opportunity to hold their employers to account if they do not deliver or invest in their education (Tweddell 2008). This demands a strong personal and political voice as well as a sense of 'personal advocacy' that continued professional and personal development will have an impact on the delivery of care.

However, this can be a reciprocal arrangement, with employers also holding staff to account to ensure that learning is occurring and practice is being enhanced. Indeed, the Knowledge and Skill Framework (KSF) (Department of Health 2004b,c) proposes to do exactly this via personal reviews which assess how an individual applies his or her knowledge and skills in practice (see below). The portfolio may be used as a means to assess and monitor this learning from both the employee's and employer's perspective. If the funding is provided then the employer may feel obliged to ensure 'value for money', monitoring the quality of the learning and development by accessing the portfolio, especially if the educational programme is provided in-house. This would replicate to some degree what currently happens within educational settings, where the mentor/facilitator/lecturer accesses and assesses the portfolio for the learning which has occurred, with its inherent problems concerning confidentiality, honesty and other ethical issues (Garrett and Jackson 2006).

Indeed, it could be argued that such a use of portfolios may be seen as a means by which to monitor practice and the quality of the care delivered. If nursing is perceived as involving the six core elements as identified by Maben and Griffiths (2008), including evidence-based practice, then it is logical that the employer will require evidence that this is occurring on a personal as well as a collegiate level. This would seem to suggest social control of learning, which is an insidious process that would stifle the creativity and dynamism inherent in children's nursing practice. It would also stifle the creativity and diversity to be found in the personal portfolio (Bowers and Jinks 2004; Endacott *et al.* 2004; Jasper 2006; Byrne *et al.* 2007).

Conversely, the portfolio may be used to demonstrate career development, critical-thinking skills, evidence-based practice and professional maturity at the annual professional review. The KSF underpins Agenda For Change and as the Department of Health notes:

> *Defines and describes the knowledge and skills which NHS staff need to apply in their work in order to deliver quality services. It provides a single, consistent, comprehensive and explicit framework on which to base review and development for all staff.*

> *(Department of Health 2004c)*

The KSF aims to facilitate the development of services which meet the needs of the public through investing in staff development. This is to be achieved by supporting individual members of staff and teams to learn and develop throughout their careers so that they can work effectively. The KSF states that all staff should have access to the same structured opportunities for learning, development and review (Department of Health 2004b,c). It is a broad, generic framework which focuses on the application of knowledge and skills to practice; it does not articulate the specific knowledge or skills that are required to undertake the role. It proposes that specific standards and competencies would need to be developed. The review process focuses on how the individual applies his or her knowledge and skills to their post, developing a personal development plan, engaging in learning and development, and evaluating and reflecting on the application of the learning to practice (Department of Health 2004b,c). The KSF sets gateways for development and career progression. Thus, the use of the portfolio is invaluable within this situation in which individual learning and development can be clearly shown and in which the maturation of the professional over time could be demonstrated to support their career aspirations and role development. This is particularly effective within the current economic climate, when financially it may not be practical to release staff from busy units onto 'expensive' courses. The portfolio is a vehicle by which children and young people's nurses can demonstrate their professional learning and development not only to satisfy the requirements for ongoing registration but also to illustrate the completion of their developmental objectives at their professional review as part of their ongoing career development. This is also beneficial to the employer, who can verify whether nurses are developing appropriately and whether their investment in educating staff is returned. The KSF focuses on what is done rather than on what staff know and can bring to the role personally. The caveat to this should be that there must be a holistic approach to the delivery of care and professional development and not one based solely on the acquisition of skills and competencies. This would lead to a reductionist approach at a time when children and young people's nursing and nursing generally are striving to exhibit a holistic approach to service development and care delivery to children and families (Storey and Haigh 2002).

Principles for practice

- Portfolios can be used to demonstrate current and future learning needs and the impact on practice and care delivery.
- Portfolios demonstrate evidence of ongoing CPD to the employer, mentor, tutor, and NMC.
- Portfolios can demonstrate competence and progression of learning, knowledge and skills to meet requirements of the KSF.

Validity and reliability

Gannon *et al.* (2001) have pointed out that the above issues and concerns, when taken together, constitute a threat to the validity and reliability of portfolios, particularly when they are being used as a method of course assessment. This concern has been shared by a number of writers, including Mallik (1993), Fergusson and Jinks (1994), Allmark (1995), Gerrish *et al.* (1997), Martin *et al.* (1997), Pitts *et al.* (1999), Calman *et al.* (2002) and Webb *et al.* (2003). However, whereas Gannon *et al.* (2001) complained about 'a paucity of literature on the use of portfolios in nursing' and suggested that there is 'a considerable amount of research waiting to be carried out into their use and utility', Webb *et al.* (2003), writing 2 years later, claimed that:

> *issues of validity and reliability in the assessment of student nurse clinical competence using portfolios have been discussed widely in the literature in the UK, USA and Australia.*

(Webb et al. *2003, p. 602)*

A full review of the literature relating to these issues up to 2001 can be found in McMullan *et al.* (2003).

As Gannon *et al.* (2001) point out, the question of the validity and reliability of portfolios, and thus of their use and utility, is to some extent dependent on how we define a portfolio. In particular, if a portfolio is seen purely as a collection of factual information and evidence, then it is a fairly straightforward process to establish its validity and reliability, whereas measuring the extent to which learning and reflection has taken place is rather more complex and complicated. However, as Webb *et al.* (2003) add, it also depends on what is understood by validity and reliability in the context of portfolio assessment. Gannon *et al.* (2001) use quantitative definitions directly from a nursing research text (Polit and Hungler 1995), and point out that, although a method of assessment 'proven to be reliable and valid in the traditional, numerical sense' might not be valued by those from the qualitative tradition, nevertheless we have to start somewhere in order to avoid inaction. Nevertheless, Pitts *et al.* (1999) warn against taking an overly technical–rational approach to portfolio assessment and warn that 'traditional' approaches to assessing portfolios are likely to prove inappropriate. Similarly, Webb *et al.* (2003) point out that many 'traditional' measures of validity and reliability, such as test–retest reliability, are not only inappropriate but practically impossible. In their place, Webb *et al.* (2003) suggest certain qualitative measures of rigour such as credibility, transferability, dependability and confirmability, based on the work of Guba and

Lincoln (1985, 1989). When applied to the assessment of portfolios, these criteria translate into the need for a wide variety of sources and types of evidence that learning has taken place, clear criteria for what constitutes a pass at different academic levels, and the need for consensus based on 'tripartite meetings' between the student, representatives from practice and representatives from the academic setting. Final decisions regarding the worth of the assignment should be based on 'a consensus judgement about the evidence in a portfolio' (Webb *et al.* 2003).

However, when portfolios are used as a means of informal continual professional or practice development, or even when they are used as a formative rather than a summative course assignment, the issues are somewhat different. For example, if the purpose of the portfolio is exclusively as a tool for enhancing personal learning from and for practice, then issues about internal and external generalizability or transferability are no longer of concern, along with the debate about who has a right or an obligation to view the portfolio. Furthermore, questions of credibility, dependability and confirmability, which all relate to whether 'data sources are identified and described accurately' (Webb *et al.* 2003), take on a somewhat different complexion. In particular, we need to question whether 'accuracy' is a relevant issue when portfolios are divorced from any requirement to present 'evidence' that learning has taken place. It could be argued, for example, that as much self-discovery and exploration of practice can occur through writing an account of a fictional event than from something that actually happened (see, for example, Rolfe 2005). The question to be asked of a portfolio kept for personal developmental reasons might be 'what has been learnt from this writing?' rather than 'how can we ensure the validity and reliability of the portfolio entries?' Once the focus shifts from the *content* of the portfolio to the *process* of writing it, then we could reasonably argue that the only person capable of providing an answer to the question is the writer her/himself. That is not to say, however, that the writer can never be deceived about the learning that is believed to have taken place; it is still possible to fool ourselves that we have learnt something when we have not, or to appear to have learnt something that is not actually true.

Further work is therefore required if portfolio use is to be appropriate and ultimately useful in practitioners' development. Portfolio use is in its infancy in nursing compared with other professions, and further research and refinement must take place if its future is to be assured (McMullan 2006; Timmins and Dunne 2009).

Key points

- Validity and reliability are recurrent issues in assessing the portfolio quality.
- Quantitative assessment of validity and reliability is not appropriate. Qualitative measures are more appropriate as they capture the richness of the portfolio entries.

Moving forward: the use of portfolios in children's nursing

We have seen that there are a number of issues that still need to be addressed in relation to the use of portfolios in nursing generally, and children and young people's nursing in particular. However, we have also suggested that portfolios can be a very powerful means of developing the learning and practice of individual nurses and the profession in general. We will now turn our attention to some of the positive uses of portfolios and explore some recent innovations in portfolio development.

There is a shortage of literature relating to the use of portfolios in children and young people's nursing. The available research relates very generally to nursing across all fields of practice, and thus principles have to be extrapolated in order to illuminate their use within children and young people's nursing practice and education. The claims made for portfolios relate to the demonstration of personal knowledge, developmental learning and competence which can be related directly to the development of practice, knowledge and critical thinking within children's nursing. Children and young people's nursing has its own specific body of knowledge and competencies associated with caring for a diverse group of children, young people and families from birth to 18 years of age and up to the early twenties (Casey 1993; Nursing and Midwifery Council 2008a,d). As identified throughout this book, children and young people's nursing covers a vast range of care situations from caring for the well child in the community (school nurses, health visitors), to sick children with complex needs who require continuing care at home or in hospice settings, acutely ill children cared for in the community, through to the sick child and young person requiring acute care within the diverse settings in hospital (Casey 1993; Department of Health 2004a; Welsh Assembly Government 2005). Children and young people's nurses, like all nurses, have a professional obligation to remain updated, to develop practice and to develop critical-thinking skills to analyse the evidence on which care is based (Welsh Assembly Government 2004; Nursing and Midwifery Council 2008b–d). The portfolio enables the practitioner to demonstrate the specific knowledge, skills and attitudes required to work with children and young people in diverse settings while engaging in reflective practice to maintain learning, develop insight and promote the development of the practice of children and young people's nursing (Welsh Assembly Government 2004; Nursing and Midwifery Council 2008a).

Portfolios and career development

Reflection points

★ Think about your career – where do you see yourself in 5 years' time?

★ How will you demonstrate your competence to follow that career pathway?

★ Will you collect evidence or use a portfolio (effectively) with reflective writing to demonstrate progression of learning, thinking and suitability for the career pathway?

Accessing specific child-oriented courses may be difficult for many reasons. The number of specific courses may be limited and based away from the workplace at a centre of learning, requiring prolonged periods of time away from practice, thus depleting staffing numbers. Because of the specialist nature of practice and the requirement for children and young people's nurses to hold specific qualifications

(Department of Health 1991; Nursing and Midwifery Council 2008a, 2010) arranging cover may be difficult, despite the NMC's requirement that from 2011 with the introduction of new educational standards and practice competencies all graduate nurses should be able to meet the essential needs of all client groups. Ultimately children and young people have a right to access and be nursed by appropriately qualified children and young people's nurses. Also, any courses that are available locally may be generic in nature. It is at this point that the portfolio proves invaluable as a tool to demonstrate the specific knowledge and practice focus that children and young people's nurses possess. The portfolio enables children's nurses to structure their learning either formally (course led) or as part of their CPD requirements for registration purposes, and to illustrate clearly the development of their practice and the application of children and young people's nursing knowledge to children and young people's practice (Welsh Assembly Government 2004; Nursing and Midwifery Council 2008a). The portfolio allows flexibility to meet the demands of the children and young people's nurses' situation academically and professionally. This flexibility meets the needs of practitioners working within diverse areas and allows for the portfolio to be eclectic in nature to reflect the often complex multidisciplinary care situations that children's nurses work in. It enables children and young people's nurses to explore their own professional values and ethics when working with children, young people and their families, and also enables them to explore issues such as multidisciplinarity, which requires integrated working, collegiate relationships and a deep appreciation of all practitioner roles, which implies that professional boundaries need to be flexible and open (Department of Health 2004a–c; Welsh Assembly Government 2005; Nursing and Midwifery Council 2008a,d).

This also has implications for the career development of children and young people's nurses. The *Post Registration Career Frameworks for Nurses in Wales* (Welsh Assembly Government 2009) and *Towards a Framework for Post Registration Nursing Careers* (Department of Health 2008a) have specified the need for distinct career pathways through which nurses may progress. This will require educational initiatives to meet the demands of the children and young people's nurses as they progress through the levels and create career pathways commensurate with their professional reviews. This is an optimum time to engage with portfolios to demonstrate development of learning, competency and critical thinking as each children and young people's nurse meets the personal objectives set within the review (Department of Health 2004b,c, 2008a; Welsh Assembly Government 2004, 2009). The frameworks demand that educational opportunities are provided and that these initiatives are flexible enough to meet the ever-changing healthcare situation. The individual practitioner's aspirations must also be accounted for within these initiatives, as some may wish to remain generalist children and young people's nurses while others may progress towards specialist areas and then on to advanced practice and beyond (Department of Health 2004b,c, 2008a; Welsh Assembly Government 2009). The frameworks, if implemented, clearly steer the development of a focused and robust career pathway within children and young people's nursing. Thus education must be flexible and rigorous enough to meet the practitioners' needs (Centre for the Development of Health Care Policy and Practice 2008).

Portfolios are an excellent medium for children and young people's nurses to develop their critical thinking, competencies and to engage in reflective writing to consolidate and demonstrate their learning and development. They provide the perfect way to illustrate and talk about the specific and specialist knowledge and competencies required to work with children, young people and families. They also provide a way to explore the care of children and young people with whom the children and young people's nurse may have had little previous experience. For example, this is pertinent to the care of children and young people with mental health problems who are encountered in settings and via routes not traditionally associated with mental health problems (Royal College of Nursing 2004a; Department for Children, Schools and Families and Department of Health 2008, 2009). Nurses are reluctant to engage with these children and young people as they feel they lack knowledge to underpin practice, confidence and skills (as discussed in Chapters 10 and 11). They feel overwhelmed by the number and complexity of problems of the children and young people they care for (Watson 2006; Wilson *et al.* 2007). The portfolio is perfect for detailing the learning journey at this point. It provides a flexible medium for practitioners to acquire knowledge, to reflect on their personal issues and professional responsibilities, while exploring the wider clinical perspective in relation to multidisciplinary liaison and working practices. Thus, the portfolio provides an excellent opportunity for personal learning objectives and opportunities to be identified and for the children and young people's nurse to study, reflect and develop competency in the care of this client group (Jasper 2006; Department for Children, Schools and Families and Department of Health 2008; Department of Health 2009; Welsh Assembly Government 2009).

The portfolio should demonstrate a maturity in its composition as the nurse's career progresses and his or her learning matures. The presentation of the portfolio should mirror this progression, providing an authentic evaluation of the personal and professional domains of practice (Rassin *et al.* 2006) until, at advanced practitioner level, the 'cake mix' model is evident and the criteria for assessment are clearly mapped to enable the clarity and maturity of thinking and practice to be apparent (Jasper and Fulton 2005).

Principles for practice

- Portfolios can be used by children and young people's nurses to map and support their career development in their chosen specialty.
- Portfolios can enable children and young people's nurses to reflect and analyse their practice in relation to children and young people with whom they have limited experience.

Reflection points

★ Is the portfolio a tool for learning or can it be used in a wider context to discuss nursing issues?

★ What is happening politically in your field of practice?

★ Could the use of a portfolio be beneficial in demonstrating your area of expertise?

Politically, the portfolio provides a voice for children and young people's nursing to demonstrate the value and importance of its speciality and the rights of the child and family to be cared for by appropriately educated, knowledgeable, skilled professional children and young people's nurses. Despite copious reports and recommendations spanning 50 years which state this point succinctly, the generalist agenda remains a threat (Ministry of Health 1959; Department of Health 1991, 2004a, 2008a; Davies 2008, 2010). Indeed, the NMC (2009) has reviewed and held a consultation on the pre-registration nursing education programme, curriculum and competencies following the publication of policy which highlighted the rapidly changing delivery of healthcare and the requirement for nursing to meet these challenges (Department of Health 2004a, 2006, 2008b; Welsh Assembly Government 2009). This consultation has resulted in the recent publication of the Standards for pre-registration nursing education, which were published in September 2010 (NMC 2010). The ethos of the standards is that all nurses should possess generic and specific competencies so that all nurses have some skills in caring for the essential needs of all client groups (NMC 2010). It could be suggested that this represents a hidden move towards generalism which children and young people's nurses must resist. Certainly, economically and managerially, a generically competent workforce is cheaper, flexible and more easily moved. However, this can be refuted on the grounds that it is not safe, that it conflicts with the ethos of children and young people's nursing and the right to access appropriate and safe healthcare. It contravenes the rights of children and young people to be valued as a specific and special client group (Welsh Assembly Government 2005; Department of Health 2004a). Subsequently it is not safe or effective to disband children and young people's nursing as a specialist branch, and research is available to demonstrate that children's nurses are cost-effective and that, when children and young people are nursed by appropriately qualified nurses, the clinical outcomes are better and hospital stay is shorter (Welsh Assembly Government 2005; Department of Health 2004a). This is also true of other clinical situations in which experienced qualified children and young people's nurses have a direct impact on the quality of care and recovery of the children, e.g. community children's nursing (Royal College of Nursing 2004b).

Portfolios can offer a voice for children and young people's nurses to resist the dangerous rise of generalism both personally and professionally. The personal portfolio can be used as a vehicle to demonstrate not only personal learning and development but also the political and interdisciplinary issues affecting the delivery of care to children, young people and their families (Jasper 2006; Byrne *et al.* 2007). Professionally, the portfolio can again be used to demonstrate the need for specialist nurses to care for this special group of patients and can be done using personal portfolios and departmental portfolios. This is applicable for all levels of children and young people's nurses but can be particularly effective in developing the critical thinking and integration of research and practice at advanced practice level. Portfolios could highlight areas for scholarly discussion, resulting in research, policy production and publication (Welsh Assembly Government 2004; Rassin *et al.* 2006).

Principles for practice

- Portfolios enable children and young people's nurses to demonstrate their value as a distinct branch of the family of nursing and to refute the move towards generic approaches to nursing.
- Portfolios give a voice to children and young people's nurses to articulate the key issues which affect children and young people's nursing.

Departmental/team portfolios

Reflection points

★ Once you have read the section below, think about your ward/department/team.

★ How would you encourage practitioners to contribute to a ward/team/departmental portfolio?

★ What would be the aims of such a portfolio in your workplace?

★ What would you include in a ward/departmental/team portfolio?

Rassin *et al.* (2006) argue that, although personal portfolios have personal benefits, the use of the portfolio could be broadened to a departmental or team level. They suggest that a departmental portfolio can be used as a managerial and evaluation tool of all activity in the department. They hypothesize that it provides insight into the team's development and achievements over time and can thus identity future goals and provide evidence of good clinical governance (Department of Health 2006, 2008a; Rassin *et al.* 2006; Welsh Assembly Government 2009). It can also be concluded from this that research could be identified and pursued, thus giving the team the opportunity to research and develop its own practice initiatives.

Departmental portfolios can be used as a collective tool to gather data, educate, evaluate functions of the department, consolidate staff knowledge and aspirations and also provide evidence of good practice. They can highlight areas where practice, research, service development, staff development and others require further work. The portfolio would provide opportunities for staff to reflect and self-evaluate their practice (Rassin *et al.* 2006). This would provide a prime initiative to develop a portfolio which contains clear, convincing reflections on the practice of children and young people's nursing, demonstrating the required practice knowledge and competencies and providing ongoing evaluation of the development of the nursing and multidisciplinary team in terms of care delivery, research opportunities and the evidence base underpinning personal and professional practice.

A departmental portfolio would provide educational opportunities for non-children and young people's nurses to access information, education and insights into the value of this specialty. Extrapolating the issues raised within educational research, it can be clearly seen that the use of a departmental portfolio would highlight the scholarship of children and young people's nursing practice with regard to practice development, critical-thinking skills, reflective skills and the use of evidence to underpin actual practice (McClellan Reece *et al.* 2001; Corry and

Timmins 2009). The departmental portfolio would build into a body of evidence to illustrate the currency and value of children and young people's nursing not just within discrete departments but also wherever children and young people are nursed and require the input of a children and young people's nurse on a 'consultancy' basis (Department of Health 1991, 2004a; Welsh Assembly Government 2005). This would act as a political voice for children and young people's nursing, children's nurses and the multidisciplinary team in putting forward convincing arguments for the value of their specialty and providing evidence refuting the move towards generalism.

Principle for practice

- Departmental portfolios provide a platform to:
  — illuminate the knowledge, skills, intricacies and nuances of children and young people's nursing
  — demonstrate scholarship within the children and young people's nursing team
  — educate non-children and young people's nursing and other professionals about the needs of children, young people and their families and the value of children and young people's nurses in terms of knowledge, research, policy and scholarship.

E-portfolios

Case study

Jayne is a children and young people's nurse and wishes to undertake a Masters degree in advanced clinical practice. Jayne is working at a hospital 50 miles from the university and cannot obtain regular study leave to attend the course. The university wishes to assess practitioners in a more innovative way.

Reflection point

★ Think about how this might be done to satisfy the academic and practice components of the course and meet Jayne's learning needs.

With the rise in access to, and the popularity of, electronic learning resources it is only logical that the move should be made from paper-based portfolios to electronic portfolios. Policy initiatives and practitioners' views point the way towards more work-based assessments which need to be flexible, responsive to need and accessible while stimulating and promoting learning and critical thinking (Department of Health 2006, 2008a; Centre for the Development of Health Care Policy and Practice 2008; Welsh Assembly Government 2009). This has implications for practitioners who, as healthcare delivery evolves in innovative ways, may find they are working in settings which are remote from traditional learning centres (Lawson *et al.* 2004). The use of an e-portfolio enables the practitioner to access educational programmes and submit work electronically.

One of the criticisms levelled at the use of the traditional portfolio was that after a period of time it became impractical to transport as it was bulky. Also, as more courses are being assessed via the portfolio, so storage of the artefacts becomes problematic (Bowers and Jinks 2004; Bogossian *et al.* 2009; Timmins and Dunne 2009). E-portfolios would appear to solve these issues. They are portable, easily accessible and, in conjunction with internet access, provide a rich, valuable learning experience (Dornan *et al.* 2002; Dion 2006; Garrett and Jackson 2006; Bogossian *et al.* 2009). They are more interactive, as the facilitator also has access to add comments and engage in a dialogue via the portfolio (Lawson *et al.* 2004; Garrett and Jackson 2006). It can be argued that to some degree this meets the concerns about confidentiality and privacy raised earlier in conjunction with traditional paper-based portfolios, since the risk of an unwanted or uninvited audience is greatly reduced. Safety of the data is ensured providing the appropriate security software is installed and monitored (Garrett and Jackson 2006; Bogossian *et al.* 2009).

Dion (2006) suggested that the ability to capture and report on nursing activities will exist almost in real time. Access to an online portfolio will enable the children and young people's nurse to capture professional development and competence activities shortly after the event and thus reduce activity that is not accounted for or degradation of information because of memory loss or distortion (Dion 2006; Garrett and Jackson 2006; Bogossian *et al.* 2009). Garrett and Jackson (2006) found those students who were given mobile devices (portable digital assistants) enjoyed using them as they could access information quickly and make notes on critical incidents and record images. This could then be uploaded to the main portfolio on their computer. However, their expected use in the clinical area did not materialize as the students felt they were too busy and that writing reflectively was time-consuming. The reality was that the students wanted a more open format to the portfolio which was structured to capture specific information and to use desktop computers to write the more complex involved reflective pieces (Dornan *et al.* 2002; Garret and Jackson 2006). The aim of keeping events and writing concurrent was not met as students completed their reflective writing at a later time, resulting in the portfolio being completed within the same timescale as for the paper-based portfolio (Garrett and Jackson 2006; Bogossian *et al.* 2009).

Bogossian *et al.* (2009), in a small study, gave three students a tablet PC (personal computer) to take into practice with the aim of maintaining an e-portfolio concurrent with events. They found that similar issues recurred. Time constraints and the busyness of the ward either made it difficult to record the students' incidents and learning experiences or the students found it difficult to find space to use their devices without disturbing anyone. The students were also reluctant to use the PC at the bedside in front of patients. Thus, students recorded their thoughts on paper and then transferred them to the PC later. The PC was used not just to record incidents but also to communicate with educational staff and other students, for teaching purposes and to access web-based information as well as storage of documents (Dion 2006; Berglund *et al.* 2007; Bogossian *et al.* 2009). There appeared to be an eclectic use of the device, which motivated completion of the portfolio. Concerns centred on security of both the information recorded and the device itself. Students needed to be vigilant in locking the screen to prevent unauthorized access to information and the physical security was an issue regarding loss or theft. Thus, students completed work at home ostensibly because it was quieter and calmer; however, this made the portfolio remote from clinical practice, which defeated the aim of its use in practice.

Thus, the use of e-portfolios would appear to be an interesting development. There are some caveats to this. Managerially and culturally there may need to be a shift in how e-portfolios and PDAs are regarded. New technology being used at the bedside is unfamiliar to practitioners, and users of such technology found that they were being judged in a negative light for using the e-portfolio or PDA (Dion 2006; Garret and Jackson 2006; Bogossian *et al.* 2009).

Although there are practical constraints in using them while working with patients, as the research has shown, their use for development and learning is apparent. The portfolio can be used to create a dialogue with the facilitator, who can enable the reflective process and stimulate the development of critical-thinking skills as an ongoing process which is in agreement with the practice situation (Lawson *et al.* 2004; Garrett and Jackson 2006; Bogossian *et al.* 2009).

The e-portfolio has advantages in that reflective writing is confidential between the facilitator and the student, adding to the privacy and trust that needs to be engendered in the process, thus possibly leading to a more honest approach to writing. The other advantages lie in being able to access the portfolio online at a time suitable to the writer in a location which is appropriate and not being constrained (Lawson *et al.* 2004; Mason *et al.* 2004). This is particularly important with distance learning, when children and young people's nurses may be some distance from their tutor. Also, with online courses gaining popularity for a variety of reasons, the online portfolio becomes an excellent means of assessing knowledge, practice issues, critical thinking and reflective writing in order to ascertain how the evidence which underpins practice is conceptualized and utilized in care delivery (Lawson *et al.* 2004; Mason *et al.* 2004).

The e-portfolio would appear to provide a secure, flexible environment in which to write, reflect and gather information, thus building a live document which captures and develops the ability to write in a cohesive integrated manner as the children's nurse progresses through his or her education and learning experiences, either within the constraints of a formal education process or as a means of ensuring personal professional development both to develop practice and to ensure continued registration. E-portfolios go well together with the notion of adult learning, which underpins the ethos of the portfolio. E-portfolios enable self-directed learning which recognizes the skill, experiences and the person who is active and dynamic and their learning (Knowles 1990).

Principles for practice

- E-portfolios are a dynamic, interactive medium for capturing experiences and learning from them at the same time.
- E-portfolios widen access to opportunities for education, reflection and critical writing.
- E-portfolios meet the concerns regarding confidentiality.

Conclusion

Portfolios have become increasingly popular as a means of assessing learning and development both professionally and within educational programmes, where it is believed the portfolio allows learners the freedom to explore and reflect upon their knowledge base, knowledge acquisition and the application to practice. Indeed, a substantial number of courses now use portfolios as assessment tools based on what appears to be largely anecdotal claims of their positive influence. Although portfolios have been perceived as a solution for developing personal and professional learning, which it is proposed develops and refines practice, it can be clearly seen that a number of tensions exist. The portfolio was originally a private enterprise designed to enable practitioners to reflect on their learning, development and practice, but soon became a statutory requirement before returning to a personal endeavour.

The construction and development of a portfolio is suggested to be an individual, personal, flexible process which relies on a level of competence that learners may not have despite exhibiting higher levels of critical thinking and analysis in other areas. Also, issues around confidentiality and honesty need to be addressed, as it is possible for the learner to feel exposed and intimidated when writing for a 'public' audience, i.e. mentor/tutor, possibly leading to the adoption of a censorious writing style. Rigour is also an issue as a debate has taken place around ensuring the reliability and validity of the portfolio in terms of its capacity to assess learning, critical thinking and analytical ability as well as the transference into and refinement of knowledge in practice.

However, the available evidence demonstrates that practitioners do value an alternative method of assessing their learning and the opportunity to reflect on their practice. Portfolios provide an opportunity to reflect on how competencies are achieved in practice, whether they are academic requirements or requirements of the KSF, as well as facilitating analysis of the complex knowledge required to deliver high-quality care. They are a valuable adjunct in career progression as they demonstrate the maturation and development of the practitioner.

Portfolios in all their forms would appear to be an adjunct to the practice of children and young people's nursing to illustrate and support the contention that children and young people's nursing is a specialist area of practice and that ongoing education is vital for its development both personally and professionally. Children's nurses can use portfolios to demonstrate the specific knowledge, competencies and skills required to deliver high-quality care to children, young people and their families, thus providing a response to the rise of the generic argument. This can be achieved through the use of personal portfolios or developing departmental portfolios which demonstrate the knowledge and expertise of the children and young people's nursing team. This provides a valuable resource for teaching and can give a political voice to children's nurses to put forward arguments related to their specialist field of practice.

Although portfolios are seen as a positive innovation with much to offer the learner in terms of flexibility underpinned by adult-learning principles, the research has focused on the use of portfolios by learners, mentors and academics. There is a lack of research evidence in relation to the claims that portfolios facilitate learning and critical thinking as well as positively influencing competence and the quality of care delivered. There needs to be robust research into this area to substantiate these claims and to clearly demonstrate that portfolios as a learning tool do influence the quality of care delivered if the portfolio is to survive as both an assessment and development tool within nursing.

Summary of principles for practice

- Children and young people's nurses need to develop a clear understanding of the purpose and structure of the portfolio for their practice.
- Children and young people's nurses need to articulate and showcase the specific body of knowledge and clinical expertise required to care for children, young people and their families.
- Children and young people's nurses must be clear that they are writing for themselves and not a perceived audience in order to develop practice knowledge.
- Children and young people's nurses need to use portfolios as a powerful tool to identify learning and professional development in order to meet the demands of the Knowledge and Skills Framework and advance nurses' careers.
- Children and young people's nursing teams can use portfolios to demonstrate expertise, innovation, research and development in clinical practice, which can inform and be used as a consultative tool.

References

Allmark P (1995) A classical view of the theory-practice gap in nursing. *Journal of Advanced Nursing* **22**: 18–22.

Berglund M, Nilsson C, Révay R, *et al.* (2007) Nurses' and nurse students' demands of functions and usability in a PDA *International Journal of Medical Informatics* **76**(7): 530–7.

Bogossian FE, Kellett SEM, Mason B (2009) The use of tablet PCs to access an electronic portfolio in the clinical setting: a pilot study using undergraduate nursing students. *Nurse Education Today* **29**: 246–53.

Bowers SJ, Jinks AM (2004) Issues surrounding professional portfolio development for nurses. *British Journal of Nursing* **13**(3): 155–9.

Brown R (1995) *Portfolio development and profiling for nurses*, 2nd edn. Lancaster: Quay Publications.

Byrne M, Delarose T, King CA, *et al.* (2007) Continued professional competence and portfolios. *Journal of Trauma Nursing* **14**: 24–31.

Calman L, Watson R, Norman I, *et al.* (2002) Assessing practice of student nurses. *Journal of Advanced Nursing* **38**(5): 516–23.

Casey A (1993) Development and use of the partnership model of nursing care. In: Glasper A, Tucker A (eds) *Advances in child health nursing*. London: Scutari Press.

Centre for the Development of Health Care Policy and Practice (2008) *Towards a framework for post-registration nursing careers: report of the outcomes from the national consultation*. Leeds: CDHPP, University of Leeds.

Corry M, Timmins F (2009) The use of teaching portfolios to promote excellence and scholarship in nurse education. *Nurse Education in Practice* **9**: 388–92.

Davies R (2008) Children's nursing and future directions: learning from 'memorable events'. *Nurse Education Today* **28**(7): 814–21.

Davies R (2010) Marking the fiftieth anniversary of the Platt Report: from exclusion to toleration and parental participation in the care of the hospitalised child. *Journal of Child Health Care* **14**(1): 6–23.

Department for Children, Schools and Families and Department of Health (2008) *Children and young people in mind: the final report of the National CAMHS Review*. London: DCSF/DH.

Department for Children, Schools and Families and Department of Health (2009) *Healthy lives, brighter futures: the strategy for children and young people's health*. London: DCSF.

Department of Health (1991) *The welfare of children and young people in hospital*. London: DH.

Department of Health (2004a) *The National Service Framework for children, young people and maternity services*. London: DH.

Department of Health (2004b) *An introduction to the NHS Knowledge and Skills Framework and its use in career and pay progression*. London: DH. See http://www.dh.gov.uk/prod_consum_dh/groups/dh_digitalassets/@dh/@en/documents/digitalasset/dh_4105472.pdf

Department of Health (2004c) *The NHS Knowledge and Skills Framework (NHS KSF) and the development review process*. London: DH. See http://www.dh.gov.uk/en/Publicationsandstatistics/Publications/PublicationsPolicyAndGuidance/DH_4090843

Department of Health (2006) *Modernising nursing careers: setting the direction*. London: DH.

Department of Health (2008a) *Towards a framework for post-registration nursing careers: consultation response report*. London: DH.

Department of Health (2008b) *A high quality workforce: NHS next stage review*. London: DH. See http://www.dh.gov.uk/prod_consum_dh/groups/dh_digitalassets/@dh/@en/documents/digitalasset/dh_085841.pdf

Department of Health (2009) *New horizons: towards a shared vision for mental health – consultation*. London: DH.

Dion K (2006) Nursing portfolios: drivers, challenges and benefits. *Deans Notes* **27**(4).

Dolan G, Fairbairn G, Harris S (2004) Is our student portfolio valued? *Nurse Education Today* **24**: 4–13.

Dornan T, Carroll C, Parboosingh J (2002) An electronic learning portfolio for reflective continuing professional development. *Medical Education* **36**: 767–9.

Endacott R, Gray MA, Jasper MA, *et al.* (2004) Using portfolios in the assessment of learning and competence: the impact of four models. *Nurse Education in Practice* **4**: 250–7.

Fergusson J, Jinks AM (1994) Integrating what is practised in the nursing curriculum: a multi-dimensional model. *Journal of Advanced Nursing* **20**: 687–95.

Gannon FT, Draper PR, Watson R (2001) Putting portfolios in their place. *Nurse Education Today* **21**: 534–40.

Garrett BM, Jackson C (2006) A mobile clinical portfolio for nursing and medical students using personal digital assistants. *Nurse Education Today* **26**: 647–54.

Gerrish K (1993) An evaluation of a portfolio as an assessment tool for teaching practice placements. *Nurse Education Today* **13**: 172–9.

Gerrish K, McManus M, Ashworth P (1997) *Levels of achievement: a review of the assessment of practice*. London: English National Board.

Guba E, Lincoln YS (1985) *Effective evaluation: improving the usefulness of evaluation results through responses and naturalistic approaches*. San Francisco: Jossey Bass.

Guba E, Lincoln YS (1989) *Fourth generation evaluation*. Newbury Park: Sage.

Harris S, Dolan G, Fairbairn G (2001) Reflecting on the use of student portfolios. *Nurse Education Today* **21**: 278–86.

Hull C, Redfern L (1996) *Profiles and portfolios*. Basingstoke: Macmillan.

Hull C, Redfern L, Shuttleworth A (2005) *Profiles and portfolios*, 2nd edn. Basingstoke: Palgrave Macmillan.

Jasper M (2006) *Professional development, reflection and decision making*, pp. 154–83. Oxford: Blackwell Publishing.

Jasper MA, Fulton J (2005) Marking criteria for assessing practice based portfolios at master's level. *Nurse Education Today* **25**: 377–89.

Johns C (1999) Reflection as empowerment? *Nursing Inquiry* **6**: 241–9.

Joyce P (2005) A framework for portfolio development in postgraduate nursing practice. *Journal of Clinical Nursing* **14**: 456–63.

Kicken W, Brand-Gruwel S, van Merrienboer J, Slot W (2009) Design and evaluation of a development portfolio: how to improve students self directed learning skills. *Instructional Science* **37**(5): 453–73.

Knowles M (1990) *The adult learner: a neglected species*, 4th edn. Houston: Gulf Publishing.

Lawson M, Nestel D, Jolly B (2004) An e-portfolio in health professional education. *Medical Education* **38**: 569–70.

Maben J, Griffiths P (2008) *Nurses in society: starting the debate*. London: National Nursing Research Unit, Kings College London.

Mallik M (1993) Theory-to-practice links. *Senior Nurse* **13**: 41–6.

Martin JM, Kinnick VL, Hummel F, *et al.* (1997) Developing outcome assessment methods. *Nurse Education* **22**(6): 35–40.

Mason R, Pegler C, Weller C (2004) E-portfolios: an assessment tool for online courses. *British Journal of Educational Technology* **35**(6): 717–27.

McClellan Reece S, Pearce C, Devereaux Melillo K, Beaudry M (2001) The faculty portfolio: documenting the scholarship of teaching. *Journal of Professional Nursing* **17**(4): 180–6.

McColgan K (2008) The value of portfolio building and the registered nurse: a review of the literature. *Journal of Perioperative Practice* **18**(2):64–9.

McMullan M (2006) Students' perceptions on the use of portfolios in pre-registration nursing education: a questionnaire survey. *International Journal of Nursing* **43**: 333–43.

McMullan M, Endacott R, Gray MA, *et al.* (2003) Portfolios and assessment of competence: a review of the literature. *Journal of Advanced Nursing* **41**: 283–94.

Ministry of Health (1959) *The welfare of children in hospital.* The Platt Report. London: HMSO.

Nairn S, O'Brien E, Traynor V, Williams G, *et al.* (2006) Student nurses' knowledge, skills and attitudes towards the use of portfolios in a school of nursing. *Journal of Clinical Nursing* **15**: 1509–20.

Neades BL (2003) Professional portfolios: all you need to know and were afraid to ask. *Accident and Emergency Nursing* **11**: 49–55.

Nursing and Midwifery Council (2008a) *Advice for nurses working with children and young people.* London: NMC. See http://www.nmc-uk.org/Nurses-and-midwives/Advice-by-topic/A/Advice/Advice-on-working-with-children-and-young-people/

Nursing and Midwifery Council (2008b) *The code: standards of conduct, performance and ethics for nurses and midwives.* London: NMC. See http://www.nmc-uk.org/Documents/Standards/nmcTheCodeStandardsofConductPerformanceAndEthicsForNursesAndMidwives_TextVersion.pdf

Nursing and Midwifery Council (2008c) *The prep handbook.* London: NMC. See http://www.nmc-uk.org/Educators/Standards-for-education/The-Prep-handbook/

Nursing and Midwifery Council (2008d) *Values for integrated working with children and young people.* London: NMC. See http://www.nmcuk.org/aArticle.aspx?ArticleID=3566

Nursing and Midwifery Council (2009) *Review of pre-registration nursing education – phase 2.* London: NMC. See http://www.nmc-uk.org/Get-involved/Consultations/Past-consultations/By-year/Review-of-pre-registration-nursing-education/

Nursing and Midwifery Council (2010) *Standards for pre-registration nursing education.* London: NMC. See http://www.nmc-uk.org/Documents/Consultations/draft%20standards%20pre%20reg.pdf

Pitts J, Coles C, Thomas P (1999) Education portfolios in the assessment of general practice trainers: reliability of assessors. *Medical Education* **33**: 515–20.

Polit DF, Hungler BP (1995) *Nursing research principles and methods,* 5th edn. Philadelphia: Lippincott.

Rassin M, Silner D, Ehrenfeld M (2006) Departmental portfolio in nursing: an advanced instrument. *Nurse Education in Practice* **6**: 55–60.

Redfern L (1998) The power of the professional portfolio. In: Quinn FM (ed.) *Continuing professional development in nursing,* pp. 121–45. Cheltenham: Stanley Thornes.

Rolfe G (2005) The deconstructing angel: nursing, reflection and evidence-based practice. *Nursing Inquiry* **12**: 78–86.

Royal College of Nursing (2004a) *Children and young people's mental health – every nurse's business.* London: RCN. See http://tinyurl.com/d3xk3r   accessed: 04/01/2010

Royal College of Nursing (2004b) *Commissioning health care services for children and young people: increasing nurses' influence.* London: RCN. See http://www.rcn.org.uk/__data/assets/pdf_file/0003/78591/002169.pdf

Royal College of Nursing and Children's Community Nursing Forum (2000) *Promoting effective teamworking for children and their families.* London: RCN & Community Children's Nursing Forum.

Scholes J, Webb C, Gray M, *et al.* (2004) Making portfolios work in practice. *Journal of Advanced Nursing* **46**(6): 595–603.

Snadden D, Thomas ML (1998) Portfolios learning in general practice vocational training – does it work? *Medical Education* **32**: 401–6.

Storey L, Haigh C (2002) Portfolios in professional practice. *Nurse Education in Practice* **22**: 44–8.

Timmins F, Dunne PJ (2009) An exploration of the current use and benefit of nursing student portfolios. *Nurse Education Today* **29**: 330–41.

Tweddell L (2008) Building a quality workforce fit for the future of nursing. *Nursing Times* **104**(27): 10.

Watson E (2006) CAMHS liaison: supporting care in general paediatric settings. *Paediatric Nursing* **18**: 30–3.

Webb C, Endacott R, Gray MA, *et al.* (2003) Evaluating portfolio assessment systems: what are the appropriate criteria? *Nurse Education Today* **23**: 600–9.

Welsh Assembly Government (2004) *Realising the potential: a strategic framework for nursing, midwifery and health visiting in Wales into the 21st century.* Briefing paper 7. *Nurturing the future: a framework for realising the potential of children's nurses in Wales.* Cardiff: WAG.

Welsh Assembly Government (2005) *National Service Framework for children, young people and maternity services in Wales.* Cardiff: WAG.

Welsh Assembly Government (2009) *Post registration career framework for nurses in Wales.* Cardiff: WAG.

Wilson P, Furnivall J, Barbour RS, *et al.* (2007) The work of the health visitor and school nurse with children with psychological and behavioural problems. *Journal of Advanced Nursing* **61**(4): 445–55.

Chapter 14

Advanced practice in children and young people's nursing

Dave Barton, Alyson Davies and Ruth Davies

Overview

This chapter will provide insight into the issues and debates surrounding the development of the advanced practitioner role within general care settings and specialist areas of practice. The chapter will provide an historical context in which to set these issues before examining them within current-day nursing practice. The tensions between that of generalist and specialist practice with regard to children and young people's nursing are articulated and analysed. That is, should advanced practitioners be generalists with an interest in and some experience of caring for children and young people or should they be educated and qualified as children and young people's nurses? The chapter is contentious, deliberately so, in order to stimulate an informed debate on this vitally important role.

Introduction

The debate on advanced nursing practice as well as its meaning, value and regulation has been actively ongoing within the UK for over two decades and continues still (Stilwell *et al.* 1987; UK Central Council for Nursing, Midwifery and Health Visiting 1998). The level of this debate has increased in recent years following the publication of the White Paper *Trust, Assurance and Safety* (Department of Health 2007), which was produced as a direct result of the Shipman enquiry (Smith 2005). The effect of this is that the government's and public's preoccupation with public protection from the potential dangers of health professionals has reached new heights. As a consequence, we have most recently witnessed the report of the Centre for Healthcare Regulatory Excellence (CHRE) on the complexity of professional regulatory issues and have noted the Nursing and Midwifery Council's (NMC) continued deliberations and new enthusiasms on advanced nursing practice with regard to definition, regulation and competencies required to practise at this level (Coe *et al.* 2005). We have also seen the activity and influence of the national *Modernising Nursing Careers*, a review that was published in January 2010 (Department of Health 2010).

It is in this climate of change and uncertainty that this chapter will critically examine the nature of advanced nursing practice both in the broad nursing context and within the specific of children and young people's nursing. It will trace the historical development of the concept and innovation of advanced nursing practice and discuss how this is currently defined and regulated. Differing levels of practice and the resultant array of roles that have emerged will also be considered and contrasted alongside the current driving policies and strategies.

The authors of this chapter have deliberately adopted a controversial stance that we hope will engage the reader in some critical and reflective debate regarding children and young people's nursing and the nature of advanced nursing practice. To do this, we have put forward different perspectives on how nurses, particularly those working with children and young people, may advance their practice. In doing so, we have recognized that the boundary between nurses' initial registrant field of practice and others is becoming increasingly blurred, and may even be deemed as irrelevant by some. Likewise, we also recognize and discuss the arguments put forward that the aspiring advanced nurse practitioner, regardless of his or her initial registrant specialist field, needs to attain a generic and generalist standard of practice for advanced practice.

The main purpose of this chapter is to explore and explain the role(s) and activities of advanced nurse practitioners who are working with children and young people. We believe that such advanced nurse practitioners may arise from any of the current four UK 'fields' or 'branches' of nursing practice to which new registrants are assigned at successful completion of their pre-registration studies (child; mental health; learning disability; adult).

The development of advanced nurse practitioners, as well as their role, activity, scope of practice, education and regulation, has a complex history and is currently an unfinished story. It is fair to say that few areas of nursing activity have been so closely scrutinized and researched (Svensson 1996; Horrocks *et al.* 2002; Carnwell and Daly 2003), and yet it remains controversial and challenging. Because of that uncertainty, and because of the main purpose of this chapter, we will begin our discussions on advanced nurse practitioners by looking at their historical context, and then applying the concepts that arise from this to the activities of children and young people's nursing.

This chapter will review and explore the definitions, history and development of advanced nursing practice and advanced nurse practitioners in the general sense and in the widest context. The concepts and principles outlined will then be applied and discussed in relation to children and young people's nursing and to the development and status of advanced nurse practitioners in the care of children and younger people. There is discussion on current issues; the relation of children and young people's field competencies to advanced practice competencies, and the modernization of career pathways; and how education must adapt to meet the needs of children's nursing in the future. We will then consider specifically the role of the advanced nurse practitioner in some key areas of children and young people's nursing practice.

The chapter will conclude with a summary of the current status of children and young people's nursing and advanced nursing practice in the UK.

Advanced practice in context

What is immediately and abundantly clear is that the advanced nurse practitioner has been, and remains, a complex and controversial concept, and an issue that has engendered enormous debate in the nursing profession. In addition it is a concept (a role, a level of practice) that has persistently been promoted by health strategists as a mechanism to overcome healthcare manpower shortages by enabling new clinical roles that can be used to promote healthcare quality and service delivery (Department of Health 1993). However, we also believe that, despite the strategists' positive promotion of advanced nurse practitioners, the education of such practitioners has been an erratic and unregulated affair that has lacked any central coherency until most recently. Consequently, the standards of practice and competence held by those who claim to be advanced nurse practitioners varies widely (Hunt 1999). It is this situation that has led to the long debate on how advanced practice may be defined and measured. That endeavour has been grounded in the professional and public concern over the profession's ability to ensure that advanced nurse practitioners are fit for practice within any of the four initial registrant fields of nursing practice, including those working with children and young people.

Key points

- Advanced practice is a complex and controversial concept that has caused enormous debate in the nursing profession.
- It is a role that has been persistently promoted by health strategists as a mechanism to overcome manpower shortages as well as promote healthcare quality and service delivery.

The concepts and vocabulary of advanced practice

First, let us consider the concepts and terminology that have evolved over time, and that are now commonly used when describing issues and themes in the world of advanced nursing practice (Fig. 14.1).

The generalist A healthcare worker/professional (doctor, nurse, support worker, physiotherapist, etc.) working with client groups that have undifferentiated or undiagnosed health needs	**The specialist** A healthcare worker/professional (doctor, nurse, support worker, physiotherapist, etc.) working with a specific client group or a specific disease or pathology
The advanced generalist practitioner is commonly, but not exclusively, titled a: **nurse practitioner**	**The advanced specialist practitioner** is commonly, but not exclusively, titled a: **clinical nurse specialist**

The advanced nurse practitioner
Some authors see both nurse practitioners and clinical nurse specialists as advanced nurse practitioners, simply with different foci of role or client group
However
Others see advanced nurse practitioners as possessing skills and attributes above and beyond those of nurse practitioners and clinical nurse specialists

This hierarchy may be linked to the 'level' of academic study and clinical preparation for these roles (undergraduate, master, doctoral) as advanced practice competencies
OR
May be linked to known competency frameworks (e.g . NMC, RCN, KSF)
OR
BOTH!

Figure 14.1 Concepts and vocabulary of advanced practice.

PART 4

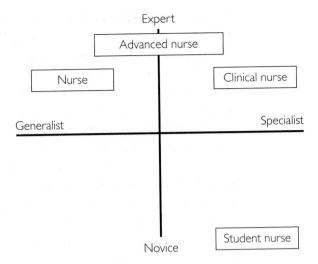

Figure 14.2 Clinical specialists and generalists – novice to expert.

Now apply these terms in a conceptual map that visually describes the dimensions of practice (Fig. 14.2).

It is now generally acknowledged in the UK that there are dimensions of practice that range horizontally from the novice student through to the most expert practitioner, and laterally from the generalist practitioner to the specialist practitioner. The Advanced Nursing Practice Toolkit (Scottish Government 2008) has arisen from the *Modernising Nursing Careers* initiative (Department of Health 2006) and has promoted this concept as a national guideline. Thus, it is entirely credible to suggest that, as we have pre-registrant fields of practice, student nurses are novice specialists, whereas advanced nurse practitioners may be working in generalist environments or specialist environments.

Key point

- Dimensions of practice range horizontally from novice student through to most expert practitioners, and laterally from generalist practitioner to the specialist practitioner. Advanced nurse practitioners may be working in generalist environments or specialist environments.

Historical perspectives and the international view of advanced practice

The first specialist nurses are referred to in the literature as early as the late nineteenth century (Manton 1971) and the use of the title 'specialist' became increasingly evident in healthcare practice in the USA during the 1930s and 1940s (Peplau 1965; Storr 1988). However, it was during the 1960s that clinical nurse specialists were widely introduced into the American nursing profession (Storr 1988; Hamric and

Spross 1989; Fenton 1992). The development of the specialist nurse in the USA was mainly an uncontroversial one and reflected a general perception of the clinical nurse specialist role as one that lay comfortably within the domains of nursing practice as they were understood at that time.

Nevertheless, the origins of modern advanced clinical roles in nursing can be traced to the introduction of the specialist nurse in the USA. The title 'specialist nurse', with all that it implied, was intimately related to the notion that nurses could develop advanced levels of clinical *nursing* expertise and skill above and beyond that of their initial registration (Hamric and Spross 1989). Thus, the clinical nurse specialist role presented no threat to the established order and stability of the boundary between nursing and medicine.

Today, clinical nurse specialists abound in all sectors of care, and they are engaged in an array of clinical areas and specialties. They represent a huge resource to care delivery and they are commonly and intimately linked to concepts of advanced nursing practice. Nevertheless, how they are prepared for their roles may vary considerably. As we have indicated in our conceptual models, 'specialist' should not be confused with 'expert' – and although there are multiple competency frameworks in use there is no one universally agreed national standard of competence for the clinical nurse specialist.

Key points

- The first specialist nurses may be traced back to the late nineteenth century with the title 'specialist' being used in the USA from the 1930s onwards.
- In the USA the role of a specialist nurse was based on the notion that they could develop advanced levels of clinical nursing expertise and skills above and beyond those of their initial qualification, a stance which did not threaten the boundary between nursing and medicine.

Nurse practitioners: the American origins

In contrast to the development of specialist nurses, the introduction of the nurse practitioner role in the USA in the late 1960s was founded not only on the principles of the specialist nurse concept but also openly incorporated traditional medical skills. This inevitably led to concerns about and scrutiny of the implications of this professional boundary transgression on the future scope of nursing practice.

Interestingly for children and young people's nursing the earliest origins of the nurse practitioner role lay in the work of Ford and Silver (1967) and their implementation of a new primary healthcare paediatric nurse practitioner role in 1965 in the USA. During this development of nurse practitioner practice in the USA, Zola and Croog (1968) commented on the professional status of nursing at that time. Zola and Croog (1968, p. 15) described nursing as having an uncertain professionalism, and that this was an 'age old question' that was difficult to resolve as the role of the nurse 'would not stand still long enough'. However, this role mobility also suggested that the professional nurse of that time was adaptable, and accommodating of new role developments. Thus, nursing was an occupation well situated, and well motivated, to extend its professional identity and authority, and Dingwall and Lewis (1985, p. 6) observed that enhancement of professionalism was possible if a profession could 'Reconstruct its license and win acceptance of an enlarged mandate'.

Ford and Silver (1967) had extended the nursing profession's mandate by their introduction of an advanced clinical nursing role that explicitly used traditional medical skills. However, this transgression of the occupational boundary between nursing and medicine disturbed some professional contemporaries, who saw this as potentially harmful to traditional nursing practice (Fondiller 1995). Some also viewed it as detrimental to the development of a unique occupational identity that would enhance the professional status of nursing (Shaw 1993; Deloughery 1995). These views reflected nurses' preoccupation during the 1960s and 1970s with their professional identity, and their preoccupation with nursing having a greater autonomy and distance from the traditional dominance of medical authority. This wish to distance nursing from medicine underpinned and directed much of the prevailing nursing ideology of the time (Walby and Greenwell 1994), although that ideology conflicted with the introduction of new clinical roles that had a significant component of traditional medical skills associated with them. Thus, the introduction of nurse practitioners was a controversial and challenging development affecting nursing and its relationship with other healthcare professions (Fondiller 1995).

However, we must also acknowledge that the development of nurse practitioners in the USA arose not only in response to a professional innovation but also in direct response to other social issues of the time:

Several social phenomena of the 1960s provided impetus for the nurse practitioner movement. Health manpower shortages especially of paediatricians and family practice physicians, lack of primary healthcare for many rural and urban poor populations, escalating healthcare costs, and the desire of nurses to achieve professional autonomy were stimuli for the nurse practitioner movement.

(Marchione and Garland 1980, p. 37)

These social, economic and professional causes all had their part to play in the development of the nurse practitioner role during its introduction into clinical practice in the USA in the 1960s. It is true to say that these influences were (are) also factors in the development of advanced nurse practitioner roles in the UK.

During the 1970s, the nurse practitioner concept gained considerable momentum and support in the USA, but it was a development with associated difficulties. Marchione and Garland (1980) had observed a proliferation of education programmes for nurse practitioners that arose during the 1970s. This typified an unregulated and fragmented expansion of the nurse practitioner role in the USA. It would take time before evidence became available that gave basis to the new role and it was not until the 1990s that regulation and standardization of nurse practitioner education became more widely introduced in the USA (Campbell-Heider *et al.* 1997):

There is now standardisation in terms of educational and certification requirements for NPs [nurse practitioners] in the United States. National certification for NPs is available for the areas of pediatric, family, adult, geriatric, school, women's health, and acute care.

(Campbell-Heider et al. 1997, p. 338)

However, Campbell-Heider *et al.* (1997) also noted that inconsistencies remained and that barriers to nurse practitioner practice persisted despite the efforts to regulate and standardize nurse practitioners' activity in the USA:

Individual state nurse practice acts dictate the degree of autonomous practice of NPs in terms of prescriptive privileges, reimbursement, and independence. The 50 states vary greatly in terms of title protection, authority over practice, autonomy of practice, and prescriptive privileges.

(Campbell-Heider et al. 1997, p. 339)

Thus, the certification and regulation of nurse practitioners in the USA during the 1990s was developing (Hodnicki 1998). By the early 2000s it was more established, although it remained a fairly complex process (Ponto *et al.* 2002). Today, to become a licensed nurse practitioner in the USA, the candidate must first be a registered nurse (RN) and meet several other criteria. Requirements to become a registered nurse vary between states, and may include an Associate Degree in Nursing (ADN), a Bachelor of Science degree in nursing (BSc Nursing) or a nursing diploma programme. In most cases, the BSc Nursing is a minimal requirement for prospective nurse practitioners, and some states require this. Once registered as a nurse, the prospective nurse practitioner must then further complete a state-approved advanced training programme, most usually a Master-level degree. After completing an advanced education programme, the nurse practitioner then has to be licensed by the state in which he or she plans to practise (Ponto *et al.* 2002).

Thus, the US state boards of nursing regulate nurse practitioners, and each state has its own licensing and certification criteria. Because state board requirements differ, nurse practitioners may also have to fulfil additional requirements, such as certification by the American Nurses Credentialing Center (ANCC). These license periods vary in duration between 2 and 3 years. After receiving state licensing, the nurse practitioner can also then apply for national certification from the American Nursing Association (ANA) or other professional nursing boards such as the American Academy of Nurse Practitioners (AANP). This rather complex process is evident in the guidelines on advanced practice nursing outlined by the American Association of Colleges of Nursing (AACN 1999):

Advanced Practice Nurse is an umbrella term appropriate for a licensed registered nurse prepared at the graduate degree level as either a Clinical Specialist, Nurse Anaesthetist, Nurse-Midwife or Nurse Practitioner. Advanced Practice Nurses are professionals with specialized knowledge and skills that are applied within a broad range of patient populations in a variety of practice settings (…). All Advanced Practice Nurses should hold a graduate degree in nursing and be certified. Each existing and future professional nursing specialty certifying entity must meet uniform national standards when certifying nurses for advanced practice.

(AACN 1999, p. 130)

Thus, it is evident that the introduction of nurse practitioners in the USA, and the related regulation and standardization of advanced nursing practice that had commenced in the late 1960s and early 1970s, was still developing and topical in the 1990s and 2000s (Dunn 1997; Ponto *et al.* 2002). Unsurprisingly, aspects of the US experience, for example the complex social background and the subsequent early lack of regulation, were mirrored in the UK in the 1990s and early 2000s as nurse practitioner roles, and clinical nurse specialist roles, became widely implemented in clinical practice (Hunt 1999; Carnwell and Daly 2003).

Key points

- From the 1960s, the introduction of an advanced clinical nursing role that explicitly used traditional medical skills became the subject of much debate.
- Some nurses viewed this role as detrimental to nursing and that it reflected nurses' preoccupation of the time with professional identity as well as their desire for greater autonomy and to distance themselves from medical dominance.
- From the 1970s onwards, social, economic and professional issues played a part in the development of the nurse practitioner in the USA, and by the early 2000s regulations were being established.
- Regulation and standardization of the advance nurse practitioner role remains contentious.
- Regulations are stringent with variation between states, but in most cases BSc Nursing is a minimal requirement for prospective practitioners.
- Nurse practitioners may also have to fulfil additional requirements including completion of a recognized specialist nursing degree programme, usually at Master level.

The UK development of advanced nurse practice

The origins of the nurse practitioner role in the UK arose from the work of Stilwell and colleagues (Stilwell *et al.* 1987; Stilwell 1988) with her introduction of a nurse practitioner role into primary healthcare in the late 1980s. Stilwell (1988) viewed the nurse practitioner role as undertaken by an experienced nurse who would use existing nursing skills in combination with health assessment and diagnostic skills in autonomous patient management. Subsequent to her landmark work, during the 1990s and early 2000s, nurse practitioner roles increasingly emerged in clinical practice (Hunt 1999; Carnwell and Daly 2003).

Stilwell's (1984) work provided an impetus for the development of nurse practitioner role competencies. The Royal College of Nursing (RCN) with a collaborative of universities took the established American competencies (Royal College of Nursing 2008) and adapted them for UK use. Those competencies were based on consultancy skills, disease screening, physical examination, chronic disease management, minor injury management, health education and counselling. Essentially, they required nurses to advance their clinical skills via an apprenticeship model based on collaborative time spent with clinically active doctors. During this clinical mentorship, the novice nurse practitioner observed and participated in consultations and learnt skills and techniques of medical history-taking and physical examination (Stilwell 1988).

From an educational perspective the RCN in the early 1990s established the first formal training/education programme for prospective nurse practitioners in the UK. The programme unequivocally demanded that the students develop advanced skills in health assessment and differential diagnosis and they were assessed on these in clinical examinations, often with medical practitioners present. This programme set the stage and universities around the UK quickly developed their own programmes of nurse practitioner education. Initially at diploma level, these evolved to full undergraduate programmes, and today many are at Master level. Indeed, today the Advanced Nursing Practice Toolkit (Scottish Government 2008) points clearly to Master-level education as a requisite for the advanced nurse practitioner.

Key points

- By the 1980s the nurse practitioner role had been introduced into primary care and they became widely accepted and established in clinical practice.
- By the early 1990s the first formal training/education programme for prospective nurse practitioners had been introduced and developed by universities across the UK; initially at diploma level, these evolved to degree level and today most are at Master level.
- The Advanced Nursing Practice Toolkit (Scottish Government 2008) points clearly to Master-level education as a requisite for advanced practitioner.

The evolution of these educational programmes was constantly confronted with a significant barrier to their development. Hockey (1983) had early on pointed to the paradoxical situation associated with the early development of specialist and advanced nurses in the UK. Although it was evident that the UK healthcare service needed and wanted specialist and advanced nurses, it totally misunderstood the nature of those roles because of the lack of a legitimate clinical career structure to accommodate them. The service providers wanted 'right here, right now' quick fixes to skill shortages. They saw little value in expensive 2 or 3 year 'academic' education programmes that took their staff out of the workplace for a day a week. What they wanted was quick, tightly focused skills training packages that would meet their needs in months, or even weeks! We remember clearly being contacted by an A&E Nurse Manager who wanted a 2 day clinical module on 'assessment of lower limbs', and her frustration and irritation when we explained that lower limbs did not exist in isolation from the rest of the body!

This problem persisted throughout the 1990s and into the 2000s. Many will recognize the concerns raised when statutory non-medical prescribing identified such little time for formal education, and the hurdles that were placed in the way of educationalists when they tried to tie non-medical prescribing to wider programmes of advanced practice to ensure a depth and breadth to the practitioners' practice.

However, a clinical career structure for nursing was developing internationally, identified from the research on nurse practitioners and their place in nursing

(Offredy 2000; Ketefian *et al.* 2001; Pearson and Peels 2002). Yet, in the UK, early research had focused mostly on client satisfaction and the workforce resource implications of nurse practitioners (Spitzer and Sackett 1990; NHS Executive South Thames 1994; South Thames Regional Health Authority 1998), and not on the demand for clear structured career pathways in the nursing profession. Consequently, and in the most basic sense, advanced clinical practice became articulated not by actual clinical role or competence but by an array of nebulous titles.

The key to the problem was not simply the result of the major organizational and structural changes to healthcare that began in the 1980s (and which continue unabated to the present day), but that the nursing profession in the UK had an undeveloped career structure. Undeniably there were attempts to restructure clinical nursing, as demonstrated by the introduction of the clinical regrading exercise of 1988. This was introduced just before other NHS reforms came into place in the 1990s (Holliday 1995), and it was an attempt to provide a clinical hierarchy based on role and responsibility. It was a framework which failed not only because employers manipulated it to control costs, ignoring the clinical rationale for the change, but also because no one was able to explain what an advanced clinical role was! Nevertheless, its failure acted as the spur for nursing to continue to seek a wider and more professionally relevant structure of clinical career development. The introduction of the Knowledge and Skills Framework (KSF) (Agenda for Change) in the 2000s was more significant and far reaching (Department of Health 2004). Yet even this comprehensive competency framework did not fully describe a clear career framework for nursing, it being still essentially service driven as opposed to professionally conceived, and in its brave attempt to be all embracing.

Three other important professional developments that had implications for advanced nursing practice in the UK occurred during the 1990s: the introduction of the Scope of Nursing Practice principles (UK Central Council for Nursing, Midwifery and Health Visiting 1992), the introduction of the Specialist Practice Award (UK Central Council for Nursing, Midwifery and Health Visiting 1996) and the exploration of the Higher Level of Practice (HLP) framework (UK Central Council for Nursing, Midwifery and Health Visiting 1998). These in different ways contributed to the slow evolution of a more refined clinical hierarchy in nursing and mirrored the parallel uptake of specialist titles by nurses (Read *et al.* 2000; Carnwell and Daly 2003) and the proliferation of clinical programmes for qualified nurses that sought to enable specialist and advanced skills. There was even an apparent political will to support such developments, which was evident in the government's promotion and funding of consultant nurses (Waller 1998).

From an educational perspective, it is important to note the emergence in the UK during the early 2000s of the Association of Advanced Nursing Practice Educators (AANPE) (advanced nurse practitioners). The AANPE was (is) an influential lobby of 47 UK universities that sought to represent the collective view of the education of advanced nurse practitioners. Their terms of reference pointed to collaborative curriculum development and standard setting, and advising and establishing the role and status of nurse practitioners and advanced practice through interface with other professions, professional and statutory bodies, commissioners, employers and relevant government bodies. The AANPE established close links with the RCN Accreditation Unit, the RCN Nurse Practitioner Association and the NMC.

The origins of the AANPE lay in the US National Organization of Nurse Practitioner Faculties (NONPF). NONPF was established in 1980 following the introduction (outline previously) of nurse practitioners to clinical practice in the USA in the mid-1960s. It arose as a direct result of the wish of American universities to ensure that there was a forum for dialogue on nurse practitioner education issues across the USA. NONPF's mission was (is) the provision of leadership in promoting quality nurse practitioner education at a national and international level. Its mission would, by the early 1990s, provide a foundation to the very early development of a UK-wide network of nurse practitioner educators. Indeed, it was in the 1990s that the first education collaborations arose as a result of the implementation and franchise of the RCN 'Nurse Practitioner' Diploma. That franchise brought together a small group of UK university representatives, and they began to meet on a regular basis, and shared their educational experiences and expertise. As the 1990s progressed, and as programmes of nurse practitioner and advanced clinical practice education proliferated, the number of universities involved in this early network slowly grew. In October 2000, the fledgling educational network called a general meeting of UK university representatives (all of whom were providing some form of nurse practitioner education) at the RCN in London. The attendees of that meeting concluded that a formal education forum was needed in the UK to facilitate the sharing of good practice and standard setting for nurse practitioner education in the UK.

The inaugural meeting of UK NONPF took place in November 2001, a decade after the first RCN Nurse Practitioner Diploma course had began. Membership of the UK NONPF slowly increased during 2002 and 2003, and by late 2003 a series of key meetings led to the establishment of a formal network link with the extensive national RCN Nurse Practitioner Association. In 2005, the UK NONPF changed its name to the Association of Advanced Nursing Practice Educators (AANPE) and was formally relaunched as a new independent association. By early 2007, the AANPE had forged a collaboration of universities that was unprecedented in scale and nature in the UK, with formal membership from 47 UK universities, and 107 academics and other senior health professionals in its membership. The NMC has publicly acknowledged the influence of the AANPE. From its beginnings in the early 1990s, the AANPE has evolved to become a national, influential and powerful voice in the world of advanced nursing practice.

Key points

- Barriers to the development of advanced nurses included a misunderstanding about their role and those of specialist nurses, and most pertinently the lack of a legitimate career structure.
- Important professional developments during the 1990s paved the way for a more refined clinical hierarchy and there was a proliferation of clinical programmes for both specialist and advanced nurses.
- By early 2007, the Association for Advanced Nursing Practice Educators, a consortium of 47 UK universities, had been established to represent the educational requirements of advanced nurse practitioners.

Reflection points

★ Do you have advanced nurse practitioners working in your healthcare setting?

★ If so, how many are there?

★ Which areas do they work in?

★ Are they generalists or specialists?

The current status of advanced nursing practice

The *Modernising Nursing Careers* initiative of 2007–2010 (Department of Health 2006) was initiated by the four Nursing Officers of the UK. For advanced practice, its most significant product was the Advanced Nursing Practice Toolkit. We would urge that you, the reader, visit this web-based resource (http://www.advancedpractice. scot.nhs.uk/home.aspx). The Toolkit's principle is that there are many entirely appropriate and accurate definitions of advanced practice, and as such it is somewhat fruitless to continue to seek the 'ultimate' definition.

Nevertheless, we will provide you with a working definition to be used later in the chapter. The International Council of Nurses (ICN) (2002) definition of advanced nursing practice states the following:

> *The advanced nurse practitioner is a] registered nurse who has acquired the expert knowledge base, complex decision-making skills and clinical competencies for expanded practice, the characteristics of which are shaped by the context and/or country in which s/he is credentialed to practice. A Master's degree is recommended for entry level.*

Skills for Health developed *A Career Framework for Health* in 2006 (Skills for Health 2006a,b). The framework placed the 'advanced practitioner' at level 7 (KSF), defining advanced practitioners as:

> *Experienced clinical professionals who have developed their skills and theoretical knowledge to a very high standard. They are empowered to make high-level clinical decisions and will often have their own caseload. Non-clinical staff at Level 7 will typically be managing a number of service areas.*

The more wordy NMC definition of advanced nurse practitioners (Nursing and Midwifery Council 2005) is as follows:

> *Advanced nurse practitioners are highly experienced and educated members of the care team who are able to diagnose and treat your healthcare needs or refer you to an appropriate specialist if needed.*
>
> *Advanced nurse practitioners are highly skilled nurses who can:*
>
> - *take a comprehensive patient history*
> - *carry out physical examinations*
> - *use their expert knowledge and clinical judgment to identify the potential diagnosis*

- *refer patients for investigations where appropriate*
- *make a final diagnosis*
- *decide on and carry out treatment, including the prescribing of medicines, or refer patients to an appropriate specialist*
- *use their extensive practice experience to plan and provide skilled and competent care to meet patients' health and social care needs involving other members of the health care team as appropriate*
- *ensure the provision of continuity of care including follow-up visits*
- *assess and evaluate, with patients, the effectiveness of the treatment and care provided and make changes as needed*
- *work independently, although often as part of a health care team*
- *provide leadership, and*
- *make sure that each patient's treatment and care is based on best practice.*

At the time of writing, the NMC is continuing its deliberations on how Advanced Practice can best be regulated despite the advice of the CHRE report. How that decision will unfold is unclear. Thus, in the meantime, it is the NMC's Scope of Practice that imposes the limits on the extent of any nurse's role or clinical activity, coupled with the local employer's governance of practice. Whether this affords sufficient public protection is a concern for the NMC and is a matter for wide debate.

It is a concern for all of us with a stake in advanced practice that it must look to competencies frameworks and metrics. We have alluded to the competency framework evolved by the RCN and collaborating universities. These competencies have been adopted and further modified by the NMC, and they serve as a measure by which advanced practitioners judge their knowledge, skill and competence. Many universities that provide advanced practice programmes use these competencies to tailor their curriculum. In addition, these competencies have been mapped to the KSF. However, we would be remiss if we did not also acknowledge the many other competency frameworks that are available, with Skills for Health, Critical Care and Emergency Care being but a few that are in use.

Modernising Nursing Careers (Department of Health 2006) has also resulted in a major review of the pre-registration nursing curriculum on a UK-wide basis. This has led to the development of generic and field-based competencies. Again this illustrates the dynamic nature of nursing at the time that this chapter was written. The link between the competency and practice of the newly qualified children and young people's nurse as a result of this new curriculum, and how this will compare and contrast with the exiting competencies that are expected of an advanced practitioner, has yet to be tested. It is to be hoped that, as these innovations establish themselves, the articulation of the transition from novice to advanced practitioner will become more transparent than it is now. In addition, the four countries of the UK have all produced their post-registration career frameworks, each usefully mapping succession planning across the KSF – from 1 to 9.

> ## Key points
>
> - The *Modernising Nursing Careers* initiative throughout the UK has led to the development of an Advanced Nursing Practice Toolkit.
> - In 2010 the NMC announced its decision to introduce regulations for advanced practice.
> - *Modernising Nursing Careers* has resulted in a major review of the UK pre-registration curriculum and the development of generic and field-based competencies which will have significant implications for all branches of the profession, including children's nursing.

Having laid out the complexity (and uncertainty) of advanced practice in its most broad sense, we move on now to apply this foundation in the context of the care of children and young people.

Children and young people's nursing

This section is structured in the following way. Although the particular nature of children and young people's nursing has been examined in detail elsewhere in this book, it is necessary to give some brief explanation of what is meant by this to be able to put into context the intimate relationship between advanced practice and children and young people's nursing. The section will move on to examine the current situation of advanced nursing practice in the provision of healthcare to children and young people in the UK. The principal question we are asking here is: Who are the advanced nurse practitioners who are treating children and young people? In responding to this question, we will examine the scope of the services being offered and evaluate the knowledge and skills required to provide a professional standard of advanced nursing care for children and young people. Incorporated into this will be the application of those concepts and principles of advanced practice identified previously.

The section will conclude with a summary of the current status of children and young people's nursing and advanced practice in the UK. It will review the status of the current issues, particularly the relation of children and young people's field competencies to advanced practice competencies, and the modernization of career pathways, and how education is adapting to meet the needs of children and young people's nursing.

At this point, it is worth noting that children and young people's nurses care for a diverse patient and client group as well as age range, which extends from neonates through to young people up to the age of 18 years, as well as those young people who are in the process of transition to adult-based services and may be in their early twenties (see Chapter 12). This is reflected in the evolution of the title 'children's nursing' to that of 'children and young people's nursing' both informally in clinical and educational practice and more formally at strategic level (Royal College of Nursing 2003a,b; Nursing and Midwifery Council 2008).

Children and young people's nursing defined

The RCN (2003a,b) has stated that children and young people's nursing should be underpinned by beliefs that are based on the nature of the child or young person and their status and rights within both the family and society. As well as the functions identified in the RCN's (2004a) definition of nursing, children and young people's nurses focus on assisting children and young people and their families in preventing or managing the physiological, physical, social, psychological and spiritual effects of a health problem or condition and its treatment (Royal College of Nursing 2003a,b).

In a book on children and young people's nursing we are bound to acknowledge that there are healthcare needs for children and young people that are different from those of adults. Indeed, according to the Audit Commission, there are a number of differences between nursing children and nursing adults (Royal College of Nursing 2003a,b; Department of Health and Department for Education and Skills 2004a,b; Nursing and Midwifery Council 2008).

Briefly, there are anatomical and physiological differences between neonates, children and young people, and this group of patients will also have conditions and disease trajectories that are quite different from those of adults. All of which children and young people's nurses must be knowledgeable about if they are to be safe and effective practitioners in actual clinical practice. Likewise, children and young people's nurses must also be knowledgeable about the different stages of physical, cognitive, psychological and emotional development across this age group if they are to meet their needs safely and effectively as well as in a caring and understanding manner. It may be stated that the present pre-registration Child Branch programme ensures that students gain competence and confidence in clinical skills across this age group as well understanding their particular needs at different stages of development and, importantly, by being mindful of the need to work closely with parents who play an important role in their child's care (Nursing and Midwifery Council 2008).

It is also important to note the significant consultancy reviews and recommendations that point to the need for children and young people to be looked after by healthcare professionals who hold a recognized qualification in caring for children, as well as relevant specialist qualifications and expertise (Bristol Royal Infirmary Inquiry 2001; Department of Health 2004; Royal College of Nursing 2003a,b, 2004). However, it is equally important to be honest and acknowledge that in the real world this is a difficult aspiration to achieve, with opponents of early pre-registration specialization in nursing pointing to the service need for competent generalists with transferable skills (Clark 1994).

The operational difficulties of having a children and young people's qualified nurse in every accident and emergency department or in every walk-in unit or community health centre has long been acknowledged. And it is in this reality that we find nurses advancing their practice and working with children when they may not have a formal children's qualification. The question that must be asked is: Is this acceptable? We suggest that the answer may be 'yes', at least when that practitioner has been appropriately prepared and assessed as competent for the advanced role that they fulfil. This argument is rooted in the belief that the advanced nurse practitioner develops a range of generic advanced skills regardless of his or her initial field registration. However, the question arises as to what constitutes appropriate preparation. If the policy guidelines are followed then an approved registration should be undertaken in order to gain insight into the needs of the child and young person on all levels – physically, emotionally and psychologically. Also, who assesses the competence of the said practitioner? For if advanced practitioners are scarce in practice generally, and in children and young people's nursing specifically, then who has the expertise to make the judgement. The answer may be the paediatrician; yet he or she may assess medically oriented skills, thus omitting the assessment of nursing competence and skills which underpin this nurse's role. The commitment to family-centred care, education and health promotion will distinguish the advanced nurse practitioner role from a medical role (Bennet and Hughes 2009).

Perhaps at this stage we now need to ask how nurses may be developed to become safe and effective advanced practitioners for the actual patient group they care for? There are hard empirical data to show that there has been a huge increase in the number of children and young people's nurses since Project 2000, i.e. direct entry Child Branch at pre-registration level, in the 1990s (Davies 2008). This seems to suggest that there is now a sufficient pool from which to develop them to become advanced practitioners. However, there is no reason why, just as nurses in all branches, they may not develop their careers horizontally or vertically (as set out in Chapters 9 and 13) or even in a 'zigzag' fashion, i.e. by undertaking other branch educational programmes. For example, an advanced practitioner with an Adult Branch qualification or Mental Health qualification who aspires to work with children and young people could access an accelerated Child Branch programme to give him or her the additional knowledge, skills and clinical experience needed to deliver safe and effective care.

Principles for practice

- Children and young people's nursing requires specific knowledge and skills in order to deliver high-quality care to children, young people and their families.
- Children and young people should be cared for by suitably qualified and knowledgeable practitioners.
- Cost and availability may preclude this becoming a reality.

Reflection points

★ Should advanced nurse practitioners who work with children or young people be generalist nurses or specialist nurses?

★ Think about your reasons for your answer.

Children and young people's/paediatric advanced nurse practitioners

We have argued above that, as the nurse advances his or her practice, the boundary between the fields of nursing practice or specialism becomes increasingly blurred and irrelevant. Although such an assertion may be controversial, and indeed fly in the face of policy, we suggest that that the interweaving of all field-specific competences at the advanced practice level benefits the user (in this case, the child or young person) and service deliverer. At an advanced level of practice, what matters most is the appropriateness and competence of the practitioners in working with their client groups, not necessarily their initial registrant field of practice. Nevertheless, this is viewed as a perceived transgression of field boundary, and a solution to that view is to provide a commonly understood framework and structure for advanced practice that enables that generic competence. We have noted that the current NMC/advanced nurse practitioner competency framework goes some way to achieve that. It can be argued that the maintenance of such competence may be difficult to sustain if a critical mass of children and young people are not seen or experienced on a regular basis to ensure that skills remain well honed and focused. This begs the question as to whether a generically qualified and experienced advanced practitioner would be able to care for children and young people who are very sick.

An alternative view is that entrenched attitudes are in reality evident and significant traits among the generalists, where their prevailing notion is that 'anyone can care for children', and that generalist skills can be easily augmented to meet the needs of children with additional extra 'specialist' knowledge. However, there is a real danger that this view diminishes and devalues the depth and breadth of knowledge and skill required when caring for children and young people, and consequently it is a risk to the delivery of high-quality, safe and effective services. A more balanced perspective is the one that acknowledges the knowledge base and clinical experience of all practitioners in the branches (fields of practice) within the profession that make up the family of nursing and finding the means and resolve to work collaboratively while accepting the demand for diversity.

To that end (overcoming traditional field boundaries) it may be useful to revisit the American model that we reviewed earlier. In the USA, prospective advanced practitioners all undertake a generalist programme of education. Usually within a Master-level clinical programme, they all learn the generic and common skills of advanced health assessment, consultation, diagnosis and patient management. Inherent in this learning are the foundations of leadership, critical thinking, research skills and evidence-based practice. Once qualified as an advanced practitioner they then 'specialize', in any of the many specialties that are commonly understood, including childcare. Indeed, they can also generalize, and deal with undifferentiated health needs at an advanced level of practice. What is important is that they have all learnt the same generic skills, and thus can communicate effectively with each other. What is even more important is that these generic competencies are the same as those used by other health professions, thus enabling interprofessional communication at a level not previously possible. Advanced practice may be seen to bring a common language.

Nevertheless, there are strong arguments against this approach. The majority of children and young people's nurses in the UK at least would argue that their branch is not a specialty but rather generalist nursing in a specialist age group (Bradley 2003). Also, there must be acknowledgement that not everyone would wish to undertake a generic nursing programme, which is really shorthand for adult nursing, so that they can then undertake a further educational programme to 'specialize' in children and young people's nursing. Indeed, this is not a good use of expensive educational resources and, as has been argued (Davies 2008), would result in a significant reduction over time in the numbers of children and young people's nurses in actual practice. In the estimation of many children and young people's nurses this would herald a return to the bad old days when the majority of children were cared for by general nurses with no real understanding of their needs. The history of the care of children in hospital (see Chapter 1) illustrates that the majority, prior to Child Branch entry, were cared for by generalist nurses who had no understanding of their psychological and emotional needs. Thus, for nearly 30 years, the Platt Report recommendation, which stated that 'Parents should be allowed to visit whenever they can, and to help in the care of the child' (Ministry of Health 1959), was firmly resisted by most nurses and resulted in an inhumane hospital environment for many children and their parents (Davies 2010).

In the final analysis, it may be argued that if children and young people are cared for by generalists there is the potential for unsafe practice, especially in acute areas of care, and may lead to more sentinel events such as the Beverley Allitt case (Clothier *et al.* 1994) or the Bristol Royal Infirmary Inquiry (2001) in the future. Perhaps the solution, or rather compromise, is to provide generic entry at undergraduate level with specialization, i.e. branch-specific education for child, mental health and, in the few parts of the country where programmes are provided, learning disabilities nursing, in the last year or 18 months of the programme. Perhaps, in view of the present NMC consultation, now is the time for educationalists to promote the message that all undergraduate or pre-registration nurses receive a generalist education underpinned by clinical practice placements *before* obtaining a 'specialism' in adult, mental health, learning disabilities or children and young people's nursing and are in effect dually qualified.

Who is looking after our children?

Earlier we posed the question: Who are the advanced nurse practitioners who are treating children and young people? The answer is predictably uncertain because, at present, there is mixed evidence available on the provision of advanced nursing care to this group. Some areas have an established body of literature, such as that available for the advanced neonatal nurse practitioner (ANNP), whereas others lack a robust portfolio of published information or evidence base. There are several reasons for this. Some advanced practice roles in children and young people's nursing are relatively well established whereas others are newly emerging. It is also possible that the success of some advanced practitioners in children and young people's nursing (success brought about by the practitioners themselves) has resulted in a proliferation (domino effect) of similar posts, leaving commentators and researchers struggling to keep up with the change.

Interestingly, the evidence base for advanced practitioners in childcare does not abound. Most textbooks on advanced nurse practitioners (or practice) provide little specific information. Perhaps a notable exception to this is Walsh *et al.* (1999), who devote an entire chapter to the issues involved. You can find evidence in the literature if you look hard and dig deep. For example, Peter and Flynn (2002) describe the introduction of two advanced nursing practice posts to a paediatric department of a district general hospital and explore some of the issues that arose. But, although much has been written in the UK about advanced nursing practice in general terms (often from an adult nursing perspective), very little has been published on how advanced nursing practice has affected children and young people's healthcare. Furthermore, within this small pool of children's literature there is limited empirical research available. Indeed, much of the literature is anecdotal in nature and mirrors those issues covered in the main body of advanced nursing practice articles. This fact in itself may be evidence of the commonality and generic nature of advanced practice skills that we mentioned above.

Nevertheless, it is essential that future research and evidence is generated with regard to the issue of advanced nursing care for children and young people for a number of reasons. There is of course a financial imperative. While many dislike the idea that the health service, and nursing, be subject to fiscal scrutiny, the fact is that the modern health service must demonstrate value for money, particularly in the midst of an economic recession. There is a real demand to develop metrics (Griffiths *et al.* 2008; Maben and Griffiths 2008) that can measure advanced practitioners' contribution to children's healthcare services, and to evaluate the roles practitioners have both financially and from the perspective of effectiveness, quality and safety. However, research also needs to be carried out to inform those who have a legal duty to regulate the nursing profession (the NMC) of the nature and evolution of advanced practice. And, of course, research informs academic institutions responsible for the education of future advanced practitioners.

Children and young people are being cared for by advanced nurse practitioners with professional qualifications from all three (current) parts of the NMC register:

- nursing (adult, mental health, children and young people's, and learning disability)
- midwifery
- specialist community public health nursing.

Many of these practitioners hold qualifications from several parts of the NMC register. Thus, we will use the register as a framework to illustrate the variety of advanced nurse practitioners who are caring for children and young people. The issue of whether they have received education or training for their role as advanced practitioners will also be discussed.

Key points

- Children are cared for by advanced nurse practitioners from various clinical backgrounds and expertise.
- There is a paucity of children and young people's advanced nurse practitioners.
- Further research and scholarship is needed to illuminate the impact of advanced nurse practitioners in children and young people's nursing and healthcare.
- Cost is an issue, and advanced nurse practitioners must be seen to provide value for money.

Adult nursing in relation to advanced nursing practice with children and young people

Children and young people may come into contact with an advanced nurse practitioner who is based exclusively or predominantly in the adult healthcare field of practice. This may be in the hospital or community sectors. For example, many young women are admitted to gynaecology wards and may be treated by the specialist advanced nurse practitioner. Similarly, a child or young person may be an inpatient on a children's ward but be cared for (at some point) by a predominantly adult ward-based specialist advanced nurse practitioner, e.g. orthopaedic advanced nurse practitioner, night nurse practitioner, emergency nurse practitioner or anaesthetic advanced nurse practitioner. Furthermore, children and young people may have to receive treatment from advanced nurse practitioners based in specialist hospital clinics, such as those for sexual health or renal dialysis. In the community, children and young people are likely to come into contact with advanced nurse practitioners working in GPs' surgeries or in out-of-hours services.

Thus, it is clear that 'adult' advanced nurses care for children! What is in question is whether this is acceptable. There are concerns, and these must be objectively noted. Although these 'adult' advanced practitioners are experts in their specialist or generalist fields, and may have considerable experience of caring for children and young people, this may be contrasted by a lack of a formal children's nursing qualification, or formal education or assessment in the foundation skills and knowledge related to the care of children. We would assert that this should not be a case to 'bar' such practitioners from their care, but more a demand to ensure their competency with appropriate education, assessment and governance, and thus make best use of the expertise that they have and the service that they offer.

Mental health in relation to advanced nursing practice with children and young people

Mental health nursing usefully demonstrates how blurring of 'roles' and 'fields' is becoming increasingly prevalent. It is now possible for children and young people's nurses to work in the mental health field, gathering the knowledge and skills for this area following registration. The children and young people's nurse contributes specific expertise, knowledge and insight into the development, care and support required by children, young people and their families. In some cases, mental health nurses are now members of the child health team, in which their knowledge, skills and expertise are welcomed. As already identified in Chapters 10 and 11, children and young people's nurses often feel ill prepared to meet the mental health needs of their patients and require the specialist input which can be provided by the mental health nurse being part of the team (Watson 2006). Child and Adolescent Mental Health Services (CAMHS) are multiprofessional and multifield. Indeed, there is evidence that some centres have included some 'mental health' training in their pre-registration Child Branch curriculum, demonstrating shared learning across the traditional branch/field boundaries (Terry *et al.* 2009). This input has been provided by mental health nurses who have specialized in CAMHS and who have become advanced nurses.

Practitioner commentary on advanced practice in Child and Adolescent Mental Health Services (CAMHS)

There are many different roles and functions that CAMHS nurses perform, which reflects the wide range of mental health problems and disorders that children and young people experience. There is often a blurring of professional roles with these children and young people, and in some instances nurses are in a prime position to lead services that meet specific needs. For example, there are a number of key assessment and treatment strategies related to attention deficit hyperactivity disorder (ADHD) that are clearly identified in the National Institute for Health and Clinical Excellence (2008) guidance. Good practice is to restrict the number of professionals in clinical pathways to a minimum. Nurses are able to assess, diagnose and treat children with ADHD providing they have developed the advanced assessment skills and advanced therapeutic skills, including that of prescribing. In Southampton, a nurse-led service was developed and subsequently evaluated. Results showed cost savings of more than 41% over 6 months compared with a traditional model of care involving a range of other (often more expensive) professionals. An ADHD pathway was developed with clear routes to the nurse prescriber and good use of expert parents/patients in support groups was included. Outcomes for children and for schools were measured as positive and this approach demonstrates very well the benefits of having experienced advanced nurses leading services. There are several other examples of nurse-led services for children with ADHD which can be found across the UK. There are other examples emerging where particular patient groups are benefitting from the use of advanced nurses leading services such as in the field of eating disorders and of emerging psychosis in young people. The following websites give details of innovations in practice: http://www.newwaysofworking.org.uk/component/option,com_docman/task,doc_view/gid,5/ and www.newwaysofworking.org.uk/option,com_docman/task.../Itemid,412/

Mervyn Townley, Consultant Nurse, CAMHS, Gwent, Wales

Learning disability and advanced nursing practice in relation to children and young people

Learning disability is by its very nature a multiprofessional, multidiscipline, multicontext-based area of care. Equally, it is an area of care that deals with a spectrum of disabilities, challenging behaviour, autistic spectrum disorders and mental health. The literature (Jukes 1996) suggests that there is a clear part to play for advanced nurse practitioners in learning disability. Strategic and professional health policies seeking de-institutionalization of people with learning disabilities also point to the role of advanced practitioners in enabling this. Consequently learning disability nurses have sought additional skills to enhance their practice in areas of 'challenging behaviour', epilepsy management, non-medical prescribing and psychotherapeutic/educational interventions. More importantly, they have advanced their practice development in the context of a lifespan approach, encompassing learning disabilities in children, adolescents, adults and older adults. Thus, the learning disability advanced practitioner role is exceedingly varied, and they have a role in the care of children and young people in secondary and primary care settings. There is a demand placed on them for case management and domiciliary care that makes use of multidisciplinary and multiagency teams at primary, secondary and tertiary levels of intervention for children and young people with learning disabilities and their families.

Practitioner commentary on advanced practice in learning disabilities

People with learning disabilities are a heterogeneous group with a wide range of health and social care needs. Learning disabilities nurses work across a range of settings and services to meet the ordinary and specific health needs that this group present. There is a reported increase in the prevalence of severe/complex disabilities among children with learning disabilities (Emerson and Hatton 2004). More infants are surviving into childhood and adolescence, often with very complex health and behavioural needs.

Learning disability nurses work with children and their families in a number of settings ranging from schools, home and respite through to multiagency children's services.

An area where learning disability nurses make a significant impact is in transition services. Children in transition are often leaving a children's service where much of their healthcare has been coordinated through a single healthcare professional (paediatrician) to an adult service which is primary care led and where access is required to a range of specialist healthcare services.

The advanced nurse practitioner in learning disabilities transition nurse provides a vital link between child and adult services and works across professional and organizational boundaries to ensure a safe and smooth transfer to adult services and provide a continuity of care. In-depth knowledge and sophisticated clinical skills are required to work effectively with children, their families and the services that support them. Learning disability transition nursing practice focuses on three broad areas. First, the promotion and maintenance of good health; second, the delivery of specialist health and behavioural interventions; and third, the coordination of service delivery. This coordination function is vital if the health and development of the individual is to be maintained.

Christopher Griffiths, Consultant Nurse, Abertawe Bro Morgannwg University Health Board, Port Talbot, Wales

The following Case study from practice sets out how the advanced nurse practitioner transition nurse in learning disabilities can make a real difference to the quality of life and care of a young man with severe learning disabilities by working with the him, his carers and all the other agencies involved.

Case study

David is a 15 year old young man with severe learning disabilities and complex health and behavioural needs. He has been diagnosed with guanidinoacetate methyltransferase deficiency, an autosomal recessive disorder characterized by developmental delay, epilepsy, failure of active speech and extrapyramidal movement disorder. David therefore has extremely limited communication, epilepsy, mobility problems, incontinence, poor sleep, self-injurious behaviour and aggression towards others. He was referred to the specialist learning disabilities nurse for management of the transition process between child and adult services, specifically in relation to his healthcare needs.

It was suspected that the self-injury and aggression were in part linked to pain, owing to a build up of air in the gut, which resulted from his behaviour of 'swallowing' air. Poor communication, mobility difficulties and lack of independence were also considered to be contributing factors. David has a special diet because of his condition, which needs to be administered through a percutaneous endoscopic gastrostomy. This was administered in a single feed over 6 hours, during which he was confined to his wheelchair, and resulted in restricted independence as well as frustration for him.

Because of the complexity of David's condition there is a plethora of professionals and agencies involved (health, social care, education, respite services). The advanced nurse practitioner in learning disabilities transition nurse provides specialist intervention and advice on healthcare and behaviour, and also coordinated his care needs through the period of transition. This involved working across traditional professional and organizational boundaries and between paediatric and adult services.

For David, specific health interventions included:

- A detailed functional analysis of behaviours: this revealed that trapped air was indeed a factor in the pain and discomfort that David experienced, together with reinforcing behaviours from staff. A multiprofessional action plan was devised to proactively release the trapped air several times a day and thus reduce the pain this caused. The 6 hour feed regime was split into two 3 hour feeds, thus allowing him more freedom and control over his immediate environment.
- Collaborative work around the management of epilepsy: specifically the completion of an epilepsy profile and Joint Epilepsy Council care plan for the management of seizures and prevention of status epilepticus.
- The main aim of the specialist nurse's intervention was to ensure the safe and smooth transition between child and adult services. To achieve this, it was necessary that all services worked collaboratively. Common guidelines were drawn up to ensure consistency of approach and all organizations were involved in joint training initiatives.

Christopher Griffiths, Consultant Nurse, Abertawe Bro Morgannwg University Health Board , Port Talbot, Wales

Children and young people's nursing in relation to advanced nursing practice

It is perhaps no surprise that the number of advanced nursing practice posts within the field of children and young people's nursing is increasing in a variety of different settings within both the hospital and community sectors. Advanced paediatric nurse practitioners (APNPs) within the hospital environment can be generalist paediatric clinicians and/or distinct specialists, e.g. in oncology, respiratory, neonatology, neurology or intensive care services.

Role outline of advanced paediatric nurse practitioner

I am a registered general nurse and registered sick children's nurse who has worked in various paediatric settings for the past 20 years. I achieved a Bachelor of Science Nursing degree followed by a 2 year diploma course at St Martin's College, Lancaster, and am also a qualified prescriber. My workplace in Scotland has been altering the boundaries of nursing and entering the field of medicine for over 4 years now. Advanced practice is aimed at providing holistic, effective, high-quality care to patients and their families. A third APNP will join our team this year. At present, we regularly replace a senior house officer within the inpatient ward and the assessment unit, working autonomously and as part of the multidisciplinary team. As APNPs we use advanced clinical skills and our in-depth knowledge base to comprehensively assess patients by physical examination and history-taking. We initiate investigations, interpret results, and assess and treat children and young people with undiagnosed and undifferentiated medical conditions which entails diagnosing, admitting, discharging, prescribing and referring to other professionals.

Jacqueline (Jacquie) Taylor, APNP, Kirkcaldy, Scotland

APNPs working in acute areas of paediatric medicine can expedite admission, diagnosis and treatment and even discharge as set out in the following Case study.

Case study

Fiona, an 11 year old girl, had had tummy pain for 2 days, and her GP referred her for suspected appendicitis to the local paediatric assessment unit, where the APNP assessed her. On arrival, Fiona was very chatty; she was apyrexial and had had no high temperatures at home. She complained that her tummy pain was sharp and only stayed in the lower part of her tummy but her lower back was also sore. The pain came and went all day and sometimes was there at night time. She did say she needed to go the toilet a few more times than usual. When she did pass urine she said it was 'nippy'.

On examination there was tenderness to lower abdomen but no guarding or rebound tenderness. Normal bowel sounds were auscultated. She had had constipation in the past, using lactulose to help her bowel movements. Fiona and her mother felt that her stools were normal and she had been passing normal stool daily. Results from a urine sample showed some nitrites, protein and leucocytes. Fiona's pain had since gone and she was 'starving' as she had missed her lunch by being at the GP's surgery. The APNP prescribed trimethoprim for 7 days for a urinary tract infection, advised regular paracetamol and ibuprofen for pain and wrote a prescription for this. Fiona was discharged home, with a view to a follow-up telephone call when the urine culture results came back. No further follow-up or investigation was required as per local and national guidelines and policies. She was also given 24 hours open access to the unit if her symptoms changed or her mother was concerned about Fiona.

Likewise, APNPs working in acute areas of paediatric medicine can expedite admission, diagnosis and treatment and arrange admission of the child and parents to the hospital ward for further observation, as in the following Case study.

Case study

Ryan, a 6 month old boy, was referred to the paediatric assessment unit at the local district general hospital by his GP. Ryan had had a cold, runny nose and cough for 4 days. Today, he developed a high temperature of 38°C at home, which paracetamol had not helped. He was not keen to take his formula milk or breast milk. His mother felt Ryan was unable to breathe and suck at the same time. On attendance, he was assessed by the APNP. Ryan was very miserable, crying, red all over and hot to touch. His vital signs were: temperature, 38°C; heart rate, 172; respiratory rate, 44; oxygen saturations were difficult to obtain but when recorded were 90–93% in air. His breathing sounded noisy and snuffly; clear discharge was coming out of his nose.

A more in-depth history was taken. Ryan had been taking breast and formula milk that morning, but half his usual amount. There was no history of ingestion of any foreign object. He was very hot to touch, but his hands and feet were very cold. He did not have any colour changes when coughing, or any sub- or intercostal recession on physical examination. Ryan had had one wet nappy. Capillary refill was less than 1 second centrally and peripherally. Ryan had no allergies and was fully immunized. He is the only child of two professional parents, never unwell and was usually very active and inquisitive. Today, he needed to be cuddled constantly.

On auscultation of his chest there were bilateral crepitations, no wheeze and equal air entry bilaterally. Ambient oxygen was given and no spots or rashes were seen. A nasal pharyngeal aspirate was sent to the laboratory to assess for respiratory syncytial virus. The APNP prescribed ibuprofen, oxygen and advised further antipyretic measures. She also took time to explain to Ryan's parents the complexities and treatments for the diagnosis of bronchiolitis. Chest infection could not be excluded, but as antipyretics had made him less miserable and able to feed he was admitted to the ward for overnight stay, with his parents, where observation and further review would take place.

Reflection points

★ Do you have any APNPs in your healthcare setting?

★ If so, what preparation (education and training) did they undergo for this role?

★ Where do they work and with whom?

★ If not, then do you think your area needs an APNP?

★ To what level should the children's APNP be educated?

★ Should they hold a specialist qualification?

★ Are they an 'expensive' luxury?

Having considered practitioners from all four of the main parts of the nursing register who may work with children and young people, we will now delve more into the detail on the role of advanced practitioners who have a more specific remit. It is important to state that, when reviewing those who provide an advanced nursing practice service for children and young people, the first distinction to be made should be between those from whatever branch of nursing who have successfully undertaken some formal advanced nurse practitioner programme, and those who have not. This is of particular importance because, currently, there is no regulation in the UK on advanced practice, and thus (technically at least) anyone, anywhere, can call themselves an advanced practitioner. As unlikely as you think that may be, and no matter how robust the local governance, and in spite of the scope of practice, the 'unconscious incompetent' can happen. Years of experience count for nothing without a good education. The old cliché 'experience without knowledge is blind, knowledge without experience is mere intellectual play' is true. Unfortunately, there is a legacy in the UK of badge swapping – staff nurse one day, clinical nurse specialist the next, and doing a course next year!

The readers of this chapter must appreciate that the authors of this chapter would expect any advanced nurse practitioner to have undertaken a rigorous and fully assessed programme of educational and clinical preparation. You will note that in this last sentence we have not specified the 'level', 'duration' or 'content', for by now you should be aware of the great uncertainties and diversity surrounding advanced practice. Currently, there is much discussion on how we can differentiate between a nurse practitioner and an advanced nurse practitioner. Advancing practice suggests a continuum, and perhaps this is a good thing – that practitioners 'advance' their practice from undergraduate to Master and Doctorate level, advance their clinical role from nurse practitioner to advanced nurse practitioner to consultant. Whichever programme of education is undertaken, we would suggest that a well-tested competency framework should be used to structure it – and several have been alluded to already in this chapter. We would expect that they had done something more than nothing! And we also believe that current 'regulation' is insufficient to protect the public from the 'unconscious incompetent'.

Having established the need for a robust education, it may be prudent to explore the nuances of definitions. Many authors writing about advanced nurse practitioner in child health identify the problem of agreeing a common definition of the role (Peter and Flynn 2002; Myers 2009). Myers (2009) refers to Stilwell (1988, p. 38), in which 'the nurse practitioner is seen as an experienced nurse who combines health assessment, diagnostic and prescribing skills to manage the patient autonomously'. There are other definitions, and we have provided these for you earlier, and perhaps we should avoid the trap of seeking the ultimate definition. The very fact that advanced practice is founded in evolution and change indicates that trying to tie it down actually defeats its purpose. The Advanced Nursing Practice Toolkit (Scottish Government 2008) that we discussed earlier deliberately avoids this by providing several examples – all of which have their merits. Thus, illuminating such roles is best met by using the example of an established advanced practice role. In this section, we focus on just one such role, although we are quick to note that there are many more. Advanced nursing practices in relation to children and young people's nursing are potentially many and varied, ranging from behavioural therapies, family- and community-based interventions (e.g. community children's nurses,

The advanced neonatal nurse practitioner

By far the most developed advanced nursing practice 'child' role (supported by an established body of evidence) is the ANNP. Dillon and George (1997) reported that the former Wessex region was the first in the UK to initiate an ANNP programme of education. A group of neonatologists, paediatricians and senior neonatal nurses came together in 1990 with the intention to develop an appropriate curriculum and subsequent ANNP appointments. The motivating factors for this development were similar to those of advanced nursing roles elsewhere: predominantly, the underutilization of nursing expertise and heavy dependency on a small number of senior house officers who worked in excess of 80 hours per week as part of a 3 or 6 month rotation which resulted in fluctuations in the quality of care. The course was jointly funded by the Wessex Regional Health Authority and the Department of Health, validated by the English National Board and recognized by the University of Southampton for 60 credit accumulation and transfer scheme (CATS) points. They defined the ANNP as 'a registered nurse or midwife with an established neonatal nurse background who has successfully completed a period of education on a recognised NNP course' (University of Southampton School of Nursing and Midwifery 1992, cited by Dillon and George 1997, p. 260).

In order to undertake this course, nurses were required to have 4 years' neonatal experience and to be recommended by a paediatric/neonatal consultant and a clinical nurse manager. The course consisted of 36 weeks of full-time teaching and then 26 weeks of clinical probation on the neonatal intensive care unit (NICU) the practitioners had been seconded from. During this period, practitioners would consolidate the theory learnt and gain proficiency in managing the clinical care of sick neonates, including the performance of interventions (Box 14.1) previously conducted by physicians.

Box 14.1   Examples of interventions

- Attending deliveries
- Examination
- Drug therapy
- Optimizing mechanical ventilation, including the insertion and removal of endotracheal tubes
- Instigating and interpreting laboratory investigations
- Arterial blood sampling
- Inserting long and peripheral venous cannulae and umbilical arterial cannulation
- Lumbar puncture procedure
- Suprapubic aspiration of the bladder
- Needle aspiration of the chest
- Insertion of chest drains

The first cohort completed the course in 1992. A follow-up survey and evaluation was undertaken after the third cohort of neonatal practitioners completed the course (Dillon and George 1997). The researchers interviewed 22 ANNPs (18 face to face and four via telephone). Although they found that, of the 22, only 11 were practising as ANNPs, the common opinion was that the introduction of the ANNP had extended the role of the neonatal nurse. They considered the primary function of the ANNP as the delivery of care to the neonate either in the labour ward or on the NICU. The ANNP determined admissions to the unit, started treatment regimens, initiated clinical interventions and ensured that changes in neonates' conditions were responded to appropriately.

Interestingly, the survey revealed that many ANNPs had developed a strong rapport with the senior doctors in the team, and that this relationship contributed to job satisfaction. However, some professional relationships with trainee paediatricians were noted as problematic, specifically when the ANNP's practice (such as taking blood specimens) had the effect of limiting clinical learning opportunities for them. Previously, the trainee paediatricians (in their initial weeks on the NICU) would have sought practical advice from the ANNP on such tasks, not competed for clinical experience. The development of advanced practice roles is often charged with deskilling medical practitioners! However, this survey also revealed that the teaching abilities of ANNPs was found to be increasingly in demand, and that their skills over time actually enhanced junior doctors' learning opportunities. Not only that – they also began for the first time to contribute to audit, the development of protocols and research with medical colleagues.

Some ANNPs noted a lack of structure within their units with regard to their role, with some feeling a sense of isolation and lacking direction. The more recent evidence indicates that this sense of isolation was entirely due to the lack of clinical career structure in the nursing profession (Barton 2006a,b). The work of *Modernising Nursing Careers*, and the individual post-registration frameworks of the four countries of the UK, have gone a long way to addressing this.

Over a decade after the Wessex group had instigated the first ANNP course, a further study by Smith and Hall (2003) examined how the role had evolved. During that time, the drivers that had brought about the original innovation had also developed, and changed. The workload and number of hours worked by junior doctors had been reduced by *The New Deal* (NHS Management Executive 1991). The Calman Report had brought about changes on the duration of training. Nurses had been encouraged to expand their practice and roles by the UK Central Council for Nursing, Midwifery and Health Visiting (1992), while in 1997 New Labour took power following a general election, and had begun to bring about change in the NHS with an agenda of improving quality, including the introduction of clinical governance. The imperative for ANNPs was now more pressing and relevant than ever before, and they have flourished in practice.

Key points

- ANNPs are currently the most visible and researched group of advanced practitioners in children and young people's nursing.
- The role has developed in response to economic factors and working time directives as well as a need to extend knowledge and skills.
- ANNPs undertake a myriad of roles, but feel isolated and lacking direction owing to a lack of career structure.
- ANNPs contribute to audit, research and the development of protocols as well as teaching/dissemination of knowledge.

The education of advanced nurse practitioners in children and young people's nursing

Despite the strategists' positive promotion of advanced nurse practitioners, in the UK the education of such practitioners has been an erratic and unregulated affair. This chapter should have illuminated why this was so: the lack of understanding of key concepts and roles, a 'right here, right now' service demand for educational quick fixes, a lack of regulatory guidance and career structure, traditional boundary hurdles and silos. Consequently, as we have already stated, the standards of practice and competence held by those who claim to be advanced nurse practitioners are unregulated and may vary widely. Thus, it must also be accepted that there may be in our population of advanced practice nurses those whose practice is 'unconsciously incompetent'.

However, all is not lost for there are many positive activities and developments under way in the world of educating advanced nurse practitioners. As we stated earlier, the revalidation of the pre-registration programme, bringing new child field competencies, should be viewed as a positive development that will underpin post-registration career pathway planning. Mapping these competencies to the current advanced practice competencies is work not yet undertaken. But that mapping exercise is crucial as it will set the career path for the future of children and young people's nursing by taking a completely new look at the options. It may be stated that the unique nature of children and young people's nursing is only secure if the profession is brave enough to step out of traditional ways of working and consider new ways.

The work of the ANNPE, the RCN and the NMC has highlighted the need for national standards for advanced practice from which the efficacy of educational programmes may be measured. We have acknowledged the multiple competency frameworks available, but are mapping these to the RCN and NMC competencies. The NMC has shown a new interest in implementing some form of national regulation, and the Advanced Nursing Practice Toolkit has provided a national information resource. More specifically, forward-thinking employers are now looking carefully at their advanced practitioners and developing mechanisms of governance and practical support.

For those caring for the child or young person, there are now many academic/clinical/professional programmes enabling practice-based learning that may be tailored to the specifics of children and young people's nursing and to the key issues of child development and child protection. Educationalists are alert and responsive to new demands for professional education that is responsive to service demand and is rooted in the workplace. Quality undergraduate, Master and Doctoral programmes are springing up in response to that demand. Finally, and most importantly, there is now an agreement that these advanced nursing practice roles can only be competently achieved by a detailed and structured programme of education.

Key points

- The emergence of new child and young person field competencies is a positive development.
- Field competencies will allow mapping of post-registration career pathways. Mapping these to current advanced practice is crucial.
- Children and young people's nurses need to consider new ways of working to meet the needs of children and young people.
- Advanced practice roles can only be achieved by a detailed and structured programme of education.

Conclusion

This chapter has sought to illuminate the complex world of advanced (nursing) practice, its origin, its current (still undecided) status, and its implication in relation to the care of children and younger people. As this chapter has identified in some detail, the reader will now understand how important, and how fraught with controversy, this subject is. We have stated that we believe that fields of practice are increasingly irrelevant as the nurse develops the generic skills of the advanced practitioner. The consultant paediatrician, the consultant pain specialist (nurse or doctor) and the consultant surgeon will all have their part to play in the care of a child with a serious injury. They all bring something special to that package of care, and it is indeed a truism that the whole is greater than the sum of its parts. Equally, the adult advanced practitioner, mental health advanced practitioner, learning disability advanced practitioner, and children and young people's advanced practitioner may all have their part to play in a particular child or young person's needs. Specialization and generalization are key to the function of a complex service such as healthcare – they reveal aspects of the necessary division of labour in a complex service. It may be seen that we need generalists – to sift and sort and prioritize – for they are the autonomous practitioners who manage undifferentiated health needs. In contrast, we need specialists to utilize their specific skills to manage particular client groups, or disease process. It is the package of care that counts, and that is sought by the service user, and once again we must state that the whole is greater than the sum of its parts.

Children, young people and their families need children and young people's nurses – we would not suggest otherwise – but the service user, i.e. the child or young person, may have many needs, and we bar practitioners from that input at our peril. As nurses develop advanced skills, the common transferability of their generic skills is an essential feature that is demanded by service users and service providers. If there are concerns on this, then those issues should be tackled: additional education, screening – all these are possible. What should not be entertained is the idea that only a children and young people's nurse can direct every aspect of a child or young person's needs. The advanced nurse practitioner, as we have suggested, is moving the boundaries, and transcending the traditional barriers between different departments and disciplines.

Summary of principles for practice

- Children and young people's nurses need to develop clarity regarding the role of the advanced nurse practitioner for children and young people's nursing.
- Advanced nurse practitioners from a generic background who work with children and young people also require completion of a recognized course in caring for this age group.
- Advanced nurse practitioners working with children and young people have a significant impact on the experience of care by assessing, expediting treatment and early discharge.
- All nurses working as an advanced nurse practitioner need to develop political awareness regarding their role and the specialist versus the generic debate.
- Children and young people's nurses must have a voice in developing national educational standards to ensure that clinically competent advanced nurse practitioners are prepared for the demands of practice across all specialties.
- All practitioners must recognize that registration of advanced nurse practitioners will protect children, young people and their families from the 'unconsciously incompetent'.
- Children and young people's nurses must regard the role of the advanced nurse practitioner as another career opportunity.

References

American Association of Colleges of Nursing (1999) Certificate and regulation of advanced practice nurses: position statement. *Journal of Professional Nursing* **15**(2): 130–2.

Barton TD (2006a) Clinical mentoring of nurse practitioners: the doctor's experience. *British Journal of Nursing* **15**: 820–4.

Barton TD (2006b) Nurse practitioners – or advanced clinical nurses? *British Journal of Nursing* **15**(7): 370–6.

Bennet J, Hughes J (2009) The advanced practitioner in emergency and acute assessment units. In: Hughes J, Lyte G (eds) *Developing nursing practice with children and young people*. Chichester: Blackwell Publications.

Bradley SF (2003) Pride or prejudice: issues in the history of children's nurse education. *Nurse Education Today* **23**: 362–7.

Bristol Royal Infirmary Inquiry (2001) *Learning from Bristol, the Report of the Public Inquiry into Children's Heart Surgery at the Bristol Royal Infirmary 1984–1995*. The Kennedy Report. Command Paper CM 5207. Bristol: Bristol Royal Infirmary Inquiry.

Campbell-Heider N, Kleinpell RM, Holzemer WL (1997) Commentary about Marchione and Garlands 'An emerging Profession?'. The case of the nursing practitioners image. *Journal of Nursing Scholarship* **29**(4): 228–9.

Carnwell R, Daly W (2003) Advanced nursing practitioners in primary care: an exploration of the developing roles. *Journal of Clinical Nursing* **12**(5): 630–42.

Clark J (1994) *Graduate status for nurses: does this create an elitist profession? (or: ten heresies about nursing education).* Enfield: Centre for Advanced and International Studies in Nursing, Middlesex University.

Clothier C, MacDonald CA, Shaw DA (1994) *The Allitt Inquiry.* The Clothier Report. London: Her Majesty's Stationery Office.

Coe J, Hetherington A, Keating FA (2005) *Comparison of UK health regulators guidance on professional boundaries.* Project Report. London: Council for Healthcare Regulatory Excellence.

Davies R (2008) Children's nursing and future directions: learning from 'memorable events'. *Nurse Education Today* **28**: 814–21.

Davies R (2010) Marking the fiftieth anniversary of the Platt report: from exclusion, to toleration and parental participation in the care of the hospitalised child. *Journal of Child Health Care* **14**: 6–23.

Deloughery GL (1995) *History of the nursing profession.* St Louis: Mosby Year Book.

Department of Health (1993) *Hospital doctors: training for the future.* Report on the Working Group of Specialist Medical Training. The Calman Report. London: DH.

Department of Health (2004) *An introduction to the NHS Knowledge and Skills Framework and its use in career and pay progression.* London: DH. See http://www.dh.gov.uk/prod_consum_dh/groups/dh_digitalassets/@dh/@en/documents/digitalasset/dh_4105472.pdf

Department of Health (2006) *Modernising nursing careers: setting the direction.* London: DH.

Department of Health (2007) *Trust, assurance and safety: the regulation of health professionals in the 21st century.* London: The Stationery Office.

Department of Health (2010) *Modernising nursing careers: achievements and future action.* London: DH.

Department of Health and Department for Education and Skills (2004a) *National Service Framework for children, young people and maternity services: core standards, standard 3.* London: DH/DfES.

Department of Health and Department for Education and Skills (2004b) *National Service Framework for children, young people and maternity services young people's version: getting it right for you. Health advice and support.* London: DH/DfES.

Dillon A, George S (1997) Advanced neonatal practitioners in the United Kingdom: where are they and what do they do? *Journal of Advanced Nursing* **25**(2): 257–64.

Dingwall R, Lewis P (1985) *The sociology of the professions: lawyers, doctors and others.* London: Macmillan Press.

Dunn A (1997) Literature review of advanced clinical nursing practice in the United States of America. *Journal of Advanced Nursing* **25**(4): 814–19.

Emerson E, Hatton C (2004) *Estimating future need/demand for supports for adults with learning disabilities in England.* Lancaster: Institute for Health Research, Lancaster University.

Fenton MV (1992) Education for the advanced practice of clinical nurse specialists. *Oncology Nurses Forum* **19**: 16–20.

Fondiller SH (1995) Loretta C. Ford: a modern Olympian, she lit a torch. *N & HC Perspectives on Community* **16:** 6–11.

Ford LC, Silver HK (1967) A program to increase health care for children: the pediatric nurse practitioner program. *Pediatrics* **39**(5): 756–60.

Griffiths P, Jones S, Maben J, Murrells T (2008) *State of art metrics for nursing: a rapid appraisal.* London: National Nursing Research Unit, King's College London.

Hamric AB, Spross JA (eds) (1989) *The clinical nurse specialist in theory and practice,* 2nd edn. Philadelphia: W.B. Saunders.

Hockey L (1983) *Primary care nursing.* London: Churchill Livingstone.

Hodnicki DR (1998) Advanced practice nursing certification: where do we go from here? *Advanced Practice Nurse Quarterly* **4**(3): 34–43.

Holliday I (1995) *The NHS transformed: a guide to the health reforms.* Manchester: Baseline Book Company.

Horrocks S, Andersen E, Salisbury C (2002) Systematic review of whether nurse practitioners working in primary healthcare can provide equivalent care to doctors. *British Medical Reviews* **324**: 819–23.

Hunt JAS (1999) Specialist nurse: an identified professional role or a personal agenda? *Journal of Advanced Nursing* **30**(3): 704–12.

International Council of Nurses (2002) *Regulation network bulletin*. Geneva: International Council of Nurses. See http://www.icn.ch/

Jukes M (1996) Advanced practice within learning disability nursing. *British Journal of Nursing* 5(5):293–8.

Ketefian S, Redman RW, Hanucharurnkul S, *et al.* (2001) The development of advanced practice roles: implications in the international nursing community. *International Nursing Review* 48: 152–63.

Maben J, Griffiths P (2008) *Nurses in society: starting the debate*. London: National Nursing Research Unit, King's College London.

Manton DJ (1971) *The life of Dorothy Pattison*. London: Methuen.

Marchione J, Garland TN (1980) An emerging profession: the case of the nurse practitioner. *Journal of Nursing Scholarship* 12(2): 37–40.

Ministry of Health (1959) *The welfare of children in hospital*. The Platt Report. London: HMSO.

Myers J (2009) Advanced practice in the management of children with eczema. *Paediatric Nursing* 21(2): 38–41.

National Institute for Health and Clinical Excellence (2008) *Attention deficit hyperactivity disorder: diagnosis and management of ADHD in children, young people and adults*. Clinical guidelines CG72. London: NICE. See http://guidance.nice.org.uk/CG72

NHS Executive South Thames (1994) *Evaluation of nurse practitioner pilot projects*. The Touche Ross Report. London: Touche Ross.

NHS Management Executive (1991) *Junior doctors – the new deal*. London: DH.

Nursing and Midwifery Council (2005) *The proposed framework for the standard for post-registration nursing*. London: NMC. See http://www.nmc-uk.org/templates/pages/Search?q=proposed%20standard%20for%20post%20registration%20nursing

Nursing and Midwifery Council (2008) *Advice for nurses working with children and young people*. London: NMC. See http://www.nmc-uk.org/templates/pages/search?q=advice+for+nurses+working+with+children+and+young+people.&btnG=Search&entqr=0&output=xml_no_dtd&sort=date%3AD%3AL%3Ad1&client=NMC_Live&ud=1&oe=UTF-8&ie=UTF-8&proxystylesheet=NMC_Live&site=NMC_Live

Nursing and Midwifery Council (2010) *Standards for pre-registration nursing education*. London: NMC. See http://www.nmc-uk.org/Documents/Consultations/draft%20standards%20pre%20reg.pdf

Offredy M (2000) Advanced nursing practice: the case of nurse practitioners in three Australian states. *Journal of Advanced Nursing* 31(2): 274–81.

Pearson A, Peels S (2002) The nurse practitioner. *International Journal of Nursing Practice* 8(4): 5–10.

Peplau H (1965) Specialisation in professional nursing. *Nursing Science* 3: 268–87.

Peter S, Flynn A (2002) Advanced nurse practitioners in a hospital setting: a reality. *Paediatric Nursing* 14(2): 14–19.

Ponto J, Sabo J, Fitzgerald M, Wilson D (2002) Operationalising advance practice registered nurse legislation: perspectives from a clinical nurses specialist task force. *Clinical Nurse Specialist* 16(5): 263–9.

Read SM, Roberts-Davis M, Gilbert P, Nolan M (2000) *Preparing nurse practitioners for the 21st century: executive summary*. Sheffield: School of Nursing and Midwifery, University of Sheffield.

Royal College of Nursing (2003a) *Children and young people's nursing: a philosophy of care. Guidance for nursing staff*. London: RCN. See http://www.rcn.org.uk/__data/assets/pdf_file/0003/78573/002012.pdf

Royal College of Nursing (2003b) *Preparing nurses to care for children and young people: summary position statement by the RCN children and young people field of practice*. London: RCN. See www.rcn.org.uk

Royal College of Nursing (2004) *Services for children and young people: preparing nurses for future roles*. London: RCN. See www.rcn.org.uk

Royal College of Nursing (2008) *Advanced nurse practitioners: an RCN guide to the advanced nurse practitioner role, competencies and programme accreditation*. London: RCN.

Scottish Government (2008) *Supporting the development of advanced nursing practice: a toolkit approach*. Edinburgh: Scottish Government, CNO Directorate.

Shaw MC (1993) The discipline of nursing: historical roots, current perspectives, future directions. *Journal of Advanced Nursing* 18(10): 1651–6.

Skills for Health (2006a) *A career framework for health.* London: Skills for Health. See http://www.skillsforhealth.org.uk/Search-Results.aspx?searchQuery=a+career+framework

Skills for Health (2006b) *A career framework for health. Section 1. Advanced practitioner roles.* London: Skills for Health. See http://www.skillsforhealth.org.uk/workforce-design-development/workforce-design-and-planning/competence-based-workforce-design/~/media/Resource-Library/PDF/Microsoft_Word-Section_1Advanced_Practitioner_Roles_web_2_v2.ashx

Smith J (Chair) (2005) *The Shipman Inquiry: the sixth and final report.* London: HMSO.

Smith SL, Hall MA (2003) Developing a neonatal workforce: role evolution and retention of advanced neonatal nurse practitioners. *Archives of Diseases in Childhood Fetal & Neonatal edition* **88**: 426–9.

South Thames Regional Health Authority (1998) *Evaluation of nurse practitioner pilot projects.* London: NHS Executive South Thames.

Spitzer WO, Sackett, DL (1990) 25th anniversary of nurse practitioners: the Burlington randomised trial of the nurse practitioner. *Journal of American Academy of Nurse Practitioners* **2**(3): 93–9.

Stilwell B (1984). The nurse in practice. *Nursing Mirror* **158**: 17–22.

Stilwell B (1988) Patients' attitudes to a highly developed extended role – the nurse practitioner. *Recent Advances in Nursing* **21**: 82–100.

Stilwell B, Greenfield S, Drury M, Hull FM (1987) A nurse practitioner in general practice: working styles and pattern of consultation. *Journal of Royal College of General Practice* **37**(297): 154–7.

Storr G (1988) The clinical nurse specialist: from the outside looking in. *Journal of Advanced Nursing* **13**: 265–72.

Svensson R (1996) The interplay between doctors and nurses: a negotiated order perspective. *Sociology of Health and Illness* **18**(3): 379–98.

Terry J, Maunder EZ, Bowler N, Williams D (2009) Interbranch initiative to improve children's mental health. *British Journal of Nursing* **18**(5): 282–7.

United Kingdom Central Council for Nursing, Midwifery and Health Visiting (1992) *The scope of professional practice.* London: UKCC.

United Kingdom Central Council for Nursing, Midwifery and Health Visiting (1996) *Standards for education and practice following registration (PREP) transitional arrangements: specialist practitioner title/qualifications.* London: UKCC.

United Kingdom Central Council for Nursing, Midwifery and Health Visiting (1998) *Higher level of practice: consultation document.* London: UKCC.

Walby S, Greenwell J (1994) *Medicine and nursing: professions in a changing health service.* London: Sage Publications.

Waller S (1998) Higher level practice in nursing: a prerequisite for nurse consultants? *Hospital Medicine* **59**: 816–18.

Walsh M, Crumbie A, Reveley S (eds) (1999) *Nurse practitioners: clinical skills and professional issues.* Oxford: Butterworth-Heinemann.

Watson E (2006) CAMHS liaison: supporting care in general paediatric settings. *Paediatric Nursing* **18**: 30–3.

Zola IK, Croog SH (1968) Work perceptions and their implications for professional identity: an exploratory analysis of public health nurses. *Social Science and Medicine* **2**: 15–28.

Index